Peace of Mind
During Pregnancy

PEACE of MIND
During Pregnancy

An A–Z Guide to the Substances That
Could Affect Your Unborn Baby

CHRISTINE KELLEY-BUCHANAN
with Ellen Thro

FACTS ON FILE PUBLICATIONS
New York, New York · Oxford, England

DISCLAIMER

IMPORTANT NOTE: This book contains general information on the impact of drugs, chemicals, infections and other exposures on the unborn child. It is not a substitute for consultation with your own physician. Readers who are or may be pregnant are urged to consult their own doctors before taking any drugs, prescription or nonprescription, and also before discontinuing any prescribed course of treatment.

Peace of Mind During Pregnancy: An A–Z Guide to the Substances That Could Affect Your Unborn Baby

copyright © 1988 by Christine Kelley-Buchanan

ISBN 0-8160-1907-X

Library of Congress Catalog Card Number 88-045295

CIP data available on request

Printed in the United States of America

10   9   8   7   6   5   4   3   2   1

For my husband, Stephen,
who has proved to me that
dreams really do come true.

ACKNOWLEDGMENT:

So much of what I have been able to accomplish in my career is the result of the position I held at the California Teratogen Registry. For this reason I am indebted to both Dr. Kenneth Lyons Jones and Dr. Gerald "Buzz" Chernoff for giving me the responsibility for developing and coordinating the Registry. Most important, I am grateful for their ideas and expertise, without which the California Teratogen Registry would never have been born. A special thank-you to my mentor and friend, Buzz Chernoff, for introducing me to teratology and for being the best academic teacher I ever had.

Because the California Teratogen Registry is so important to me, I cannot overlook the efforts of Peter Korn and State Senator Gary Hart, who were instrumental in securing ongoing state funds for the program. Beginning without formal funding and initially serving only the San Diego area, state money enabled the Registry to flourish and expand its services to residents through California.

An incredible number of medical journal articles had to be obtained in order to write this book. In searching for help for this task I had the good fortune of finding June Huang, a graduate student at the University of California at Santa Barbara. June became invaluable to me; she gathered the papers I requested, set up a filing system, and generally made it possible for me to concentrate on writing.

Before this book, writing for me was limited to letters to my grandmother, notes to friends, and cards at Christmas. So I am grateful to my collaborator, Ellen Thro, who helped me compose the first four chapters. Throughout the book Ellen cleaned up poor grammar, polished my sentences, and helped my words talk to you.

I am often asked how I ended up not only writing a book but actually getting it published. This would not have been possible without several people: Win Cox in Public Information at the University of California Medical Center in San Diego, who referred me to the Sandra Dijkstra Literary Agency. I am grateful to Sandra Dijkstra, my talented literary agent who was determined I should write a book and was even more determined to sell it once I did. To Judith Riven, the editor at Dell who originally bought my manuscript, thank you for sharing my vision. To my fabulous editors at Dell, Marilyn Abraham and Sheila Curry, I am grateful for their brilliant insight and guidance which shaped my ideas into a "user friendly" format that got to the point! I also want to thank Marilyn and Sheila for their kindness and support which kept me smiling through the editorial process.

The people who were chosen to review this book, Dr. Gerald F. Chernoff, Dr. Richard H. Finnell, Dr. Duncan J. Turner, Dr. Eugene Hoyme, and Dr. John C. Carey are widely known and respected for their work. I am very fortunate that these men took time out of their busy schedules to read *Peace of Mind During Pregnancy* in its entirely (no small feat!). I am grateful to each one of them for their words of advice and encouragement which were not only a tremendous help to me, but also served as a great source of inspiration. A special thank-you to Gene Hoyme for writing the foreword to *Peace of Mind During Pregnancy* and for his continued support over the years.

I also appreciate the efforts of two genetic counselors, Barbara Dixon and Susan Winokur, for their review of the section on genetics and for all of their knowledgeable suggestions.

I am indebted to Dr. Robert E. Carrel for his generosity in giving me time off work to complete this project.

There would be no need for this book without all the wonderful pregnant women out there. So many have touched my life in unique ways, making me feel needed and helpful. They have also taught me how to communicate effectively, which, I believe, has made this book special.

Last, I want to thank the most important people in my life. My parents, Neil and Dorothea Kelley, for teaching me what really matters in life—how to love others and to always do your best. And to all my family and friends who cheered me on through the long process of composing this book. But most of all, to my husband, best friend, and biggest fan, Stephen, for creating an environment that encourages me to pursue my goals.

Contents

Foreword

Behold, thou shalt conceive, and bear a son;
and now drink no wine or strong drink . . .

JUDGES 13:7

For centuries it has been recognized that maternal environmental exposures or ingestions have the potential for causing fetal malformations. This fact is the basis for the science of teratology, the study of environmental causes of birth defects. Recognition of teratogenic causes of birth defects is particularly important because, as opposed to many genetically determined birth defects, those due to adverse maternal ingestions or environmental exposures are potentially preventable through public education and awareness.

Those of us involved in some way with the provision of health care to pregnant women are keenly aware of the anxiety that exposure to a potential teratogen may engender. Unfortunately most pregnant clients rely on the popular press or "word of mouth" information from friends for guidance with respect to this important issue. Such information may be misleading at best. A recent survey of fifteen popular magazines revealed that fifty-five percent of articles regarding teratology are inaccurate.* Even if advice is sought from health care providers, the answers to questions posed may not be readily available. This lack of available information is due to many factors:

1. Medical schools and nursing schools in the past have not included principles of teratology in their curricula.

2. There is no single, authoritative, scholarly source for information about potential human teratogens.

3. Available sources are often written in a manner which is not directly or practically applicable to the questions posed by pregnant clients.

4. Data applicable to human pregnancy are simply not available for hundreds of common environmental exposures.

*S.A. Gunderson, L.P. Martinez, J.C. Carey, N.K. Kochenour, and M.G. Emery. Critical review of articles regarding pregnancy exposures in popular magazines, *Teratology* 33: (1986) 82C.

To address these issues, Drs. Kenneth Lyons Jones and Gerald Chernoff at the University of California, San Diego, School of Medicine, designed the California Teratogen Registry in 1979. That service has served dual functions: providing a single scholarly, authoritative, confidential source for the provision of information about potential human teratogens and serving as a vehicle for researching potentially "new" human teratogens. The California Teratogen Registry has proved to be immensely successful in achieving these goals. It has also been the template from which many similar services across the nation have been fashioned (see Helpful Information Resources, page 352).

Christine Kelley-Buchanan was the Coordinator of the California Teratogen Registry from 1979 through 1985. In that role, Christine did not deal with questions relating to human teratology on a theoretical plane. Rather, she supervised the counseling of thousands of pregnant clients, dealing in a very practical way with issues relating to environmental exposures and pregnancy. This book is the fruit of those years of teratogen counseling.

Many texts are available in teratology. Few, however, are as easily applicable to an individual human pregnancy as is *Peace of Mind During Pregnancy*. Christine has successfully translated her methods for interpreting available data regarding potential human teratogens into an easily comprehensible and usable text. This text should be extremely valuable to all physicians, nurses, and other health professionals dealing with pregnant women. It should also be widely utilized by pregnant women and concerned family members as an adjunct to regular prenatal care with their health care providers.

The promotion of healthy pregnancy is a joint goal of pregnant women and their health care providers. This important text should truly help in the promotion of fetal well-being and "peace of mind during pregnancy."

H. Eugene Hoyme, M.D., Medical Director,
Arizona Teratogen Information Program
Chief, Section of Genetics/Dysmorphology
Department of Pediatrics
University of Arizona College of Medicine
Tucson, Arizona

Peace of Mind
During Pregnancy

✶ ONE ✶

You and This Book

YOU, ME, AND THIS BOOK

Of course you want to have a normal, healthy baby. Everyone does. And because of today's science and medicine, most babies *are* born healthy. But there are exceptions that we all worry about. Some children are born with abnormalities. Their parents' suspicion that they might have done something to prevent the tragedy—whether true or not—is a tragedy in its own sense.

Some birth defects occur spontaneously and are beyond anyone's control. However, birth defects caused by physical states in the mother, such as diabetes, and by drugs, chemicals, infections, pollutants—substances called *teratogens* (tuh-rat′-o-gens)—are largely preventable.

The word *teratogen* may be new to you, but it is the subject of a growing field of medicine, and one in which I have considerable experience. I was one of the founders of the California Teratogen Registry at the University of California, San Diego, Medical Center—the first such program in the United States. The California Teratogen Registry is a research and telephone counseling service for California residents, providing the latest scientific information on substances that might be harmful to pregnant women. The idea for the Registry came from two faculty members of the University of California, San Diego, Medical School: the renowned Dr. Kenneth Lyons Jones, a pediatric birth defect specialist who first identified the fetal alcohol syndrome in the United States, and the outstanding researcher Dr. Gerald Chernoff, a teratologist, now at Washington State University.

From 1979 until 1985 I served as coordinator of the Registry and taught continuing education classes in teratology for health care professionals—physicians, nurses, and others. My responsibility was to develop the program and to create a data base from

1

which to counsel concerned individuals—physicians and other professionals, as well as pregnant women.

During my years at the Registry, I was aware of the mountains of available information about the emotional and physical experience of pregnancy and childbirth. I was also made increasingly aware that this type of information didn't relieve or even address the many concerns pregnant women have about potentially harmful substances. Pregnant women want to have the best available information about the various drugs, chemicals and other agents they are exposed to. *I know that teratogen-caused birth defects can be virtually eliminated by educating pregnant women to avoid substances identified as harmful.*

Unfortunately, I also learned that a portion of the information on teratogens in circulation was misleading, incomplete, or simply wrong. Some of the worries pregnant women have about hazards to their unborn children are well founded. But many of their fears arise from misinformation gleaned from a variety of sources—"experienced" friends, the media, and, in some cases, their own health care providers.

Some of these fears are well founded, and others concern remote possibilities. But they are all *real*—the fears that come from actual situations, and fears of unknown origin that wake you up in the middle of the night. I take every one of these fears seriously, just as you do, and I believe the way to conquer fear is through education.

This book is an extension of that belief. Few practicing obstetricians are able to keep up with the rapidly growing literature on the subject of teratogens. This book is designed to provide up-to-date information. It differs from other books on the topic in that it is written specifically for the parent-to-be. This is usually the mother, but I am heartened by the growing number of expectant fathers who exhibit equal concern. This book provides tangible answers to their questions.

Its goal is twofold:
• prevention of those abnormalities that science teaches us can be avoided;
• prevention of your unnecessary fears about the responsibilities and decisions your pregnancy requires.

If the book achieves this goal my reward will be in knowing that it has truly contributed to your peace of mind during pregnancy.

WHY THIS BOOK WILL HELP YOU

Peace of Mind During Pregnancy is designed to help you evaluate the safety of a substance you may have used or ingested. It will also help you avoid potentially harmful substances. It will explain what is considered safe and what is harmful, what is known and what is *not* known, about dozens of substances, ranging from common household materials to those encountered in the environment and the workplace.

Most women ask these questions *after* the fact. So if you have already been exposed to a substance, please read the section on it *before* you continue to worry. If a risk is associated with an exposure during pregnancy, bring this to the *immediate* attention of your physician! It is particularly helpful to consider the emotional consequences of an exposure *before* it occurs, rather than worry about it afterward. If you even *think* that cleaning the oven might expose your unborn baby to harmful chemicals, then don't clean the oven!

While the ideal is to avoid all potentially dangerous substances during pregnancy, the fact is that accidental exposures do happen. Not all pregnancies are planned, nor are all exposures! A woman might not recognize that she is pregnant until weeks after conception. It is during this time that many accidental exposures to teratogens occur. However, as you will discover, being exposed to a known teratogen does not in itself constitute an increased risk above the small expected risk all pregnant women face for having a baby with an abnormality.

At times it is not possible to avoid exposure to certain substances during pregnancy. Women may not be able to avoid completely various chemicals because of where they live or work. Women who become sick during pregnancy cannot simply wish the illness away. In fact, treatment is advised for certain conditions—fevers and urinary tract infections are two examples—rather than allowing the illness to run its course.

HOW TO USE THIS BOOK
TO ANSWER YOUR QUESTIONS

The entries on individual agents and substances follow a uniform format to make their use as easy as possible. Each entry begins with an overview of the agent's name or names, its risk categories, and the time during pregnancy, if any, when the risk occurs.

The entries are listed alphabetically, usually by their generic names:

Generic Name. The scientific name of a drug or chemical, like diazepam for Valium.

Common Name. Some entries, such as "microwaves," do not have a generic name. In these cases, the agent's common or popular name is used.

Medication Classification—Most of the agents are listed under their generic or common names, but in some cases a number of drugs belonging to the same medication classification—for instance, corticosteroids—are grouped together for discussion. Such drug groups are found in the alphabetical listing of entries. Each drug in a group—in this case cortisone, prednisone, and others—is listed individually in the index.

Brand Name. The name provided by the manufacturer.

Chemical Name. Some entries are not drugs and do not have brand names. In these cases, the chemical name is used. For example, Agent Orange is composed of two chemicals: 2, 4-D and 2,4,5-T.

FDA Pregnancy Category. These are the U.S. Food and Drug Administration (FDA) risk categories provided by manufacturers of drugs. If a rating is available, it is listed here. A dash (—) means a rating has not yet been assigned to the drug. (The FDA risk categories can be found in Chapter 2, Table 2–1.)

Estimated Risk Summary

This is based on Table 2-2, page 22, and includes:

Time of Exposure—the period during pregnancy in which the risk potential is described.

Risk—the risk to the unborn baby

Pregnancy Outcome—favorable, adverse, or uncertain

Documentation—the quality and volume of scientific information available.

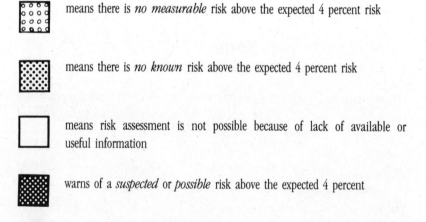

means there is *no measurable* risk above the expected 4 percent risk

means there is *no known* risk above the expected 4 percent risk

means risk assessment is not possible because of lack of available or useful information

warns of a *suspected* or *possible* risk above the expected 4 percent

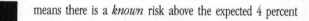

means there is a *known* risk above the expected 4 percent

pre-conception ←	All or None		Organ Development – (in weeks)						Maturation – (in weeks)				
←	1	2	3	4	5	6	7	8	9	10	12	20-36	38

conception ←— Time of Greatest Risk —→ birth

The graph provided for each entry indicates the time and degree of risk for the term of pregnancy. It is shaded for the relevant weeks of prenatal development. Shadings indicate the degree of risk. When the shading undulates it indicates that the specific time of exposure is uncertain. (The differences between these risks are explained in Table 2-2 on page 22.) It is important for you to realize that the estimated risk summary and the risk chart are not meant to be substituted for reading the entire entry; they are provided to aid you in understanding the risk.

The Estimated Risk Summary is followed by a more detailed explanation of the effect of the substance, if any, on an unborn baby. References are listed at the end of the entries. All relevant research papers were examined on each topic, including those evaluated in review articles. To simplify matters for the readers, the individual papers included in these reviews are not cited separately in the reference section.

Many entries include the reasons that obsolete risk information and common misunderstandings persist. Where possible, I have provided reassurance that a previous concern is no longer warranted.

Where appropriate, entries will also list safe alternatives to prescribed and over-the-counter medications. These are natural remedies that can be used safely for treating illnesses during pregnancy and for alleviating some of the discomforts that pregnant women normally experience.

Following select entries are actual stories from women like you, with special concerns. It's my hope that their experiences will help you realize that your worries are perfectly natural and are shared by others.

A Few Words About Absolutes

It is not the purpose of this book to tell you what to do. I firmly believe that the decision that is best for you should be reached by you. You may use what you learn here as the basis for making a decision, or simply to increase your knowledge.

But don't take your health care entirely into your own hands. Please keep in mind that this book is *not* a prescription for health care. That is the province of your health care provider, who knows your particular circumstances. There is no substitution for individual health care by a qualified practitioner. By all means bring this material to his or her attention. Its information is current as of the time of publication, but your physician may have very recent information that alters what is written here.

For your well-being and for the health of your unborn child, please check with your physician before taking a medication or exposing yourself to a chemical or other environmental agent during pregnancy. And by all means, consult with your physician before discontinuing any medication that has been prescribed for you.

Patients' expectations of an absolute yes or no from physicians on their unborn child's normality have expanded more rapidly than have the actual improvements in diagnosis. Few people are aware of this. It is important for parents to realize that even with the latest information and the most accurate of diagnostic procedures, no one can guarantee a perfect baby.

✳ TWO ✳

Risks

The voice of the woman on the telephone was filled with panic and concern. Suzette had not realized she was pregnant at the time she had diagnostic X rays. Her pregnancy was unplanned, but very much wanted.

Accustomed to situations like this, I counseled Suzette about some of the misconceptions surrounding X-radiation and its risk during pregnancy. Then I presented the current data and explained how it related to her particular exposure. I told her that based on the available scientific information, her exposure to X rays would not increase the risk to her unborn baby, beyond the small risk all pregnant women face.

Seven months later came the happy news. Suzette's baby was a beautiful, normal, healthy girl. Suzette and her husband had named her Christina.

As Suzette's story indicates, most of the thousands of women I have counseled have focused their concern on the *agents* or *substances* they may have been exposed to. My first interest is always to alter their direction from the substance itself to something else—the *risk* the substance presents as a consequence of their particular exposure.

We all take risks in our everyday lives. Some risks are voluntary, such as choosing to drive on a crowded highway or going to work on a cloudy day without an umbrella. Other risks we take automatically, just by living—such as breathing the air of a big city.

Pregnancy, too, involves certain risks. You should be aware that pregnancy, even in the United States, with the best of medical care, is not totally risk free. As with other aspects of life, some of these risks come from everyday living—everyone shares them. Other risks relate to our ancestry or to substances we use or come in contact with.

But having said that, I also want you to realize that of the more than 3.5 million babies born in the United States each year, the great majority are perfectly normal and healthy. The odds are overwhelming that your baby will be normal and healthy too!

7

Once pregnant women understand the idea of risk during pregnancy, they usually have other questions:

- How can I minimize my risk?
- Will the risk translate into a problem?
- Can birth defects be predicted before the child is conceived?
- Is there any way of detecting birth defects during pregnancy?

From my counseling experience, I know these questions can be both confusing and frightening. But they needn't be. Knowledge can provide peace of mind.

THE NORMAL RISKS INVOLVED IN PREGNANCY

Every pregnant woman faces a small risk of giving birth to a child with some type of problem. While no one can receive a 100 percent guarantee, pregnancy does result in a normal, healthy infant about 96 percent of the time. This means that the expected risk for abnormalities apparent at birth or soon after—ranging from medically serious malformations such as heart defects and cleft palate to less significant problems such as club foot—is about four percent.*

Predicting Risks

In only a limited number of situations can the probability for specific birth defects actually be predicted *before* you become pregnant. Some of these situations are:

- an abnormality in a previous child, Down syndrome, for example;
- a known defect in either of the parents, or in blood relatives (this could be a type of physical defect or a defect in the chromosomes or genes);
- when women are age 35 or older (or when the father is 50 years or older); and
- when women know they will be exposed to a known teratogen (such as a prescription drug) during pregnancy.

While these situations are associated with a risk for birth defect, only a test during pregnancy (prenatal diagnosis) can reveal if an abnormality has actually occured, in other words, whether the risk translates into a problem. While prenatal diagnosis is a way of learning about such errors in the baby's development before birth, these procedures are not 100 percent accurate and can not yet detect all types of birth defects. (Prenatal diagnosis is also valuable when circumstances arising during a routine pregnancy signal the need for exploring the unborn baby's condition. These

---

*The incidence of risk will vary depending on the population surveyed and the definition of birth defects used. The expected risk most frequently quoted is 3–5 percent. The average is 4 percent.

circumstances are discussed later in this chapter under the prenatal diagnostic procedures, page 21.)

Fortunately, for most pregnant women there is no reason to suspect that the 4 percent risk will be realized.

Causes of Birth Defects

For your peace of mind, you should understand something about the different causes (etiology) of birth defects. Today we know that birth defects are biological responses to altered genetic material or to certain environmental substances, or to a combination— influences that are expressed in the newborn child.

Genetic Causes

Genetics refers to the biological information in each of us that determines our hair and eye color, blood type, nose shape, sex, and other traits and characteristics. This information is carried in the body on *chromosomes* and their subunits, which are called *genes*.

Each of us normally has twenty-three pairs of chromosomes, forty-six in all. Each parent contributes to the child one chromosome from each pair. The father's comes from the sperm cell and the mother's from the egg cell. One pair of chromosomes, called "X–Y," determines the sex of the child. (Females have two X chromosomes, males one X and one Y.) The other chromosomes are called "autosomes."

A birth defect may result when something goes wrong with the chromosomes or the genes. Such genetic misinformation can be inherited from previous generations, or it can occur spontaneously.

Genetic factors account for about 15 percent of all known causes of birth defects.

Approximately 10 percent of genetic defects are caused by *chromosomal abnormalities*. But this number is deceptively small, since such defects are usually major. A chromosomal error can arise from the sperm, the egg, or the newly fertilized egg (zygote). It is estimated that up to 60 percent of all early miscarriages are the result of chromosomal defects. The most common chromosomal disorder seen at birth is Down syndrome (formerly called mongolism), which occurs when the baby has an extra twenty-first chromosome and forty-seven chromosomes in all.

Gene mutations account for about 5 percent of all genetic disorders. These are sometimes refered to as "Mendelian" conditions, after Gregor Mendel, the Austrian naturalist (and monk) who discovered the laws of heredity through his experiments with plants.

A gene mutation is either dominant or recessive. *Dominant* means the mutation can be passed to the child by just one parent. Passing on a *recessive* disorder requires each parent to carry the trait.

An example of an *autosomal dominant disorder* is a form of dwarfism called achondroplasia (a-con-dro-play'-zia). When a parent has such an autosomal dominant disorder, there is a 50 percent chance with each pregnancy that the condition will be passed on to the child.

Everyone carries between four and eight recessive genes for genetic disorders. "Recessive" means that the carrier of an abnormal gene does not have the disease. Only when two of the same altered genes come together, one from each parent, will the disease occur. When two people who carry the same faulty gene conceive a child, the baby has a 25 percent chance of having the disease, and a 50 percent chance of carrying one altered gene. Some conditions resulting from *autosomal recessive disorders* include PKU (phenylketonuria), cystic fibrosis, sickle-cell anemia, and Tay-Sachs disease.

Sex linked or *X-chromosome-linked* mutations are another type of genetic disorder; and as can autosomal mutations, they can be either dominant or recessive. In X-linked recessive disorders, the normal mother often carries an altered gene on one of her X chromosomes. The normal gene on her other X chromosome protects her from having the disease. But, she can pass the abnormal gene on to her children, and this happens 50 percent of the time.

If the child receiving the X chromosome containing the abnormal gene is a girl, she will also be a carrier. If the child who inherits the X chromosome with the abnormal gene is a boy, he will actually have the disease. This is because males have only one X chromosome, which they receive from their mothers. Examples of X-linked conditions include hemophilia, Duchenne muscular dystrophy, and red-green color blindness.

Genetically caused birth defects are not preventable in the true sense of the word. We cannot yet prevent the conception of a child with a genetic defect. Fortunately, though, with advancing technology we are able to detect more and more genetic defects in the baby before birth. (For more information about genetics, ask your health care provider to refer you to a genetic counselor.)

Environmental or Teratogenic Causes

Fortunately, many environmentally caused abnormalities can be prevented. Once teratogens are identified, they can be avoided.

The environmental substances, or *teratogens*, that cause birth defects are drugs, chemicals, infections, pollutants, or physical states in the mother, such as diabetes, that can bring about a variety of alterations in an unborn child. The medical study of such substances and their effects is called *teratology*; the ability of these substances to cause abnormal development is referred to as being *teratogenic*.

Environmental or teratogenic causes are responsible for about 5 percent of birth defects. However, this category may actually be larger, as some birth defects may result from a subtle, but as yet unidentified, environmental agent. Teratogens are agents that interfere with the normal development of an unborn baby. Some examples of identified teratogens are alcohol, rubella (German measles), Dilantin (an anticonvulsant), and the pollutant methylmercury. The way these substances harm the developing baby depends on several things:
• the genetic background of the mother and her child
• the time during pregnancy when the exposure takes place
• the amount of the teratogen that actually reaches the unborn baby
The abnormal development can end in death, malformations, functional defects (mental retardation and learning disabilities), and the subtle effect of growth retardation.

You should remember, however, that *being exposed to a known teratogen does not in itself constitute an increased risk.*

An increased risk is one that exceeds the expected 4 percent population risk. However, even this is not a statement of certainty.

It is not unusual for expectant parents to misinterpret a suggested risk as a definite outcome rather than an *increased chance* of a problem occurring. Like a weather service prediction of rain, it is an evaluation of the probability that an event will happen.

In addition, one *cannot assume that an increased risk exists* when a woman is exposed to many things, either at once or at various times during her pregnancy. Little is known about the effect of multiple exposures, simultaneous or not. Sometimes substances encountered at the same time alter each other's effect on the body, or on the fetus. This alteration may increase a harmful or beneficial action. Or it may actually decrease it. This "additive effect" is possible with teratogens encountered in combination, just as certain drugs could lessen or perhaps enhance the effects of other drugs.

At this state of the art of human teratology, we cannot examine such cumulative effects and define their risks. Our current knowledge only makes it possible to estimate prenatal risks for *individual* compounds.

Risk information in teratology is essentially a sophisticated guess—one based on documentation of the outcomes in women with similar exposures during a common time in pregnancy.

Once informed, most women will choose to avoid exposures to teratogenic substances. In some cases, however, a prescribed, but teratogenic, drug is needed to maintain health, making avoidance of the substance during pregnancy impossible. Erica had such a situation to face:

"Having a baby was very important to me. Like many other women, I wanted to do everything I could to insure that my baby would be healthy. Good nutrition and exercise were already a part of my health care. The only thing I was worried about was the medication I took daily. Ever since the age of sixteen, I have been taking Dilantin, a drug which controls my seizures—I have epilepsy.

"Before I became pregnant, I asked both my obstetrician and my neurologist about how the Dilantin would affect my pregnancy; I was surprised to receive two different answers.

"My neurologist told me that though some people think Dilantin causes cleft lip [harelip] and cleft palate, there was no definitive proof of cleft lip or any other birth defects in children born to women on Dilantin. My obstetrician told me that Dilantin use during pregnancy has been linked to cleft lip, cleft palate, growth retardation, mental deficiency, and heart defects.

"Before reacting, I sought other opinions, and found that most doctors agreed that Dilantin had the ability to harm an unborn baby.

"My first reaction was to stop taking Dilantin and risk having a seizure; I didn't want to take any chances! However, after thinking about how a seizure could be dangerous to both myself and my baby I decided to find out if there was a safer medication to take. Happily, an alternative drug, thought to be safer, was suggested and even though it isn't effective for everyone, it was for me." (For more information about Dilantin, see Hydantoins, page 191.)

As Erica's story shows, facing such an increased risk during pregnancy is a difficult and complex decision, best discussed with a physician or trained counselor. It is imperative to have a clear understanding of the teratogenic risk, including:
• the probability of its occurring
• what the defects are
• how these defects will limit the child
• the potential emotional and financial impact on your family

It is also important to recognize that for certain health conditions, pregnancy itself could present a risk. So when contemplating a pregnancy, it is always a good idea to discuss it with your doctor, particularly when daily medication must be taken.

Multifactorial Causes

About 20 percent of all abnormalities result from multifactorial causes, which are a combination of genetic and environmental influences.

Disorders which are multifactorial in origin tend to run in families but are not inherited in the simple Mendelian fashion. Rather, family members possess a strong genetic predisposition toward the malformation. This combined with environmental factors encourages the abnormality to appear. The extent to which genetic and environmental factors influence the occurrence of a malformation varies from case to case.

Multifactorial disorders include cleft lip (harelip) and cleft palate, the central nervous system conditions called "neural tube defects" (spina bifida and anencephaly), a constriction in the stomach's outlet (pyloric stenosis), congenital hip dislocation, and various heart defects.

Unidentified Causes

Unfortunately, the largest number of birth defects—60 percent—result from unidentified causes. Many of these are probably multifactorial in nature.

Unexplained abnormalities can be particularly distressing and can cause guilt feelings in the parents of affected children. It is common for such parents to search for their own reasons if told by experts that there is no explanation. Some parents will conclude that a drug or chemical exposure during pregnancy was responsible for the child's misfortune, even if there is no such medical evidence.

As one expert has said, people tend to look for an explanation for any problem. If no reasonable one exists, they may find a fantasy explanation. They may think they have done something wrong or failed to do something right. They believe the problem might not have happened had they acted differently. The worst part of such behavior is that it may cloud their judgment and keep them from making the best decisions for the child.[1]

Parents in this situation must come to believe in their own best intentions and to dispel this unnecessary guilt. Many times one of the most important things counsellors can do is to help parents accomplish this.

Minimizing the Risk

The main thing is to concentrate on the 96 percent for having a normal, healthy baby! There are many things you can do to maximize your chances of everything going well:

- seek medical counseling *before* becoming pregnant if you have any medical problems (diabetes for example), if you regularly take medication, or if there is a family history of birth defects or mental retardation,
- *before* you are pregnant find out if you have had rubella (German measles, p. 289), if you haven't, make certain you receive a rubella vaccination (p. 290) (the vaccination is contraindicated during pregnancy),
- follow a course of conscientious prenatal care, including seeing your doctor or other health care provider early in the pregnancy and making regular visits,

- eat a well-balanced diet,
- remember to exercise—walking is good for you, unless your doctor or other health care provider has specifically advised against it,
- take prenatal vitamins, if prescribed, and
- avoid known and suspected teratogens, such as alcohol and cigarettes, and any unnecessary medications.

Finally, *enjoy the pregnancy.* Know that you're doing all you can!

RISKS FROM EXPOSURES
IN THE BABY'S FATHER

It is important to realize that fathers have a role to play in maximizing the chances for a normal pregnancy outcome, just as mothers do.[2,3] Teratogens affect the unborn child directly through the mother's exposure, but scientists are finding that environmental agents encountered by the father also can affect reproduction. However, this is a new area of concern, and information is most often incomplete or sparse.

The role of fathers in the health of their unborn babies has recently been brought to the public's attention by the Agent Orange controversy. Several Vietnam veterans who have fathered malformed children have sued the Veterans Administration and the manufacturers of Agent Orange because they are convinced their exposure to the herbicide was responsible (see Agent Orange, page 55).

While a father's exposure to some environmental agents causes infertility or early miscarriage, other potential effects of the father's exposure are less certain. It is mainly the results of animal studies that have raised concern about men's possible role in causing birth defects. Very few potential "male teratogens" have been studied in both humans and laboratory animals, so there is very little experience in comparing effects of any one agent among various species.

Theoretical effects from environmental exposures in males could include low birth weight, birth defects, growth retardation, and developmental disabilities. *None* of these have been conclusively proven to occur in human beings as the result of an exposure in the father *alone.* Despite this, prospective fathers should not risk unnecessary exposures.

Drugs, chemicals, and physical agents can act through the father in three ways:

1. They can alter the man's sex drive and sexual performance, resulting in temporary or permanent infertility. According to one source, for example, 15 percent of the most often used prescription drugs can change men's reproductive ability.

2. They can be transferred from the sperm to the pregnant woman through sexual

intercourse, and theoretically from her to the unborn child. There have been instances of drugs being detected in seminal fluid. But the chances of their actually causing a birth defect are *extremely* remote, primarily because of the very small quantity of drug involved. In addition, if the drug were present in the semen at the time of fertilization, timing would make it unlikely for a birth defect to occur. It is at the "all or none" stage of teratogenic effects—when the embryo either repairs any damage or is unable to and dies (see The First Two Weeks—the "all or none" phenomenon, page 34.)

3. They can alter the sperm cell either before or after it is mature, resulting in cell, chromosome, or gene damage.

- Cellular damage can decrease male fertility through: lowered sperm count, decreased movement by the sperm, a smaller number of healthy sperm, or a larger number of abnormal sperm.

- Chromosome damage, changes in either chromosomal number or structure, can lead to infertility, miscarriages, or, theoretically, birth defects. In many such cases, however, the abnormalities are lethal. The result is no pregnancy or else a pregnancy loss. In some cases the miscarriage occurs so early that it is confused with a late menstrual period.

- Gene damage causes mutations that can be either dominant or recessive. Only mutations to dominant disorders would most likely be evident because only one dominant gene is necessary for the disease to appear. Recessive mutations would not be apparent for perhaps generations, because the disease can occur only when two individuals with the exact same abnormal gene conceive a child. On average, recessive diseases tend to be more incompatible with life (or limit reproductive potential) than dominant conditions, although a great number of dominant gene mutations are severe enough to be incompatible with life. The results are similar to those for chromosomal abnormalities.

For any of the information provided in this section, you should recall two teratogenic principles: (1) Animal studies cannot be used to predict human effects, and (2) people respond uniquely to drugs or other agents.

Here is a review of what is known about the effects on the unborn child of a variety of substances encountered by men.

Environmental and Occupational Chemicals

Lead. A heavy, toxic metal, lead has long been known to interfere with reproduction in both women and men. It is present in the environment from many sources, including old house paint, polluted soil and drinking water, and automobile emissions. Some people also encounter it in the workplace. Lead affects a man's fertility. Several studies have associated fathers' exposures to lead with increased incidence of miscarriage. Other studies have linked it to more stillborn children and higher death rates of newborn babies, but these effects are the likely result of the mother's exposure. Much of this information was gathered by investigations conducted in the early part of this century when workers were exposed to higher levels of lead and for a longer time than is permitted today.

Vinyl chloride. This chemical is widely used in manufacturing and is known to cause cancer. Men exposed to it have exhibited abnormal chromosomes and diminished sex drive. The rate of miscarriages among wives of men exposed to vinyl chloride is higher than expected. Animal studies have found that the toxic effects of the chemical do not appear in the male reproductive system, and so cannot be transferred to the fetus.

Carbaryl (Sevin). This and several other pesticides are known to damage the chromosomes of men who work with them for long periods. However, no link has been found between them and abnormalities in unborn children.

Dibromochloropropane (DBCP). The wives of men who work with this pesticide were found to have higher rates of spontaneous abortion than expected.

Agent Orange. Exposure of service men to Agent Orange, a defoliant used in the Vietnam War, has been claimed as the cause of an increased risk of abnormality in their children. Despite such claims, scientific studies have found no such association. The issue of Agent Orange is comprehensively reviewed in Chapter 5 (see Agent Orange, page 55).

Kepone. This pesticide (also known as chlordecone) was widely used in the United States until the mid 1970s, though it is no longer manufactured. It is known to have caused sperm abnormalities.

Methylmercury. Another toxic metal found as an environmental pollutant, methylmercury has been linked to abnormal sperm and altered sex drive among men exposed to it. Methylmercury is also an identified teratogen (see mercury, page 231.)

Diseases and Medical Treatments

Epilepsy and Anticonvulsants. Diminished fertility and changes in sperm have been found in some men who have epilepsy. The anticonvulsant medication Dilantin (phenytoin) at one-fifth of its original dose has been found in the sperm of men who use it to control seizures. In addition, Dilantin has been associated with a higher than expected rate of birth defects in the children of men who are taking it. But the malformations probably are related to either the epilepsy or some other factor, rather than to anticonvulsant drugs.

Anesthetic gases. There has been considerable publicity about the possibility that anesthetic gases can cause problems during pregnancy. Several studies have associated these gases with an increased rate of both miscarriages and birth defects among a number of groups: women who are exposed to them on the job and the wives of anesthetists, anesthesiologists, and dentists who are occupationally exposed. Scientific studies have found only one main link between exposure on the job to anesthetics and pregnancy problems: Women who work with the gases under certain conditions have an increased risk of miscarriages (see anesthetics, inhalation, page 76).

Chemotherapy. Various substances used in cancer treatment are known to damage sperm. Return of the sperm to normality may take some time. It would therefore be wise to delay pregnancy until a few months after such therapy is discontinued. It is reassuring to know however, that there is no known association between chemotherapy in the father and birth defects.[4] This is true irrespective of the time of the exposure and the time of conception.

Substances for Nonmedical Use

Alcohol. Despite common beliefs, no well-conducted human studies have found that large amounts of alcohol taken by fathers causes birth defects or other pregnancy problems. As one expert has pointed out, men who abuse alcohol are often married to women with similar problems, so it is difficult to separate the two roles in determining the cause of birth defects. However, some associations have been found in laboratory animals. And long-term male alcoholics exhibit sperm abnormalities of various types, lowered sex drive, and infertility. When cirrhosis of the liver is also present, more extreme reproductive problems occur.

Caffeine. Caffeine is widely available in soft drinks, tea, and coffee, and in various prescription and nonprescription medications used as stimulants and for headache relief. There is a questionable link between its *excessive* use in men and higher than expected rates of miscarriages, prematurity, and stillbirths. But there is no conclusive proof. Animal studies have shown some of these same effects.

Nicotine. This component of tobacco has been associated with newborns of low birth weight and increased rate of death among newborn babies. This effect might be related to the effects of "secondhand" smoke (see cigarette smoking, page 112).

Mind-altering Substances

These drugs may have some adverse effects on men's sexual activity, but their role is not clearly defined.

Physical agents

Radiation. Exposure to ionizing radiation at work or as a medical treatment for cancer may cause damage to sperm, depending on the dose involved. Return of the sperm to normality may take some time. For this reason, men undergoing radiation therapy are recommended to postpone fathering a child until several months after the treatment is concluded. It is reassuring to know, however, that low or even high doses of radiation in males are not linked to malformations. And children who are conceived during their father's recovery phase after radiotherapy for testicular cancer are *not* at a higher risk for birth defects.[4]

Heat. There are few studies of the effects of high temperature, including working in hot environments, on men's reproductive systems. But several have seen an association with various sperm abnormalities. One study found that the effects lasted for three months after the exposure.

In summary, there is very little information currently available on the potential hazards from environmental exposures in men. Risks can be accurately assessed only after more research is conducted in human males.

TOOLS FOR EVALUATING RISKS FROM ENVIRONMENTAL, MEDICINAL, AND OTHER SUBSTANCES (TERATOGENS)

Despite all the uncertainties of determining teratogenic risk, it is possible, of course, to classify risks in a way that can be useful to as many people as possible. The best known classification is that developed by the U.S. Food and Drug Administration (FDA), which rates some drugs on a five-category scale for teratogenicity: A, B, C, D, and X. The purpose of this scale (Table 2–1) is to give physicians information beyond that found on drug package inserts, for counseling their patients. Since it is designed primarily for health professionals, it holds certain problems for interpretation by the general public, so I have designed an alternative—a series of risk statements for use specifically in teratogen counseling, whether for people I speak to personally or for you reading this book.

A word of caution: Health care providers sometimes rely on drug package inserts to provide information on possible teratogenicity. Many of these inserts contain only a phrase such as "safe use of this drug has not been established and it should be used only if the anticipated benefits outweigh potential risks." Animal studies are often the basis for the pregnancy risk information contained in these inserts, which are prepared by the pharmaceutical manufacturers. As a result, the information provided may not be the most current or the most accurate for counseling patients. You should read the package insert for any medication you take. If it isn't provided, ask your pharmacist for one. After you read it, it's a good idea to seek more detailed information on the medication's effects during pregnancy.

Estimated Risk Statements

Semantics are an important consideration in teratogen risk counseling. I have found that individuals in an anxious state may listen selectively and interpret information based on their fears or on what they want to hear. Even individuals in their most lucid moments may be confused by factual presentation of teratological data. To circumvent any misconceptions, five statements have been developed for use as guidelines in summarizing risk counseling, given in Table 2–2.

These statements were developed with pregnancy outcome and documentation in mind.

Pregnancy Outcome—Defined

A pregnancy can have one of three outcomes, based on evaluation of published information about a particular substance:

Favorable

This means that normal pregnancy outcomes have been observed.

Uncertain

The outcome cannot be predicted because:
• there is no information available on human pregnancies, or
• the little information available is not useful, or
• there are conflicting reports of favorable and adverse pregnancy outcomes.

Adverse

A pregnancy outcome is considered adverse if any of the following are observed:
1. pregnancy loss (miscarriage or fetal death)
2. disabilities in the baby after birth, including
   • structural (physical) defects
   • mental retardation
   • learning disabilities
   • growth retardation (including low birth weight)
   • complications at birth, such as withdrawal symptoms, alterations in heartbeat and rhythm or low blood sugar

Documentation—Defined

As you will see in Chapter 4, scientific studies on teratogens have varying degrees of usefulness, depending on their design. In counseling, documentation falls into one of three categories:

Conclusive

Conclusive documentation means that
• well-conducted studies have yielded consistent or similar results; or
• consistent outcomes have been documented (through clinical experience) over time for a large number of pregnant women who shared a similar exposure.

(Here it must be understood that while *risk can* be scientifically measured, total *safety can never be conclusively proven.*)

Inconclusive

Documentation may be inconclusive because
• some knowledge has been gained through clinical experience, but more research is needed;
• the studies may be abundant, but methodologically inadequate, such as biased retrospective studies;
• data may be based on limited number of well-conducted studies, such as prospective studies with only a small number of exposed cases; or
• only minimal human data are available (case reports, for instance) although the results are similar to well-documented animal studies.

Unavailable or insufficient

This means that either no information is available on human pregnancies or that the information available is not useful (insufficient) and conclusions cannot be drawn. As I have said before, data from animal studies cannot be used as the *sole* source of information for assessing a human risk.

A Final Thought on Risk Assessment

I have found that some pregnant women become worried when they hear that "Risk assessment is not possible." This statement should not be interpreted as meaning an increased risk exists. Essentially it means that no published information is available on a particular exposure during human pregnancy. It is basically the same as saying, "I don't know," or stating, "currently the answer to your question is not known." And "I don't know" does not mean we should guess the answer, or that there is no risk.

Just because science has not documented a "problem" does not mean that one couldn't actually exist.

Knowing that there is no available information is, in fact, receiving information. Even though it may seem a bit frustrating, at least you know two things: First, the scientific literature has been reviewed and relevant information concerning your question has not been located. Second, you don't have to search for information any further.

DIAGNOSING AND TREATING PROBLEM PREGNANCIES

Diagnostic Methods Used Before Birth

While the specific *causes* of many birth defects remain unknown, today an increasing number of them can be diagnosed during pregnancy. The state of the medical art does not permit prenatal diagnosis for every defect. When diagnosis before birth *is* possible, it has several benefits.

First and best, it can usually show that the suspected defect is not present. Even when the defect is found, the information is valuable to both parents and child. In an extremely small number of situations, the condition can be treated before birth. In other cases, the knowledge can give the parents time to come to terms with the situation, allowing for emotional adjustments to be made prior to the infant's birth. If necessary, they and the physician can plan courses of treatment and care to be followed after the baby is born. Such information will also help doctors to better manage the pregnancy and birth. In some cases this involves having a medical team ready to handle the special—even lifesaving—needs of the child. And in some instances it can provide the information that will help the woman decide whether to terminate the pregnancy.

Most prenatally detectable abnormalities are genetic in origin. Teratogens often cause subtle patterns of abnormalities and growth retardation rather than the more dramatic malformations. For this reason, prenatal diagnosis is occasionally but not usually an option for women exposed to a known teratogen. Certainly, the arm and leg malformations caused by thalidomide were not subtle. If today's diagnostic procedures had been available twenty years ago, such defects could certainly have been discovered before birth.

Table 2–3 provides an overview of the prenatal diagnostic procedures and the reasons they are used.

Table 2–1: **FDA RISK CATEGORIES**

Category A means that drugs tested through controlled studies of pregnant women do not demonstrate a risk to the fetus during the first three months, and that there is no evidence of a risk later in pregnancy.

Category B includes two possibilities related to animal studies: (1) Studies on pregnant animals have not demonstrated a risk to the fetus, but there have been no controlled studies in women. Or (2) animal studies have shown some risk; however, controlled studies of women in the first trimester have not confirmed the risk, and no risk has been found to women in later stages of pregnancy.

Category C covers two alternatives. (1) Animal studies indicate a risk to the fetus, but no human studies have been performed. (2) No studies in either animals or women are available.

Category D includes drugs that have been associated with a risk when used in humans, but whose potential benefits to the pregnant woman may outweigh the risks—for instance, if the drug is used in the treatment of a life-threatening condition.

Category X is for drugs that have been shown, through either animal or human studies, to cause abnormalities, and which pose a risk that outweighs any possible benefit.

Table 2–2: **ESTIMATED RISK STATEMENTS**

No measurable risk*
PREGNANCY OUTCOME favorable
DOCUMENTATION conclusive, based on current knowledge

No known risk*
PREGNANCY OUTCOME appears favorable
DOCUMENTATION inconclusive; based on minimal data, more studies needed

Risk assessment is not possible
PREGNANCY OUTCOME uncertain
DOCUMENTATION unavailable or insufficient; either no information is available or the available information is not useful (insufficient)

Suspected or possible risk*
PREGNANCY OUTCOME uncertain: favorable and adverse outcomes observed
DOCUMENTATION inconclusive; based on minimal data, more studies needed

Known risk*
PREGNANCY OUTCOME adverse
DOCUMENTATION conclusive, based on current knowledge

*above the expected 4 percent background risk

Table 2-3 PRENATAL DIAGNOSIS (For the most current information, contact a genetic counselor).

Procedure	Estimated Risk of Procedure to the Unborn Baby	Types of Defects Detected	How Often Procedure Is Performed
Ultrasound — Level I	None known (see page 24)	Level I does not scan for defects (but it can detect anencephaly and abnormal amounts of amniotic fluid—too much or too little)	Very frequent
Ultrasound — Level II	None known (see page 24)	Spina bifida, anencephaly and hydrocephalus, also some kidney, bladder, skeleton, and gastrointestinal defects	Fairly often, but only when circumstances indicate it necessary
Amniocentesis	Risk for miscarriage = 1 in 200	Neural tube defects (anencephaly and spina bifida) Various inherited or sporadic chromosome and gene defects (examples: Down syndrome, hemophilia, sickle-cell anemia, and Tay-Sachs disease)	Frequent
Chorionic Villus Sampling	Increased risk (less than 1 in 20) for miscarriage and spontaneous rupture of membranes	Various inherited or sporadic chromosome and gene defects	Under careful study. Maybe more widely available in the near future
Maternal Serum Alpha-fetoprotein	No increased risk	Neural tube defects (anencephaly and spina bifida) Abnormal alpha-fetoprotein levels can also be used as a marker for other types of problems, including some genetic defects (primarily Down syndrome)	Very frequent and routine in some states
Fetal Echocardiography	None known	Arrhythmias (abnormal heartbeat rhythms) Various structural heart defects	Fairly new procedure. Not widely available.

Ultrasound (sonography)

Ultrasound is probably the most commonly used prenatal diagnostic procedure. It involves taking a picture of the baby by means of high-frequency sound waves (similar to sonar scanning of the ocean floor for treasure), and displaying the information on a TV-like monitor. The purpose of this procedure is to obtain information that will help the physician make a diagnosis and provide better care. The intensity of ultrasound used in these diagnostic procedures is very low, and is not known to do any harm to the unborn child or the mother (for more information, see ultrasound, page 329). The person who administers these tests is a *sonographer*.

Ultrasound Level I

This level of ultrasound is used in the "standard" ultrasound examination. *It is not intended to scan for birth defects.* Even so, it should not be used routinely, but only when medically indicated. Some of these indications are:

• to evaluate the age of the fetus when there is a discrepancy between its actual and expected size;
• to locate the placenta when there is vaginal bleeding;
• to determine a multiple pregnancy (twins, triplets, or more);
• to monitor fetal growth when growth retardation is suspected;
• to determine fetal size in breech presentation (when the baby is born buttocks or feet first);
• to evaluate the amount of amniotic fluid surrounding the baby.

Ultrasound Level II

Level II ultrasound is used to help in special procedures such as amniocentesis and chorionic villus sampling. It is also used to search for structural defects in the unborn child. These include neural tube defects (spina bifida and anencephaly), hydrocephaly (enlargement of the cerebral ventricles related to the accumulation of fluid within the baby's brain), malformations in various internal organs (heart, kidneys, bladder, and gastrointestinal tract), and some defects of the bones. The procedure is similar to Level I ultrasound, but the equipment is more sophisticated. This allows for a more detailed examination of the fetus. Level II ultrasound should be performed only by a trained examiner with experience in prenatal diagnosis of birth defects.

Level II ultrasound is *not* routine and is performed only when a problem in the pregnancy is suspected. The test is usually performed between the sixteenth and twenty-fourth weeks, although it can be done earlier or later in pregnancy, depending on when the concern arises.

Amniocentesis

Amniocentesis involves inserting a hollow needle into the mother's abdomen to remove a sample of the amniotic fluid, commonly called the "bag of waters," in which the child "floats." Some of the fluid, along with the fetal cells it contains, is then analyzed in a laboratory. Ultrasound is used along with this procedure in order to reveal the position of the placenta (the organ that connects the child to the mother), the amount and location of the amniotic fluid, fetal age, and various aspects of fetal growth.

Amniocentesis is used primarily to detect chromosomal abnormalities (such as Down syndrome) and certain genetic disorders (such as hemophilia, sickle-cell anemia, thalassemia, and Tay-Sachs disease). In fact, because chromosomal abnormalities increase with advancing maternal age, this test is most often performed on women age 35 and over.

Amniocentesis also reveals the child's sex. This is helpful information for families with Duchenne muscular dystrophy and other X-linked (sex-linked) disorders that affect only male children. The procedure is also used to detect neural tube defects (spina bifida and anencephaly).

In addition to diagnosing various birth defects, amniocentesis is also used to determine the severity of the blood disorder known as "Rh disease." For an expected premature birth, it can also provide valuable information about the maturity of the baby's lungs.

Amniocentesis is usually performed sixteen to seventeen weeks after the first day of the woman's last menstrual period. It carries a 1 in 200 risk of miscarriage above the background risk for pregnancy loss at this point in pregnancy.

Maternal Serum Alpha-Fetoprotein (MSAFP)

This maternal blood test is currently used to screen for defects in the neural tube—the beginning of the central nervous system. Such defects arise from an error in the prenatal development of the brain (anencephaly) and spinal cord (spina bifida). The incidence of these defects in the United States population is about 1 per 1,000 live births. Spina bifida and anencephaly occur with equal frequency.

Alpha-fetoprotein (AFP) is normally produced by the growing fetus. If the neural tube is abnormal, AFP is often present in the amniotic fluid in large amounts. Since AFP crosses the placenta, it can be measured in the mother's blood. Consequently, with a simple blood test most neural tube defects can be detected early in pregnancy.

The test is performed during the second trimester, between the fifteenth and twentieth weeks of pregnancy, preferably at sixteen to eighteen weeks. It poses no health threat to either mother or baby.

Besides neural tube defects, abnormal AFP levels can indicate:
• multiple births (high levels),
• defects in the abdominal wall (high levels),
• fetal death (high levels),
• low birth weight (high levels),
• the possibility that the age of the unborn baby has been underestimated (high levels) or overestimated (low levels), and
• Down syndrome and possibly other types of chromosomal abnormalities (low levels). However, MSAFP is not an adequate substitute for amniocentesis when information on chromosomes is needed.

Chorionic Villus Sampling

This test is performed during the end of the first trimester (weeks nine to eleven), in order to detect chromosomal (genetic), rather than teratogenic problems. It involves removing a small bit of tissue from the chorion (early placental tissue, which is outside the amniotic sac or "bag of waters"). The sample can be taken either through the abdomen (as in amniocentesis), or by entering through the vagina and cervix. Unlike amniocentesis, chorionic villus sampling can be performed in the first trimester of pregnancy, so it provides concerned parents with much earlier information on fetal well-being. Unfortunately, it involves a higher risk for miscarriage in its present stage of development.

The safety and reliability of this test are still under study, and it is currently performed only at a limited number of medical centers in this country and abroad.

Fetal Echocardiography

This is the use of ultrasound to diagnose problems in the unborn baby's heart, either structural or in the heartbeat ("arrhythmia"). Like other forms of prenatal diagnosis, fetal echocardiography is used only when a problem is suspected, specifically, fetal cardiac complications. Fetal echocardiography is usually performed at about twenty weeks gestation and it can detect some serious heart defects. One in 100 newborn babies exhibit abnormal heartbeats, so this procedure could permit treatment before birth. Echocardiography has another use as well. It gives parents and the physician time to arrange for the birth to take place at a hospital that can care for the special needs of a newborn with heart complications.

A Final Thought on Prenatal Diagnosis

Prenatal diagnosis is not for every pregnant woman—and it is not reasonable for every pregnancy to be screened by all available methods of prenatal diagnosis. Many birth defects still cannot be detected. More important, the procedures are not without risks to both mother and unborn child. The woman and her physician must weigh the possible benefits against such risks.

Treatments Used Before Birth

Just as diagnosis of a problem in an unborn child may not show its cause, diagnosis does not guarantee that treatment is possible.

Ideally, correctable problems discovered in unborn children are best treated *after* birth. This is true even if early delivery must be induced to prevent the disease from progressing further. On the other hand, one of the most innovative developments in contemporary medicine is the growing number of techniques for treating unborn babies. Some treatments take place within the womb. Others involve temporarily removing the unborn child, treating the problem, and returning the baby to the womb for further development before delivery. You should be aware that the consequences of fetal surgical treatment are not without potentially life-threatening complications to both mother and child.

Less invasive treatments involve administering medications to the mother, for natural diffusion to the child.

Available Treatments

Treatment before birth can be tried in *only a few* of the instances where prenatal diagnosis has revealed a problem. Even so, the fact that these techniques exist does not necessarily mean they are successful.

One successful treatment is a fetal blood transfusion when mother and child have blood with incompatible Rh factors.

Treatment before birth can be in the form of medications administered to the mother in order to benefit the fetus. Steroids are used to prevent breathing problems (respiratory distress syndrome) in immature lungs, when it is known that the child will be born prematurely. Drug therapy before birth is also an effective means of treating certain heart and thyroid problems.

In some instances bladder obstructions may be surgically treated before birth by placing a drainage tube (or "shunt") in the fetal bladder to allow drainage of fetal urine into the amniotic fluid. Once the child is born, further surgery will be required.

Are Such Techniques Advisable?

Should you take advantage of such a technique, if the situation arises? The question has no simple response.

Treatments before birth ("in utero") are becoming more available, and earlier in pregnancy. As such, they enter a stage of pregnancy when the only previous alternatives were continuing to term, delivering the baby early, or choosing to have an abortion. The availability of these treatments also further highlights the ethical considerations of the rights of the mother and those of the unborn child. One researcher/philosopher has pointed out several of the ethical issues involved.[5]

• Will the treatment actually improve the life of the unborn child, or prevent premature death?

• Will encouraging the possibility of treatment conflict with the parent's possible desire to terminate the pregnancy?

• Is the possibility of treatment based on solid research, or on the physician's enthusiasm?

• What are the economic and social costs if treatment during pregnancy results in the birth of an individual who will need lifelong special care?

Since many of these techniques are still experimental, such questions must be answered in terms of the laws governing medical experimentation. For the parent, the most important provision is that of requiring informed consent before the procedure is performed. To make such a decision, the best information is needed, often requiring diagnostic procedures that themselves might involve some risk.[6]

If you are in such a situation, I have no clear-cut answers for you. No one does. You and your medical advisors must combine your knowledge and your expertise. With this, you will be able to make the best possible decision—one you can live with.

References:

[1]E. Y. Hsia, The genetic counsellor as information giver, *Birth Defects*, 15, Original Article Series (1979): 169–86.

[2]F. L. Cohen, Paternal contributions to birth defects, *Nursing Clinics of North America* 21 (1986): 49–64.

[3]J. M. Joffee and L. F. Soyka, Paternal drug exposure: Effects on reproduction and progeny, *Seminars in Perinatology* 6 (1982): 116–24.

[4]Y. D. Senturia, C. S., Peckham, and M. J. Peckman, Children fathered by men treated for testicular cancer, *Lancet* 2 (1985): 766–69.

[5]J. C. Fletcher, The Fetus as Patient: Ethical Issues, *Journal of the American Medical Association* 246 (1981): 772–73.

[6]S. Elias and G. J. Annas, Perspectives on fetal surgery, *American Journal of Obstetrics and Gynecology* 145 (1983): 807–12.

THREE

How Substances Cause Birth Defects

Abnormal births have occurred throughout history; it is only recently, however, that scientists have begun to understand the real reasons abnormalities occur, as well as to develop ways of predicting their extent.

Certainly you must understand how the conclusions of scientific studies affect pregnant human beings in general. But more important, you need to know under what circumstances the conclusions apply to you as a pregnant individual. This is the essence of teratogenic risk assessment.

Although much remains to be investigated and learned, today teratologists have a method of evaluating all the new information about potentially harmful substances. The answers to your questions come from this evaluation process. These answers depend on a series of generalizations or principles that help define present knowledge about harmful substances and about birth defects.

Once you understand these principles, you will be better able to judge the information you are receiving—whether from the news media, well-intentioned friends, or health care providers.

BIRTH DEFECTS: A HISTORICAL PERSPECTIVE

Early Beliefs About Birth Defects

The word *teratogen* is derived from the Greek word *teras*, meaning "monster." So a teratogen in the literal sense is something that makes monsters. Today we do not refer to a child with an abnormality as a monster, but this was not always true.

Science, religion, tradition, morality, ethics, and the law are some of the cultural ingredients that form people's attitudes toward birth defects and their cause. What people think is the "truth" about the origin of birth defects has changed dramatically over time. Dr. Josef Warkany, one of the pioneers of teratology, has said that, throughout history, attitudes toward deformity have ranged from adoration to hostility. The unexplainable was described as a miracle or wondrous event, or as a portent for good or evil.

In the ancient world, priests combined the functions of healer, moralist, and philosopher. Such priests in sixth century B.C. Chaldea, a province of ancient Babylonia, were among the most famous of the early teratologists. They perceived abnormal births as omens, and made predictions about the future based on a particular defect; the child was seen as a messenger. For example, if a child was born missing its right ear, then the days of the king would be prolonged.

Early Christian Europeans thought some malformed children were hybrids. Children who were thought to resemble nonhuman animals were killed, sometimes along with their mothers. In fact, societies around the world have practiced infanticide of the malformed, sometimes as sacrifices to various gods.

During the fifteenth and sixteenth centuries, Europeans believed that the world was populated by demonic creatures who plagued human beings. Deformities of hands, feet, and ears, and even birthmarks were said to resemble features of the Devil, meaning that the child was probably of satanic origin.

There is a common belief held even today that a pregnancy's outcome may be influenced by the mother's thought and emotions. Originally this idea was used for eugenic purposes—the improvement of the species, or the "fruit of man," for instance, through positive thoughts. At various times during the twentieth century, the popularity of this idea has encouraged expectant mothers to listen to "good music" or read out loud uplifting literature, specifically to give their children an edge in life.

The idea of maternal impressions was also formerly used to explain malformations. If a pregnant woman looked at a rabbit, her baby might be born with a "harelip," the lay term for the malformation known as cleft lip.

The biological basis for understanding the true origins of birth defects dates from the turn of the twentieth century, when the earlier genetic research of Gregor Mendel was rediscovered. Mendel studied the principles of heredity in plants, which later scientists applied to humans and other animal species as well. Thus, scientists came to believe that genetic misinformation was responsible for causing all birth defects—a total turnaround from medieval attitudes.

The picture was not actually complete until the medical community recognized the role of drugs and other substances in causing birth defects.

This did not happen until the thalidomide disaster of the 1960s.

Thalidomide and the Nature of Birth Defects

Between 1959 and early 1962, several thousand malformed babies were born in Germany, Britain, Australia, and other countries. Typically, they had incompletely developed or absent arms and/or legs, and other malformations, also appeared. Two astute clinicians, Dr. Widukind Lenz in West Germany and Dr. W. G. McBride in Australia, linked the children's problems to a sedative drug their mothers had been given to prevent nausea. The drug was called thalidomide.

Lenz and McBride independently reported their suspicions in papers submitted to a well-known medical journal, which rejected it because of the preposterous suggestion that a drug could cause birth defects. At that time scientists believed that the unborn child, protected by the "placental barrier," was secure from all outside influences. After evidence continued to accumulate, the drug thalidomide was finally accepted as the cause of the severe limb malformations.

In 1961 the drug was quickly withdrawn from use.

Thalidomide had been tested for safety by the manufacturer, through studies on laboratory animals. As it turned out, the laboratory animals used in the study did not react to the drug in the same way humans do—they displayed no abnormalities. Thalidomide was never approved for general use in the United States, due to the skepticism about its safety of just one researcher—Dr. Frances O. Kelsey, at the U.S. Food and Drug Administration.

The discovery of thalidomide's effects on unborn babies, combined with other research, led to a revision in understanding the role of the placenta in pregnancy.

Ironically, from this tragedy, hope was born—hope that scientific research and medical observations could help us prevent future mishaps. The fate of the unborn was not, after all, entirely genetically sealed.

HOW SUBSTANCES REACH THE UNBORN CHILD

The thalidomide episode is a stark reminder of how important it is to know how various substances affect the developing human baby. Part of this involves knowing the means by which substances—including teratogens—transfer from the mother's body to that of the unborn child. The principal route of drug and chemical transfer to the developing baby is via the placenta.

Teratogens and the Placenta

The placenta is an organ within the mother's uterus during pregnancy that transfers substances in both directions between mother and her developing child.

As recently as the early 1960s, the placenta was thought of as the "placental barrier" against harmful substances. Its primary function was considered to be the transferring of nutrients from the mother to the baby. To do this, it was believed, the placenta acted as a screen, allowing only good things to enter into the baby's system. Such a concept made it reasonable for physicians to prescribe medications to pregnant women, confident that the drugs would not reach the developing baby.

We now understand that rather than being a barrier, the placenta is really a transfer point, where substances move from the mother's arterial blood to the blood in the baby's veins. So the effect of any substance on the unborn child also involves its interaction with two other dynamic organisms—first, the mother's body, and second, the placenta. As one expert has said, the placenta acts as a mediator between mother and child.

A substance's ability to pass through the placenta depends on its chemical characteristics, but most substances do get across. If the concentration is high enough and the exposure is over a long enough time, appreciable amounts can accumulate in the unborn baby's system.

Several uncertainties are involved in this process. First, as the mother's body changes during the course of a pregnancy, so does its capacity for moving substances to the placenta. In addition, each woman is unique in her specific ability to metabolize substances. This means that some babies will receive more of a substance than others do. And then each individual fetus may react differently to the various substances that reach it across the placenta.

The placenta does something else: It produces various enzymes that react with substances it receives, breaking them down or changing them. And environmental agents it receives from other parts of the mother's body can affect the way the placenta works. (Cigarette smoke is one such agent.) In other words, the placenta's reaction to any substance presented to it can affect the developing fetus in one of several ways:

• The placenta can produce materials that directly act on the baby, causing abnormalities,

• the substance can disrupt the placenta's normal activity, creating an abnormal environment for the baby, or

• it can reduce the ability of the placenta to function effectively.

Any of these might disrupt the normal course of prenatal development. This is why physicians often caution women to avoid using any unnecessary substances.

As you may realize by now, all these uncertainties mean that there are no yes–no answers in teratology. How then do teratologists determine whether substances are indeed harmful or not?

The basis for their decision involves four fundamental principles, against with which they compare the available research. I want you to be equipped to make the best use you can of the information on specific substances presented later in the book. Knowing the principles of teratology and understanding the role they play in the decision process are the best tools you can have for doing this.

THE PRINCIPLES OF TERATOLOGY

These are the principles[1] that I, and other trained counselors, follow in order to assess and estimate the risks a substance or condition might pose to your unborn baby. As such, they also serve as guidelines for use in interpreting the significance of scientific studies. There are various scientific approaches for evaluating the teratogenic potential of a substance. The extent to which a study follows the principles of teratology will determine how dependable the conclusions of the investigation are.

THE FIRST PRINCIPLE: PEOPLE DIFFER. CONSEQUENTLY, ALL TERATOGENS DO NOT AFFECT ALL INDIVIDUALS EQUALLY. AND THEY AFFECT SPECIES DIFFERENTLY.

Similar exposures to teratogens will affect different fetuses differently.

This is because each person's genetic makeup—the traits and characteristics that have been passed from generation to generation—are unique. The genetic makeup, then, of both the mother and the fetus influences the extent to which a given substance affects the developing baby.

Beyond this, genetic differences between species are far greater than any genetic variation among members of a single species. The difference between humans and other species is reflected in the differing responses to potential teratogens. Certain drugs cause abnormalities when given to pregnant animals, but do no harm when given to pregnant women. With other substances, the harm occurs in humans, but not in other species. This was the case with thalidomide, which was tested in rodents without any ill effects, while human prenatal exposure resulted in severe abnormalities.

What these differences between species mean is that studies conducted solely on laboratory animals may not be useful in predicting human effects.

THE SECOND PRINCIPLE: THE POTENTIAL FOR A SUBSTANCE TO INTERFERE WITH A BABY'S NORMAL DEVELOPMENT DEPENDS ON THE STAGE OF PREGNANCY IN WHICH IT IS ENCOUNTERED/TAKEN.

In other words, *timing*.

Keeping in mind the fetus's genetic makeup, and its possible predisposition to react to a substance, the time at which the substance is encountered is critical.

There are specific times during a baby's development when a teratogen has an increased potential to do harm. The most sensitive period is the early part of pregnancy, during organ formation. However, the potential for danger is not over after the first trimester, because other parts of the fetus, the brain, for one, continue to develop throughout pregnancy. As pregnancy advances, the unborn child becomes more resilient in withstanding foreign substances—a teratogen cannot malform a part of the baby that has already formed normally! Learning about the stages of pregnancy will better enable you to understand how the risks for birth defects are estimated. (Fig. 3–1 provides an overview of prenatal development.)

For this discussion, I have divided pregnancy into three stages—*predifferentiation ("all or none"), organ development,* and *maturation.*

The First Two Weeks: The "All or None" Phenomenon

All or None		Organ Development						Maturation			
		1 mo					2 mo	3 mo			term
1wk	2wk	3wk	4wk	5wk	6wk	7wk	8wk	9wk	12wk	20-36wk	38wk

conception

Figure 3–2. "All or None"

This stage is also known as *predifferentiation* (see Fig. 3–2)—the time before cell differentiation. It is the period from conception to the time when the placenta begins to function, allowing substances in the mother's blood supply to be shared with the baby.

The events of the first two weeks of pregnancy provide the basis for what is referred to as the "all-or-none" phenomenon. This assumes that the exposure to a substance will have either

• *no effect*—the child will not be harmed by it—or
• *a total effect,* resulting in a miscarriage.

The "all or none" theory is based on three observations:

1. There is no direct "communication" between the mother's system and that of the embryo. The embryo does not directly encounter the mother's blood supply or

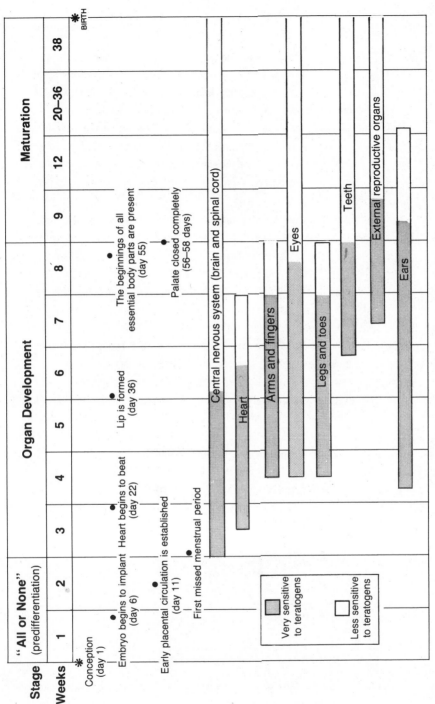

Figure 3–1. Human Prenatal Development

much of anything else from her until the placenta begins to function. This is when the embryo has become *implanted* or attached to the inner wall of the uterus, establishing what will become the placenta. Implantation occurs between days six and eleven and primitive placental circulation is established by around day eleven.

Before implantation, any drug that would affect the embryo would have to be excreted into the mucous blanket of the maternal genital tract, or otherwise independent of the mother's blood supply. One agent that is potentially teratogenic prior to implantation is a very high dose of radiation—far more than received during a normal dental or chest X ray.

2. The embryo is extemely small, composed of only a few cells. Because of this, it is very vulnerable, since a substance that enters the system and destroys too many cells can result in the death of the embryo, and a miscarriage. If the damage is not too extensive, however, the embryo can recover and continue to develop normally.

3. The baby's cells are still all of the same type—referred to as *undifferentiated.* Most people are surprised to discover that an embryo can recover even if its development is disturbed. In the very early embryo, this is possible because the cells are alike. They haven't received their role assignments yet, and do not know what part of the body they will be when they "grow up." In other words, damage to one or more cells will not result in abnormal development of specific organs or systems.

For these three reasons, the "all or none" phenomenon should be good news for those of you worried about exposures that took place during those first two weeks of your pregnancy. (Still, it is important to be aware that this is a theory, and is not a guarantee that if the pregnancy continues, everything will be perfectly fine.)

Weeks Three–Eight: Organ Development

All or None		Organ Development						Maturation			
		1 mo					2 mo	3 mo			term
1wk	2wk	3wk	4wk	5wk	6wk	7wk	8wk	9wk	12wk	20-36wk	38wk

conception

Figure 3–3. Organogenesis

The medical term for the period during which most of the baby's organs develop is *organogenesis* (Fig. 3–3). *Genesis* means the beginning, and *organogenesis* refers to the beginning of organ formation. As Figure 3–1 shows, the first organ to develop is the central nervous system, followed by the heart, arms, eyes, and legs. Though some organs, such as the brain and external genitalia, continue to develop beyond this period, most structures are basically complete by the fifty-fifth day after conception.

Organogenesis describes the stage during which the embryonic cells receive their role assignments, the beginning of cell differentiation. As the cells take on specific roles, they group together to form organs, each with its *critical period of formation*— the specific time frame in which formation begins and ends. Since most organs experience their critical period of formation during the first three months, the first trimester is often referred to as the most important time of pregnancy. But this is true only for organ development.

Weeks 9–36: Maturation

All or None		Organ Development						Maturation			
		1 mo					2 mo	3 mo			term
1wk	2wk	3wk	4wk	5wk	6wk	7wk	8wk	9wk	12wk	20-36wk	38wk

conception

Figure 3–4. Maturation

Maturation (Fig. 3–4) is the last stage of an unborn baby's development. It is the time when the cells in each organ mature and begin to function. In some cases, organ development continues. The brain, for example, remains sensitive to environmental influences throughout pregnancy. The first organ to begin development, the brain is the last organ to finish. In fact, the brain and the rest of the central nervous system are not complete until about eighteen months after the baby is born. As one expert says, birth is just another step in development.

In addition to cell maturation, the last six months of pregnancy are characterized by growth. The baby becomes bigger in terms of length, weight, and head size. A child who is born full term and yet is significantly smaller than it should be in these measurements—meaning 90–97 percent of full-term babies are larger—is considered to be growth retarded. This is referred to as prenatal onset growth deficiency.

Most people do not consider growth retardation to be an abnormality. But intrauterine growth retardation is an abnormality of fetal growth. And it is the most frequent and sensitive indication that a teratogen has been present. Prenatal exposure to alcohol is a good example of this point, as intrauterine growth retardation is one of the most consistent outcomes of drinking during pregnancy. Children with the fetal alcohol syndrome have retarded growth after birth too. This is a consequence of fewer cell numbers in certain parts of the body, including the brain and liver.

This is not the same as being a short/small person or as "dwarfism," which for the most part are genetically determined.

Growth retardation can occur any time during pregnancy. The time when the embryo/fetus is negatively affected will determine the pattern of altered normal growth. Occurring early in pregnancy, the pattern is symmetrical, characterized by a smaller head and body. Uneven or asymmetrical growth retardation, in which the head and brain are growing but body growth is inhibited, occurs in response to interference later in pregnancy (beyond thirty-two weeks).

During the later part of this period, the maturing fetus also begins to respond to certain drugs in a manner similar to that of children and adults. Thus some substances are associated with central nervous system effects, such as lethargy, jitteriness, addiction, and withdrawal. Other drugs can alter fetal breathing movements or interfere with clotting time associated with bleeding.

While it can be compromising to the newborn, one advantage of this fetal reaction is that drugs can be administered to the pregnant mother specifically to treat the fetus, as discussed in Chapter 2.

The Importance of Timing

Now you can appreciate why the stage of pregnancy is important when estimating a risk from an exposure. A number of teratogenic agents, including tetracycline and cigarette smoking, do their damage in the latter part of pregnancy. Since the baby's organs and systems develop at very specific times, knowing when the exposure occurred is vital for understanding whether a particular substance caused a malformation. For example, an agent demonstrated to increase the risk of heart defects, taken during the heart's period of development (the first eight weeks) could very well encourage the expression of that defect. By the same token, a substance suspected of causing cleft lip (harelip) and introduced into the baby's system after the seventh week of pregnancy would be unlikely to cause that defect since the critical period for it (thirty-five days) has passed.

In other words, *exposure to a known teratogen increases risk of malformation only at particular times for particular organs or developmental events.* It is so important that teratologists are very skeptical about the conclusions of studies that fail to document accurately *when* during pregnancy the exposure took place. And it is one reason why not all scientific studies are relevant to risk assessment.

THIRD PRINCIPLE: A SPECIFIC AMOUNT OR DOSE OF A TERATOGEN IS REQUIRED BEFORE THE UNBORN BABY IS DAMAGED.

The key idea here is *dose,* specifically the *dosage threshold,* or the lowest dose of a substance at which irreparable damage is done. For every teratogen there is a dose that will cause no damage, and there is a dose that will cause more damage than the unborn child can recover from. Therefore, it is not *whether* a substance transfers across the placenta that implies teratogenicity, but *how much.*

There are two possible ways for a dangerous dose to be received—a large concentration of the agent in a single dose, or an elevated concentration over a given period of time. We do not know which of these alternatives is more important in terms of interference with normal embryonic development.

The dose for which an agent is known to be teratogenic is usually below the amount that causes toxicity (poisoning) in adults. And many substances when given to the right species, at the right time, and in large enough doses, are capable of adversely affecting development.

The risk to the developing baby will rise with an increase in the amount of the teratogen present in its system. For example, a baby's risk for having the fetal alcohol syndrome, characterized by various developmental abnormalities, increases with the amount of alcohol the mother consumes and the frequency of consumption. But in each case, the dosage threshold is dependent on other factors. The amount of alcohol necessary to cause malformations (dosage threshold) will also depend on the mother's and the fetus's susceptibilities—their own *genetic* makeup (First Principle)—as well as on the stage of pregnancy during which she drinks (Second Principle). The same is true of any teratogen.

For these reasons, science is not yet able to determine individual human dosage thresholds.

FOURTH PRINCIPLE: ABNORMAL DEVELOPMENT RESULTS IN DEATH, STRUCTURAL ABNORMALITIES, GROWTH RETARDATION, AND FUNCTIONAL DEFECTS.

I mentioned earlier that the fetus has some ability to recover from damage caused by a teratogen. However, if too many of its cells are destroyed, the fetus will not be able to recover. Instead, it will develop abnormally, with a potential spectrum ranging from death to several kinds of damage. These include physical malformations, growth

retardation, and such functional abnormalities as mental retardation, learning disabilities and hyperactivity, and other behavioral problems. The spectrum of defects
corresponds to the time of exposure and the systems undergoing major development at
that time.

Typically, the abnormalities produced by teratogens are characteristic *patterns of
malformation,* rather than single defects. Such patterns tend to appear over and over
again, indicating that teratogens have a preference for interfering with certain aspects
of development. It is this consistency that leads investigators to implicate a particular
substance as teratogenic. A good example is the characteristic facial appearance,
central nervous system problems, and growth retardation all seen in children with the
fetal alcohol syndrome.

But these abnormalities are not always unique to a single teratogen, as different
substances can produce similar effects. For instance, several teratogens are known to
interfere with normal central nervous system development. Finally, despite the drama
of thalidomide, many of the teratogen-caused malformations we know about are subtle
in appearance, making their effects more difficult to recognize. Unfortunately, some
problems, such as mental retardation and learning disabilities, are difficult to
recognize at birth.

Reference:

[1] J. G. Wilson and F. C. Fraser, *Handbook of Teratology, Principles and Etiology,* vol 1. (New York:
Plenum Press, 1977), pp. 49–62.

✳ FOUR ✳

Evaluating Scientific Information

Teratology is a relatively new field, and the ways in which substances interact with developing babies are just beginning to be discovered. For instance, scientists cannot yet predict a substance's possible harmful effect simply by examining its structure or its expected behavior in the human system. Also, a substance's ability to pass to the fetus does not automatically mean it will be harmful.

Tests of possibly harmful materials in pregnant laboratory animals are not satisfactory, because the reactions may differ from one species to another—as the thalidomide episode showed. However, if a substance causes defects in several animal species, it is viewed with suspicion for human use.

As a result, a substance's teratogenicity is determined mostly by its track record in human babies inadvertently exposed to it. This is usually done through studies of the incidence of various defects among selected groups of babies.

Once the studies are completed, teratologists can begin to evaluate the significance of their findings. As you have seen, there are no yes–no answers to the question "Is the substance harmful?" Teratologists use the Principles of Teratology* as guidelines in making informed judgments about the safety or harmfulness of any substance. In other words, the scientific studies become the raw material to which they apply the principles.

For this reason, I want you to understand the Principles of Teratology. I want you to be able to do the same thing the professionals do—evaluate information you read or hear that state "such-and-such causes birth defects."

As an informed person, you can add your intelligent judgment to the evaluations you obtain from others, using the same scientific principles they use (or should).

*people differ; importance of timing; dosage; abnormal development results in several possible defects

41

The origin of any information about teratogenic effects is one of the several types of scientific study. I am going to go into some detail about this because these studies have varying degrees of appropriateness for assessing and estimating the risk of birth defects. Because there are several important points to remember about all of this, here is a list of questions to ask yourself when evaluating the reliability of a study's results:

- "What type of study is this?"
- "Is there a human study of this substance, as well as the animal study?"
- "Is this the result of a large-scale study, or an isolated case?"
- "Was the study group's size appropriate for the presumed risk?"
- "Did a trained observer personally examine each child?"
- "Were the normal as well as the abnormal exposed children studied?"
- "How long after the births was the information collected?"
- "Were medical records the only source of information on exposed children?"
- "How accurately did the study pinpoint the time during pregnancy of the exposure?"
- "Did the study consider other possible causes of the defects?"
- "Is there more recent information about this substance?"

HUMAN STUDIES

There are three different types of investigation into human health problems: the prospective study, the retrospective study, and the case report.

Prospective Studies

The most accurate type of scientific study for determining the teratogenicity of a drug or chemical and for calculating the degree of risk involved is "prospective." Prospective means looking toward the future. A prospective study begins by gathering all necessary information from a population of pregnant women who share a common exposure. This type of study can end at birth, or the investigators can follow the "exposed" and "unexposed" children over a long period of time. Certainly, the longer the study continues, the more valuable the results are because the outcome in terms of growth, behavior, and motor and intellectual development can be better evaluated.

The reason prospective studies are more accurate is that the timing (Second Principle) and dosage (Third Principle) of an exposure can best be documented by interviewing the mother while she is pregnant. Data can be gathered on exposures that are difficult to document later, after the child is born. For example, information on nonprescription and illegal drugs can be recorded along with the details of her exposure to chemicals at work or to pesticides.

Another bonus of prospective studies is that the magnitude of the risk can be calculated, because the number of women who were exposed is known. This permits determination of the number of children born both normal and abnormal (First Principle).

A control group (pregnant women who were not exposed), if used, is also followed in a similar manner. Only at the end of the study period can the results of a prospective study be known. If the study is well designed and carried out—if the population studied is large enough and if other risk factors are taken into account—then the results are highly reliable.

While the majority of the studies found in the medical literature on the effects of drugs and chemicals on the unborn are not conducted in this manner, those that are usually provide the most accurate data for human risk counseling.

In any study, the size of the population under investigation should be appropriate to the presumed risk: The lower the anticipated risk, the larger the study population should be. If the presumed risk is, say, 50 percent, then the study group need not be too large, since the results should be readily apparent. However, if the anticipated risk of a teratogen is considered to be low, say 1–2 percent over the ordinary 4 percent risk of birth defects, then the study group should be large. Here, if the group is small, the defects, particularly the rarer malformations, might not show up. Under these circumstances, not detecting an increase in abnormalities may result in a false sense of security.

On the other hand, lack of supporting evidence that an agent is teratogenic does not rule out its potential to be a "low-level" teratogen. This is one reason why it is so difficult to say with any certainty that a substance is "safe."

Finally, it should be asked whether the study has revealed a consistent pattern of malformation (Fourth Principle), especially the frequently subtle ones, for example, the small eye openings, thin smooth upper lip, and flat mid-facial area seen with the fetal alcohol syndrome. Unless each child in a study is examined by a trained observer, the subtle pattern of abnormalities caused by a teratogen might not be noticed.

Retrospective Studies

A common but often less effective type of study is the *retrospective*, meaning going back in time. In a retrospective study, the group is defined by the outcome, so it often begins with a group of children who were born with an abnormality. By examining medical records or through interviewing the mothers, the study attempts to identify the cause of the problem. Such studies allow formulation of hypotheses about cause in a relatively short period of time. The primary limitation of this approach is that it is very difficult to collect accurate information on drugs, chemicals, and infection after the fact. If a study looks only at medical records, then nonprescription drugs and chemical exposures might be overlooked.

If the information for a retrospective study is collected by interviewing the abnormal child's mother, she might not remember exactly *what* the drug or chemical was. Even more difficult than remembering what substance she took is attempting to recall the exact *time* (Second Principle) of the exposure during her pregnancy. If the child is ten years old, the mother must search her memory for events that occurred more than a decade ago.

Knowing when an exposure occurred (Second Principle) is important when interpreting the results of any study, and is crucial to your understanding of why all studies are not relevant to risk assessment. To imply that an agent caused a particular birth defect, the time of the exposure needs to coincide with the time of development for that particular structure. Retrospective studies, for example, often fail to adequately document the exposure information. This makes them not worthless but of less value. At times, this course is the only one available, because the approach is very cost-effective.

Most women want to know how high their risk is for having a child with a problem. Risks are calculated by knowing how many women had an exposure, during a particular time of pregnancy (Second Principle), and how many of these women had normal or abnormal children. Retrospective studies are also deficient for this purpose, because the magnitude of a risk can only be guessed. If a retrospective study investigates the prenatal drug and chemical exposures only of abnormal children, then no one can determine how many other children who had the same exposure were born normal (First Principle).

Retrospective studies often fail to include an examination of the exposed infants. Instead they may identify abnormal children through medical records where only very obvious abnormalities can be noted. Early pregnancy loss and the less dramatic defects, which teratogens often cause, are not usually recorded on hospital birth records or on death certificates.

Case Reports

Case reports, are presentations of *single instances* in which an abnormal pregnancy outcome follows an unusual exposure. Case reports can be a result of either prospective or retrospective observation. While such reports call attention to suspicious events, it is inappropriate to conclude, particularly from an isolated event, that the exposure caused the defect. As every pregnancy faces a small risk for an adverse outcome, observing this after exposure to an agent could simply be a chance occurrence. When several case reports describe similar exposures and pregnancy outcomes, actual risks are suspected.

Stories about birth defects that appear in the daily and weekly press often stem from case reports, since there are many more of them than of fully developed prospective or retrospective studies. The concern these stories cause among parents-to-be has several negative effects. They create undue fears, since they represent isolated events. And the press rarely gives equal time to the later investigations that often disprove the original suspected cause. In addition, the unproven fears such stories trigger may lead to lawsuits that must be evaluated by jurors who may be equally misinformed.

The teratogenic effects discovered in some case reports have later been found accurate. However, it is important to realize that most of the possible effects reported in this manner in medical journals have not been substantiated.

Whatever the outcome, it is vital to remember that case reports do not *prove* anything. They only *suggest the possibility*.

Limitations of Human Studies

It is very important to understand some of the inherent limitations of all human studies.

In order to be useful, a human study should clearly link the teratogen to the defect (Fourth Principle). For instance, if a teratogenic effect is reported for a drug prescribed for a medical condition, it may be difficult to separate its effect on the fetus from the effect of the illness for which it was prescribed.

As another example, behavioral problems in a child may be linked to the teratogenic effect of substance abuse by the pregnant mother. Yet the child's difficulty may just as well have been caused by one or more other factors, which are difficult to sort out. These may include poor maternal nutrition, the mother's age, difficulties during delivery, infections, poor parenting, or many other social factors. If the study does not investigate *each possible alternative* to a teratogenic effect, its results should be accepted cautiously. Because of the difficulties in sorting out the constellation of factors that influence childhood behavior, most studies cannot provide conclusive results.

Studies examining performance and development beyond the newborn period and early infancy unfortunately are infrequent. As most signs of central nervous system disability may not be apparent until later, usually not until the child is of school age, long-term follow-up studies are required.

Certain studies only demonstrate that a drug or chemical can pass into the baby's system. Based on the Third Principle, in order to cause harm, the substance must be present at a particular level. But if we don't know what the substance does to the developing baby, its mere presence doesn't tell us anything. The study must demonstrate that a baby who is prenatally exposed to a drug is either born normal or born with a defect.

Or the reporting of birth defects in the study group may imply a cause-and-effect that does not actually exist—a statistical fluke of just a chance occurrence. In other words, seeing an association between a drug and a birth defect does not prove the drug caused the problem. Just as failing to find an association does not prove that the drug is safe.

As one well-known expert has said, "We will never be in a position to state that an environmental agent has no teratogenic potential. The most we can say is that the agent presents no measurable risk."[1]

ANIMAL STUDIES

Many animal studies are designed to provide an understanding of the basic principles of abnormal developmental biology. Animal studies are required by the U.S. Food and Drug Administration for preclinical evaluation of the safety of pharmaceutical drugs. Often large numbers of abnormal offspring are required, so pregnant animals are treated with high doses (way above the human therapeutic range). Such levels can cause maternal illness and death, as well as fetal abnormalities.

As stated earlier, the results of animal studies are not always useful in predicting teratogenic effects in humans. This is illustrated beautifully by research conducted by the U.S. Food and Drug Administration (FDA) on the effects of the drug caffeine, a component of coffee. Typical of animal studies, the FDA's investigation involved administration of large amounts (Third Principle) of caffeine to pregnant rats, the equivalent of drinking up to eighty cups of coffee at one time. The caffeine was administered through a tube into the rats' stomachs—a manner quite different from the way we consume coffee. In addition, the FDA researchers chose an animal, the rat, that metabolizes caffeine in a completely different manner than humans do (First Principle). The end result? The FDA's conclusions on the relationship between caffeine and birth defects cannot be used to understand the effect of the drug on a human embryo or fetus.

On the other hand, some drugs may cause malformations in human children, but do no damage to the offspring of pregnant animals. The prime example here was the tragedy of thalidomide, in which the studies of pregnant rodents did not reveal it to cause any abnormalities. In humans, however, approximately 20–30 percent of the children (First Principle) whose mothers took thalidomide 24–36 days after conception (Second Principle)—the time of limb development—were born with severe limb abnormalities (Fourth Principle).

These are only two illustrations of the unsuitability of animal studies for predicting what might occur in a human pregnancy. Because of this, *animal studies will be addressed in this book only when they illuminate the answers to questions in human studies,* or when their conclusions have misrepresented or confused the true situation. The reason for this is that some anxious pregnant women have difficulty maintaining a perspective on the limitations of experimental studies and their results.

My most memorable instance of this is the occasion when I had to explain the significance of a study showing that a substance caused infant mice to be born minus their tails. My pregnant caller became very upset, and I had to remind her that it was, in fact, desirable to have a human child without a tail!

Conclusion

In sum, keep these things in mind when evaluating any information you encounter:
- No single approach will either prove or disprove that a substance is safe or harmful during pregnancy.
- Despite what you read or see in the news about "authoritative evidence" implicating an agent as a teratogen, be skeptical! One study proves nothing, and any definitive conclusions based on it are premature. The best scientific evidence comes when several independent studies reach the same conclusions. When in doubt, seek the opinions of medical experts.
- Case reports are important in alerting clinicians to suspicious agents. But alone, they are not appropriate for predicting risk for pregnant women.
- Abnormal pregnancy outcomes are more likely to be reported in medical journals than normal ones. So the uncritical reader may infer from such reports a degree of risk that does not in fact exist.
- Some individuals mistakenly use the results of animal studies to predict the outcome of a human pregnancy.
- Be especially careful in accepting calculation of risk, even if you read it in a drug package insert. It may have originated in an animal study, from poor analysis of statistical data, or from an error in data collection.
- There are also quite a few well-established rumors that even health professionals don't recognize as myths. For instance, the vaccine to prevent rubella (German

measles) has mistakenly been considered teratogenic because it contains a version of the live rubella virus (see rubella vaccine, page 290). So, even if it is something that you are "sure is true," check it out with your doctor or an expert in the field.

• It is important to know how up-to-date the information behind a conclusion or recommendation is. With the rapid influx of new data, the risk counseling on a particular substance may change or be supplemented.

• Last, but not least, remember *always to consult your health care provider* with any questions you might have!

Reference:

[1]Brent, Editorial comment on comments on "Teratogen Update: Bendectin," *Teratology* 31 (1985): 429–30.

∗ FIVE ∗

Can This Substance Harm My Unborn Baby?

Many women have questions about substances that might harm their unborn children. For you, such questions may arise from your obstetrician's warnings, after reading a magazine article about an over-the-counter medication, or after seeing a news story about a local air or water pollutant. Whatever the substance involved and the way you learned it, the answer you of course want to hear is, "No, it's not dangerous, and it's not going to hurt your baby."

Scientists rarely give yes–no answers, and for good reason. They recognize the difference between the general and the particular. And teratologists recognize the limitations on what is known about the effects of individual substances on an unborn baby.

If you keep such limitations in mind, this chapter will provide you with useful information about many substances. It will enable you to avoid harmful and questionable substances. And it will set your mind at ease about substances with no known increased risk to your baby. The entries are written to be as easy as possible for you to use. However, if you have any doubts about the precise meaning of the risk statements, be sure to review the discussion on Tools for Evaluating Risks, pages 18–21, 22.

The entries for the individual substances are listed in alphabetical order. If the entry is for a medication, the generic name is listed. If there is no generic name, the agent's common or popular name is used. If there is a brand or a chemical name, this is also listed. In some cases, related substances are grouped under their medication classification. Though they are grouped in the entry, each is listed in the index, for easy referral.

The FDA pregnancy category is a letter rating of risk provided by the drug's manufacturer, based on guidelines established by the U.S. Food and Drug Administration. This is a fairly new system, and not all drugs have been rated by their manufacturers. If no rating is available, a dash (——) is used. The estimated risk summary is my evaluation of the agent, according to Table 2–2 on page 22. It relates the time of exposure, the estimated risk itself, the observed pregnancy outcome, and the documentation or quality and volume of information on which the risk assessment is based. The chart gives the degree of risk, if any, for various times during the pregnancy. The key on this page explains what the shadings indicate. It is imperative that you realize the estimated risk summary and the risk chart are not meant to be substitutions for reading the entire entry; they are meant only to aid your understanding of the risk. The remainder of the entry is a detailed description of the agent, the ways it is used, and its effects, if any, on an unborn child. References to the scientific studies are listed at the end of the entry. Following select entries are actual stories from women like you, with special concerns. It's my hope that their experiences will in some way help you realize that your worries are perfectly natural and are also shared by others.

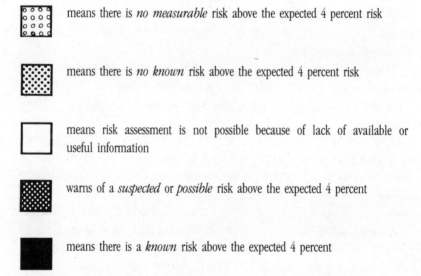

means there is *no measurable* risk above the expected 4 percent risk

means there is *no known* risk above the expected 4 percent risk

means risk assessment is not possible because of lack of available or useful information

warns of a *suspected* or *possible* risk above the expected 4 percent

means there is a *known* risk above the expected 4 percent

GENERIC NAME: **ACEBUTOLOL**

Brand Name: (Sectral)

FDA Pregnancy Category: B

ESTIMATED RISK SUMMARY:

Time of Exposure first 3 months
Risk Risk assessment is not possible
Pregnancy Outcome uncertain
Documentation insufficient

Time of Exposure last 6 months of pregnancy
Risk No known risk*
Pregnancy Outcome appears favorable
Documentation inconclusive

Time of Exposure near the time of delivery
Risk Suspected risk* for slower than normal heartbeat (bradycardia)
Pregnancy Outcome uncertain: favorable and adverse outcomes observed
Documentation inconclusive, based on minimal data

pre-conception	All or None		Organ Development – (in weeks)						Maturation – (in weeks)				
	1	2	3	4	5	6	7	8	9	10	12	20-36	38

conception ←—— Time of Greatest Risk ——→ birth

Acebutolol belongs to a group of drugs that are classified as beta-adrenergic blocking agents (beta blockers). It is used to treat high blood pressure (hypertension) and certain abnormal heartbeat rhythms (arrhythmias). While birth defects have not been linked to the use of acebutolol by pregnant women, information relative to its use during the first three months of pregnancy is lacking.

A slight decrease in average birth weights of acebutolol-exposed infants has been reported. The mother's illness along with other medications she might also be taking could have contributed to an observed effect on birth weight.

Acebutolol has been associatd with slower than normal heartbeat (bradycardia) and low blood pressure (hypotension) in some newborn infants whose mothers took this drug near the time of delivery.[1] For this reason, babies born to women using this drug should be observed for a couple of days for any evidence of these symptoms.

Long-term follow-up studies of children exposed before birth have not been located.

*above the 4% background risk

Reference:

[1]Y. Dumez, C. Tchobroutsky, H. Hornych, and C. Amiel-Tison, Neonatal effects of maternal administration of acebutolol, *British Medical Journal* 283 (1981): 1077–79.

GENERIC NAME: **ACETAMINOPHEN**

Brand Names: **(A Cenol, Acephen, Aceta, Actamin, Amphenol, Anacin-3, Anuphen, APAP, Banesin, Bayapap, Bromo Seltzer, Children's Anacin-3, Children's Panadol, Children's Tylenol, Conacetol, Dapa, Datril, Dolanex, Febrinol, Genebs, Halenol, Liquiprin, Medatab, Mejoral, Mejoralito, Mejoral without Aspirin, Neopap Supprettes, Oraphen-PD, Panadol, Panex, Pedric Wafers, Peedee, Phenaphen, St. Joseph Aspirin-Free, SK-APAP, Sudoprin, Suppap, Tapanol, Tapar, Tempra, Tenol, Tylenol, Tylenol Extra Strength, Ty-tabs, Valadol, Valorin)**

FDA Pregnancy Category: —

ESTIMATED RISK SUMMARY:
   Time of Exposure before conception and throughout pregnancy
   Risk No known risk*
   Pregnancy Outcome appears favorable
   Documentation inconclusive

pre-conception	All or None	Organ Development – (in weeks)						Maturation – (in weeks)				
	1	2	3	4	5	6	7	8	9	10	12	20-36	38

conception   ←——Time of Greatest Risk——→   birth

Acetaminophen is used to relieve pain and reduce fevers. As an alternative to aspirin, acetaminophen is less irritating to the stomach and does not prolong bleeding time (see salicylates, page 293). However, it lacks the anti-inflammatory effects of aspirin.

*above the 4% background risk

Acetaminophen's lack of side effects had made it increasingly popular since the 1950s as a pain reliever during pregnancy. Studies have failed to demonstrate that the use of acetaminophen during pregnancy causes birth defects.[1] Considering the extensive use of this drug, the few isolated cases of birth defects in women taking it appear to be coincidental.

If medication is needed to reduce pain or a fever in the latter part of pregnancy, particularly near delivery time, acetaminophen is the drug of choice. Unlike aspirin, it does not promote maternal or fetal bleeding or affect the incidence of intracranial hemorhage (bleeding in the head) in newborns.

In adults, overdoses of acetaminophen have produced severe liver damage. Theoretically, similar damage could occur in an unborn child if the pregnant mother took an overdosage. In three known cases of acetaminophen overdosage during pregnancy, two infants had no apparent drug affects[2,3] and one fetus, shown to have poisonous concentrations of acetaminophen in its system, died.[4]

*Natural remedies for headaches:***

The bodily changes and emotional stress of pregnancy cause headaches. While an occasional headache might be anticipated, if you have frequent or severe headaches, consult your health care provider. And do not take *any* headache medications, either prescription or over-the-counter, without the approval of your physician.

The better-safe-than-sorry approach to dealing with headache would be to avoid any kind of medication. Here are some commonsense methods of dealing with headache and with the stress that may cause it:[5]

Avoidance. If you can determine which situations or substances—such as eyestrain, fluorescent light, and stuffy rooms—cause your headache, make an effort to avoid them.

Empty stomach. Eat often during the day, but be certain not to overeat.

Fluids. Don't allow yourself to become dehydrated. Drink adequate amounts of fluid.

Fresh air. Try to spend part of each day outside if the air is fresh.

Stress reduction. Rest during the day and get enough sleep at night.

Massage. Muscle relaxation is a good way to avoid or reduce headaches. Massage (or have someone else massage) your scalp, face, neck, and shoulders.

References:

[1]E. Collins, Maternal and fetal effects of acetaminophen and salicylates in pregnancy, *Obstetrics and Gynecology* 58S (1981): 57S–62S.

**None of these commonsense remedies have been medically proven. They are listed here for you because I have found them useful.

[2]A. J. Byer, T. R. Taylor, and J. R. Semmer, Acetaminophen overdose in the third trimester of pregnancy, *Journal of the American Medical Association* 247 (1982): 3114–15.

[3]I. M. Stokes, Paracetamol overdose in the second trimester of pregnancy, *British Journal of Obstetrics and Gynecology* 91 (1984): 286–88.

[4]H. Haibach, J. E. Akhter, M. S. Muscato, P. L. Cary, and M. F. Hoffman, Acetaminophen overdose with fetal demise, *American Journal of Clinical Pathology* 82 (1984): 240–42.

[5]The Over-The-Counter-Drug Committee of the Coalition for the Medical Rights of Women, *Safe and Natural Remedies for Discomforts of Pregnancy* (San Francisco, Calif., January 1981; rev. 1982).

GENERIC NAME: **ACYCLOVIR**

Brand Name: **(Zovirax)**

FDA Pregnancy Category: C

ESTIMATED RISK SUMMARY:
   Time of Exposure throughout pregnancy
   Risk Risk assessment is not possible
   Pregnancy Outcome uncertain
   Documentation insufficient

pre-conception	All or None		Organ Development – (in weeks)						Maturation – (in weeks)				
	1	2	3	4	5	6	7	8	9	10	12	20-36	38

conception   ← Time of Greatest Risk →   birth

Acyclovir is an antiviral agent used primarily to treat initial episodes of genital herpes infection (see herpes, page 187). It is only marginally effective in suppressing and treating recurrent episodes.

Acyclovir has not been shown to be teratogenic in laboratory animals. In humans there is evidence that it crosses the placenta, but information on its potential to cause birth defects is unavailable.

In extreme cases of herpes infection, women in the third trimester of pregnancy have received acyclovir.[1] Currently there is no evidence of adverse effects in either the mothers or their children when the drug is used this way. Whether acyclovir could be used to treat or prevent infection in the unborn remains to be determined.

Because of the way acyclovir works against herpes infection, some researchers think it might be a mutagen (produce changes in genetic material). Research suggests that these concerns are related to doses far above what is needed for treatment. Also, acyclovir seems to be selective in its action, killing the virus in infected cells but leaving uninfected cells alone.[2] In general, acyclovir seems to be of low toxicity, and investigations do not show it to be a mutagen.

Long-term follow-up studies of children exposed before birth have not been located.

References:

[1]S. A. Berger, M. Weinberg, T. Treves, P, Sorkin, E. Geller, G. Yedwab, A. Tomer, M. Rabey, and D. Michaeli, Herpes encephalitis during pregnancy: Failure of acyclovir and adenine arabinoside to prevent neonatal herpes, *Israel Journal of Medical Sciences* 22 (1986): 41–44.

[2]G. B. Elion, P. A. Furman, J. A. Fyfe, P. De Miranda, L. Beauchamp, and H. J. Schaeffer, Selectivity of action of an antiherpetic agent (9-(2 hydroxyethoxymethyl) guanine. *Proceedings of the National Academy of Sciences of the United States* 74 (1977): 5716–20.

COMMON NAME: **AGENT ORANGE**

Chemical Names: **(phenoxyherbicides, dioxin (TCDD), 2,4,5-T and 2,4-D)**

FDA Pregnancy Category: not applicable

ESTIMATED RISK SUMMARY:

Time of Exposure before conception
Risk No known risk*
Pregnancy Outcome appears favorable
Documentation inconclusive

Time of Exposure throughout pregnancy
Risk Risk assessment is not possible
Pregnancy Outcome uncertain
Documentation insufficient

pre-conception	All or None		Organ Development – (in weeks)						Maturation – (in weeks)				
	1	2	3	4	5	6	7	8	9	10	12	20-36	38

conception   ←—Time of Greatest Risk—→   birth

*above the expected 4% background risk

Agent Orange,[1,2] named for the color of its container barrels, was a herbicide used in Vietnam to clear jungle vegetation and destroy crops. Its widespread use there (potentially millions of people were exposed) has caused extreme public concern over its possible health effects, particularly among Vietnam veterans and their families. Exposure to Agent Orange has been suspected of causing a variety of physical problems, but the following discussion will be confined primarily to its effect on reproduction in men who saw military service in Vietnam.

For more information on male exposures in general, see Risks from Exposures in the Baby's Father, page 14. Risks for both males and females from exposures to herbicides, either before or during pregnancy, can be found under herbicides, page 182.

Agent Orange is an equal mixture of two herbicides: 2,4-D and 2,4,5-T. During the manufacturing of 2,4,5-T it is unfortunately contaminated by unwanted by-products, called dioxins. The most toxic and most studied of the dioxins is TCDD (2,3,7,8-TCDD).

Experimental studies using rodents have shown 2,4-D, 2,4,5-T and TCDD to be teratogenic, with TCDD ("dioxin") by far the most harmful.

It is unfortunate, but very limited data exists on the effects of direct Agent Orange exposure to the Vietnamese population. One investigation inquired about Agent Orange exposures in the parents of fifty-seven children with malformations who were born in a heavily sprayed area. The research design was flawed by not including a control group of normal children. But the results did show that both parents were exposed to Agent Orange in thirty-two cases, and neither parent was exposed in four cases.[3] While definitive conclusions cannot be made from one study conducted in this manner, it does alert us to possible complications from *direct* Agent Orange exposures *during pregnancy.*

Aside from the Vietnam studies, there have been various investigations into human reproductive risks from exposure to 2,4-D, 2,4,5-T, and TCDD. However, they have failed to link exposure to an increased frequency of abnormalities in their children. Attempts to evaluate miscarriage and stillbirth rates have produced conflicting results, warranting further investigation (for more information, see the entry on herbicides, page 182).

Studies focusing specifically on Vietnam veterans have not proven that exposures to Agent Orange are free from risks of birth defects, but they do imply it. Unfortunately, none of these studies are flawless, and can be criticized on two points: whether the men studied were actually exposed, and the exact dose they received.

The greatest criticism concerns exposure: Investigations usually assumed rather than proved that the men being studied had been exposed to Agent Orange. As a result, some studies ended up addressing whether or not *serving* in Vietnam increases the risk of having a child with birth defects, rather than whether *serving* in Vietnam *and* being *exposed to Agent Orange* increases the risk of having a child with birth defects.

Another problem with these investigations is the difficulty in determining dose— how much Agent Orange a man came in contact with. Knowing the extent of the exposure would help separate the potential risk of a very minimal exposure from that of a severe exposure.

At this time, it is safe to say that *service* in Vietnam is *not* associated with an increased risk of having children with birth defects. Some scientists will go so far as to say that available studies also do not support the belief that male *exposure* to Agent Orange increases risks for having a child with an abnormality; however, other scientists are less convinced.

Anecdotal reports attributing malformations in children to Agent Orange exposure have come to the attention of the medical community. Such reports have also led to law suits filed against the Veterans Administration, the Department of Defense, and several herbicide manufacturers. Yet the scientific information still does not support an association between birth defects and Agent Orange—how can these cases be explained?

One likely explanation is based solely on the number of Americans who served in Vietnam and the expected incidence of birth defects in our population. From this, an estimated 150,000 children with birth defects could have been born to Vietnam veterans by chance occurrence alone. It is therefore not surprising that a veteran who could have been exposed to Agent Orange might question whether a child with a birth defect resulted from that exposure.

In addition to all of the above information, you should keep in mind that to date, *no* exposure in a man has been proven conclusively to cause birth defects in his children. Traditionally, the only effects expected are failure to conceive or an early miscarriage.

References:

[1] J. H. Pearn, Herbicides and congenital malformations. A review for the paediatrician, *Australian Paediatric Journal* 21 (1985): 237–42.

[2] J. M. Friedman, Does Agent Orange cause birth defects? *Teratology* 29 (1984): 193–221.

[3] S. Fabro (ed.), Agent Orange and dioxin: Reproductive toxicology, a medical letter, 3(2) (1984): 6.

COMMON NAME: **AIDS (acquired immunodeficiency syndrome)**

Brand Name/Chemical name: **not applicable**

FDA Pregnancy Category: not applicable

ESTIMATED RISK SUMMARY:

   Time of Exposure before conception, throughout pregnancy, during delivery, and while breast-feeding

   Risk Known risk*

   Pregnancy Outcome adverse

   Documentation conclusive, based on current knowledge

pre-conception	All or None		Organ Development – (in weeks)						Maturation – (in weeks)				
	1	2	3	4	5	6	7	8	9	10	12	20-36	38

conception   ← Time of Greatest Risk →   birth

AIDS (acquired immunodeficiency syndrome)[1] is caused by a virus that scientists have named human immunodeficiecy virus (HIV). The virus interferes with the body's immune system, leaving it vulnerable to certain infections and various life-threatening illnesses. AIDS is a deadly disease for which we have no cure.

The AIDS virus is spread by certain types of sexual contact, by sharing unsterilized needles when injecting drugs, and now we know that an infected mother can pass it to her unborn baby. AIDS *cannot* be casually transmitted. The virus is not passed through the air when someone coughs or sneezes. One cannot get AIDS by swimming in public pools; by eating in restaurants; by shaking hands; or by sharing towels, drinking glasses, or toilet seats. And there is no evidence that it can be transmitted through kissing.

Not everyone infected with the AIDS virus actually develops AIDS. Some people will remain alive and well, but nevertheless, they can still pass the virus on to others. Others might develop AIDS-related complex (ARC), a disease which is less severe than AIDS. And a portion of the people infected with the AIDS virus will go on to develop

*above the 4% background risk

frank AIDS, which is often characterized by pneumonia, tuberculosis, and/or a form of cancer, Karposi's sarcoma.

AIDS is a major public health problem in the United States. The only way to contain the AIDS epidemic is by reducing the rate of transmitting the virus. The U.S. Surgeon General has advocated "safer sex"* as a means of reducing sexual transmission, IV drug users are being told not to share needles, and now women infected with the AIDS virus are being discouraged against becoming pregnant. This source of transmission, from mother to unborn baby, will be discussed here.

According to the U.S. Public Health Service, the AIDS virus is passed from the infected mother to her baby during pregnancy, during delivery, or after birth through breast milk. But no one yet knows how often the virus is transmitted before birth. Preliminary studies have reported rates as high as 65 percent. Giving birth to one child infected with the AIDS virus increases one's chances of passing it on to children born subsequently.[2] But passing the virus to the unborn is not inevitable. Unaffected infants born to women with the AIDS virus have been reported.

Some researchers have observed that babies infected in the womb display some degree of growth retardation and have a characteristic facial appearance.[3,4] (Features include: abnormally small head size [microcephaly]; a flat nasal bridge; wide-spaced eyes, which mildly slant upward or downward; large wide eyes; prominent, boxlike appearance of the forehead; and a full upper lip.) In one study, children with the most severe facial changes developed symptoms of the AIDS disease earlier (within six months of birth) than did moderately or mildly affected children.[5] Other problems, such as a higher rate of preterm delivery, premature rupture of membranes, and low birth weight have also been reported.[6] Additional investigations are needed to confirm these suspicions and to rule out other possible contributing factors, such as poor maternal health habits and the use of drugs and alcohol during pregnancy. To further complicate matters, becoming pregnant might make a woman who is infected with the AIDS virus more likely to develop ARC or frank AIDS.[2,7,8] But this too needs further confirmation.

In order both to protect the mother and to reduce the incidence of AIDS transmission during pregnancy, the Centers for Disease Control recommend that women belonging to high risk groups should be tested for the antibody to the AIDS virus before becoming pregnant. Women who are not at risk do not need to be tested, but certainly should be if they wish.

---

*"Safer sex" refers to using a condom during sexual intercourse (vaginal, anal, and oral). When used properly, condoms will reduce but not eliminate the risk of transmitting the AIDS virus. (Condoms made out of latex offer the most protection against AIDS.) There is also some evidence that the over-the-counter spermicide nonoxynol 9 will inactivate the AIDS virus. It should be used in addition to a condom.

High risk factors for women include:

- having the AIDS infection or testing positive for the AIDS antibody,
- using intravenous drugs (for recreational not medical purposes),
- being born in a country where heterosexual transmission is thought to play a major role (Haiti or Central Africa), and
- having unprotected sex (not using a condom) with intravenous drug users, men with hemophilia, bisexual men, men who were born in countries where heterosexual transmission is thought to play a major role, men who have AIDS, or men who test positive for the AIDS antibody.

Women who test positive for the AIDS antibody are recommended to postpone conception until more information is available about the virus's effect during pregnancy and the incidence of viral transmission to the unborn.[1] The woman who has negative test results needs to know that sexual intercourse with an infected partner will increase her chances of infection and that proper use of condoms will offer her some protection against acquiring AIDS.

Guidelines for infection control in caring for patients with AIDS have been published by the Centers for Disease Control.[1]

References:

[1] Centers for Disease Control. Recommendations for assisting in the prevention of perinatal transmission of human T-lymphotropic virus type III/lymphadenopathy-associated virus and acquired immunodeficiency syndrome. *Morbidity and Mortality Weekly Report* 34 (1985): 722–26, 731–32.

[2] H. Minkoff, D. Nanda, R. Menez, S. Fikrig. Pregnancies resulting in infants with acquired immunodeficiency syndrome or AIDS-related complex: Follow-up of mothers, children and subsequently born siblings. *Obstetrics and Gynecology* 69 (1987): 288–91.

[3] R. W. Marion, A. A. Wiznia, R. G. Hutcheon, A. Rubinstein. Human T-cell lymphotropic virus type III (Htlv-III) embryopathy. *American Journal of Diseases of Children* 140 (1986): 638–40.

[4] S. Iosub, M. Manji, R. K. Stone, D. S. Gromisch, E. Wasserman. More on human immunodeficiency virus embryopathy. *Pediatrics* 80 (1987): 512–16.

[5] R. W. Marion, A. A. Wiznia, R. G. Hutcheon, A. Rubinstein. Fetal AIDS syndrome score. Correlation between severity of dysmorphism and age at diagnosis of immunodeficiency. *American Journal of Diseases of Children* 141 (1987): 429–31.

[6] H. Minkoff, D. Nanda, R. Menez, S. Fikrig. Pregnancies resulting in infants with acquired immunodeficiency syndrome or AIDS-related complex. *Obstetrics and Gynecology* 69 (1987): 285–87.

[7] G. B. Scott, M. A. Fischl, N. Klimas, et al. Mothers of infants with the acquired immunodeficiency syndrome: Evidence for both symptomatic and asymptomatic carriers. *Journal of the American Medical Association* 253 (1985): 363–66.

[8] H. Minkoff, deRegt R. Haynes, S. Landesman, R. Schwarz. Pneumocystis carinii pneumonia associated with acquired immunodeficiency: A report of three maternal deaths. *Obstetrics and Gynecology* 67 (1986): 284–87.

COMMON NAME: **AIR TRAVEL**

Brand Name/Chemical Name: **not applicable**

FDA Pregnancy Category: not applicable

ESTIMATED RISK SUMMARY:
   Time of Exposure throughout pregnancy
   Risk No known risk*
   Pregnancy Outcome appears favorable
   Documentation inconclusive, based on minimal data

← pre- conception	All or None		Organ Development – (in weeks)						Maturation – (in weeks)				
	1	2	3	4	5	6	7	8	9	10	12	20-36	38

conception   ← Time of Greatest Risk →   birth

Commercial *air travel* is not hazardous to the unborn baby in a healthy, uncomplicated pregnancy. Several concerns about air travel have been raised—altitude, cabin noise, vibration, jet lag, and low-level radiation among them.

Commercial jet airlines are pressurized because no one can tolerate the low amount of oxygen at the altitude where ordinary jet aircraft cruise. Cabin pressure is usually the equivalent to that of 5,000 to 8,000 feet, while symptoms of hypoxia (oxygen deprivation) become most marked at altitudes above 10,000 feet (3,048 m).[1] The effects of high altitude on pregnancy are discussed elsewhere in the book (see altitude, high, page 68). Suffice it to say that the rather-safe-than-sorry approach would be for pregnant women to avoid flying above 10,000 feet in *un*pressurized aircraft.

A study evaluating mothers and their unborn children during air travel found no reason to restrict healthy pregnant women from flying in pressurized commercial aircraft.[2] While some moderate heart rate and breathing changes were documented in pregnant women, significant reactions were not observed in their unborn babies. Fetal heart rate monitored during air travel was within normal limits. Based on this measurement, there was no reason to believe that oxygen supply to the fetus was compromised during flight. Most airlines do restrict passengers from traveling during the final weeks of pregnancy, because of the undesirability of giving birth in flight. Few people would argue against this commonsense regulation.

*above the 4% background risk

In addition to the slight altitude exposure, pregnant flight attendants have the added burden of their work load during flight. This activity is associated with an increase in heart rate, which in the absence of other risk factors (such as cigarette smoking) should pose no increased risk to the fetus. Their active duty in the later stages of pregnancy is obviously impaired by increasing body size. However, this is simply increased difficulty in moving around the plane, rather than a health hazard.

Occasionally, someone will ask me if there is any truth to the rumor that flight attendants have increased risks of miscarriages and abnormal children. I have never found any scientific evidence to support such concerns, although I think these worries probably have two bases: (1) news of isolated instances of problems that circulate among workers and are misinterpreted as cause and effect, and (2) information culled from studies evaluating pregnancy outcome in inhabitants of high-altitude regions (see altitude, high, p. 68).

Other issues in air travel during pregnancy include noise and vibration, low-level solar radiation exposure, low humidity, and jet lag. Noise and vibration at the current low levels in modern commercial aircraft have no known adverse effect. Radiation exposure in an airplane is *extremely low* and far below that which is associated with an increased risk (see X rays, page 347). There is no information suggesting that even very-high-altitude air travel will significantly increase the natural background radiation dose you normally receive (which varies depending on where you live).

Low humidity in the aircraft causes you to experience a small loss of body water. This can be best handled by increasing your *water* intake. I've even heard that drinking six to eight glasses of water on long flights will help reduce the effects of jet lag. This is only anecdotal evidence, but I've tried it and it seems to help me feel better. Jet lag has no known effects on the developing fetus, although it obviously has a temporary effect on how well you personally feel. To help you adjust to the new time zone, you should go to bed upon arrival and sleep until the normal morning there.

Pregnant women are encouraged to move about on the airplane, particularly during long flights, because being immobile can impair blood flow to the legs and pelvis. Walking around every forty minutes or so should be sufficient.

A final word

Airport security machines emit low-energy *non*-ionizing radiation. It is similar to radar, microwaves, radio waves, and even color television sets (see also microwaves, page 241). From a biological standpoint, this radiation has little in common with the ionizing radiation emitted by X-ray machines.

Currently there is no scientific evidence suggesting that "routine" exposures to non-ionizing radiation are hazardous during pregnancy. Despite such reassurances, some pregnant women may still not feel comfortable about going through airport security machines. In such cases, they can request to be searched by a female security officer.

References:

[1]P. Scholten, Pregnant stewardess—should she fly? *Aviation, Space and Environmental Medicine*, 47 (1976): 77–81.

[2]R. Huch, H. Baumann, F. Fallenstein, K. T. M. Schneider, F. Holdener, and A. Huch, Physiologic changes in pregnant women and their fetuses during jet air travel. *American Journal of Obstetrics and Gynecology* 154 (1986): 996–1000.

COMMON NAME: **ALCOHOL**

Chemical Name: **(Ethanol, Ethyl Alcohol)**

FDA Pregnancy Category: not applicable

ESTIMATED RISK SUMMARY:

Time of Exposure throughout most of pregnancy
Risk Suspected risk* for moderate drinking
Pregnancy Outcome uncertain: favorable and adverse outcomes observed
Documentation inconclusive, based on minimal data

Time of Exposure anytime during pregnancy
Risk Risk assessment is not possible for rare and "binge" drinking
Pregnancy Outcome uncertain
Documentation insufficient

Time of Exposure throughout most of pregnancy
Risk Known risk* for heavy drinking
Pregnancy Outcome adverse
Documentation conclusive, based on current knowledge

pre-conception	All or None		Organ Development – (in weeks)						Maturation – (in weeks)				
	1	2	3	4	5	6	7	8	9	10	12	20-36	38

conception ← Time of Greatest Risk → birth

*above the 4% background risk

While not formally recognized as a major cause for abnormal prenatal development until 1973, *alcohol*-related birth defects[1,2,3,4] have been a medical concern for more than 250 years. Initially the constellation of abnormalities, termed the "fetal alcohol syndrome" (FAS), was associated with heavy drinking throughout pregnancy. Now we know that lesser amounts of alcohol can also be damaging to an unborn baby.

The fetal alcohol syndrome is the third most commonly recognized cause of mental retardation and it is the only one that is *completely* preventable! (Down syndrome and spina bifida are, respectively, the first and second most commonly recognized causes.)

The severity of alcohol-related birth defects depends on *when* during pregnancy you drink, *how much* you drink, *how often* you drink, and on you and your baby's *individual response* to alcohol.

When?

As with any teratogen the time of exposure determines what part of development is disturbed. And, like most teratogens, alcohol is most damaging during early pregnancy, when rapid development of all systems takes place. But alcohol also interferes with the normal development of the baby's brain. The first organ to begin development, the brain is also the last organ to complete its development (which continues into the infant's first years of life). Thus, this vital organ remains sensitive to the effects of alcohol throughout pregnancy. Growth, too, is adversely affected by alcohol, and all stages of prenatal development are characterized by growth. For these reasons, there is no time when drinking during pregnancy is without some potential risk. But risk is also determined by a combination of other factors.

How much? and How often?

These questions cannot be specifically answered. In general terms we know: The more you drink, the higher the risk; and the longer you continue to drink, the higher the risk. It is important to realize that it's not what you drink, but how much of what you drink that matters. Drinking one beer is the same as drinking four ounces of wine or 1.2 ounces of hard liquor (all of these are equivalent to about one-half ounce of absolute alcohol). There has even been a case where a child with features of FAS was born to a mother who throughout her pregnancy consumed large amounts of a cough syrup containing alcohol. Basically there is no specific amount of alcohol known to be safe during pregnancy. This is partly because equal amounts of alcohol affect different people differently.

Individual response:

Your individual makeup determines how your system handles or metabolizes alcohol. Some people drink very little and feel "high," others drink large amounts and appear unaffected. This is related to the amount of alcohol in your system (blood alcohol levels). The higher the blood alcohol level, the more intoxicated you feel. Research suggests that high blood alcohol levels in the mother are associated with alcohol-related birth defects in the child.

The full-blown fetal alcohol syndrome is associated with heavy drinking throughout pregnancy. FAS has three main characteristics:

- growth retardation—occurring before and continuing after birth,
- improperly functioning central nervous system, including intellectual impairment, developmental delay, and behavioral problems such as hyperactivity, and
- abnormal facial characteristics, including: very small head size (microcephaly); small eye openings; thin smooth upper lip; and a flat look to the midface area (maxillary hypoplasia)

Other associated abnormalities include: joint, limb, heart, and genitourinary (genital and urinary organs) defects. Dental problems, including teeth that do not meet properly, have been observed in older children with FAS.[5] One of the most serious consequences of FAS is mental retardation. Intellectual levels among affected children show considerable variation, as shown in one study of twenty children born to chronically alcoholic mothers. One severely affected 18-month-old in an institution had an IQ of 15, while a mildly affected 9-year-old had an IQ of 105.[6] Exposure to alcohol before birth has been associated with hyperactivity in children—characterized by lack of attention, ease of distraction, impulsive behavior, and lack of self-discipline. Normally intelligent children with FAS have also been diagnosed as hyperactive.[6]

The severity and the extent of FAS varies from child to child. Some infants don't have the actual fetal alcohol syndrome but have components of the syndrome. These are referred to as fetal alcohol effects (FAE).

The incidence of FAS in our population as a whole is between 1 per 700 and 1 per 2,000 live births. The prevalence of FAE in our population is more difficult to determine because various criteria are used to identify such effects, the estimates range from 1.7 per 1,000 to 5.9 per 1,000 to 90.1 per 1,000 live births.[3]

The reported incidence of FAS among children of mothers who are chronic alcoholics varies depending on the type of study conducted. Prospective studies suggest between 2.5 percent and 10 percent of the children are affected. Retrospective case studies, which tend to overestimate the incidence of abnormalities, have reported that up to 50 percent of children born to chronic alcoholics have FAS.

My experience dictates that the concerns of most pregnant women are related to the effects of rare (less than one drink per month), moderate (variable definitions), and "binge" (excessive on occasion) drinking during pregnancy. (Two definitions of moderate drinking include [1] drinking one or two ounces of absolute alcohol per day for at least the first three months, and [2] drinking more than once per month but less than forty-five drinks per month and five drinks on some occasions.) Unfortunately, there is no scientific consensus on the effects of lesser amounts of alcohol. Consistent moderate drinking is likely to pose some, as yet undetermined, increased risk. Evidence of an increase in miscarriages, features of the fetal alcohol syndrome, growth retardation, lower birth weight, behavioral problems, and a slight decrease in mental development scores have been reported among the children of moderate drinkers. A large prospective study observed twice the expected rate of miscarriages in women who took one to two drinks daily for the first two months; the rate was higher in those who took more than two drinks daily.[7] Another prospective investigation into moderate drinking gathered information on alcohol consumption from pregnant women *during* their first trimester.[8] No increase in the overall malformation rate or in major malformations were found in newborns whose mothers drank one to two drinks or less per day. However, when the frequency of malformations in specific organ systems was examined, an increase in genitourinary defects was linked to increasing alcohol consumption. Further studies are needed before these findings can be fully interpreted.

Drinking one small glass of beer or wine a day has not been associated with a measurable risk, but there is absolutely no proof that it is safe, either. Certainly the safest recommendation is not to drink at all during pregnancy. If you are pregnant and have been drinking, you need to know that your chances for a normal, healthy child will be much better if you stop. Stopping does make a difference! And the earlier the better, since alcohol poses an increased risk to the unborn child during every stage of pregnancy. If you have been drinking heavily, even reducing your consumption will improve your unborn baby's chances.

Finally, you might wonder how drinking by the baby's father will affect your pregnancy. While birth defects have not been reported, a man's heavy drinking can interfere with his ability to perform sexual intercourse as well as decrease his fertility.

Mary's Story:

Dinner is a very social time for my husband and me—it gives us a chance to unwind and discuss the day's activities. We both enjoy drinking wine. Over the last couple of years I've been in the habit of having a few glasses almost every night with dinner. Sometimes, my husband and I end up sharing the whole bottle.

I continued this habit until I discovered I was pregnant. I stopped as soon as I found out, because I had heard that drinking can be harmful to a developing baby. But I wasn't certain that wine was as dangerous as hard liquor. Most of my friends drink a lot of wine and somehow it doesn't seem the same as drinking martinis.

When I first found out I was pregnant, at six weeks along, I worried about what damage might have already occurred, and I wondered how much wine I could safely continue to drink.

I learned that any type of alcohol—whether it be beer, wine, wine coolers, hard liquor like vodka and Scotch, or even types of cough syrup that contain alcohol—can be potentially harmful. I guess this didn't really surprise me— alcohol is alcohol!

Some of my friends said that they heard drinking one glass here and there would be okay. But I was told that when you drink, your baby drinks too. I imagined how ridiculous it would be to give a baby a bottle containing alcohol and not milk—even doing such a thing every once in a while would be dumb. Hearing that eliminating alcohol altogether would be the best thing for my baby, made it easier to say no.

I have to admit that I was worried about the effect of the wine I drank in my early weeks of pregnancy. No one could tell me for sure if my baby was at an increased risk. The doctors and nurses I spoke to were all very supportive and focused on the positive side of my baby having a better chance if I didn't drink anymore. I know that stopping makes a difference—so I did just that!

References:

[1]K. L. Jones, D. W. Smith, C. N. Ulleland, and A. P. Streissguth. Pattern of malformation in offspring of chronic alcoholic mothers, *Lancet* 1 (1973): 1267–71.

[2]A. P. Streissguth, S. Landesman-Dwyer, J. C. Martin, and D. W. Smith. Teratogenic effects of alcohol in humans and laboratory animals, *Science* 209 (1980): 353–61.

[3]E. L. Abel, Prenatal effects of alcohol, *Drug and Alcohol Dependence* 14 (1984): 1–10.

[4]H. L. Rosett and L. Weiner, Alcohol and pregnancy: A clinical perspective, *Annual Review of Medicine* 36 (1985): 73–80.

[5]A. P. Streissguth, S. K. Clarren, and K. L. Jones, Natural history of the fetal alcohol syndrome: A 10 year follow-up of 11 patients, *Lancet* 2 (1985): 85–91.

[6]S. E. Shaywitz, D. J. Cohen, and B. A. Shaywitz, Behavior and learning difficulties in children of normal intelligence born to alcoholic mothers, *Journal of Pediatrics* 96 (1980): 978–82.

[7]S. Harlap and P. H. Shiono. Alcohol, smoking and the incidence of spontaneous abortions in the first and second trimester, *Lancet* 2 (1980): 173–76.

[8]J. L. Mills, B. I. Graubard. Is moderate drinking during pregnancy associated with an increased risk for malformations? *Pediatrics* 80 (1987): 309–14.

COMMON NAME: **ALTITUDE, HIGH**

Brand Name/Chemical Name: **not applicable**

FDA Pregnancy Category: not applicable

ESTIMATED RISK SUMMARY:

Time of Exposure throughout pregnancy

Risk Possible risk*

Pregnancy Outcome uncertain: favorable and adverse outcomes observed

Documentation inconclusive

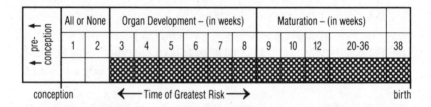

pre-conception	All or None		Organ Development – (in weeks)						Maturation – (in weeks)				
	1	2	3	4	5	6	7	8	9	10	12	20-36	38

conception   ← Time of Greatest Risk →   birth

High altitude causes a variety of effects on the human body stemming from the lower level of oxygen available. For this reason, residing at high altitudes and vacationing or visiting such regions might pose a risk to pregnancy and its outcome (see also air travel, page 61).

For this discussion, high altitude is loosely defined as 8,000 feet (2,400 m) and above. Published information reveals that symptoms of hypoxia (oxygen deprivation) and adverse reproductive outcome become most marked at altitudes above 10,000 feet (3,048 m).[1,2]

Residing at High Altitude

Babies born to women living at high altitude are generally smaller than those born closer to sea level. Recent data seems to confirm the long-held belief that hypoxia retards fetal growth.[3]

A retrospective study conducted in Aspen, Colorado (about 8,000 feet above sea level), found that babies born there were, on the average, about half a pound (8.5 ounces or 240 g) lighter than the average birth weight for babies born in the United States.[4] The investigators believed that the white, middle-class background of the

*above the 4 percent background risk

mothers (nonsmoking, good nutrition) made the differences less obvious. This is because nonwhites of low socioeconomic status, smokers, and women who do not eat properly are at greater risk of having low birth-weight babies. Low birth weight can lead to other medical complications in the baby, so this is a significant indicator of health.

The Colorado study also found other complications that they attributed to residing at high altitude during pregnancy, including greater frequency of pregnancy-induced hypertension (high blood pressure) and hyperventilation in the mother. It also can cause increased amounts of bilirubin (a pigment from red blood cells, too much of which can lead to jaundice) in babies within four weeks after birth—a disease known as neonatal hyperbilirubinemia.

Hyperventilating, or breathing faster, is greater at high altitudes and even more so for pregnant women. In a pregnant woman, this can decrease the amount of carbon dioxide in her blood, which can in turn compromise the health of her baby by producing metabolic changes (respiratory alkalosis and metabolic acidosis) in her fetus. Though other investigators have observed a higher death rate among such newborn babies,[5] this study did not.

Many studies conducted on the effect of high altitude on pregnancy outcome have been on populations living in predominantly rural areas, such as the Peruvian Andes, far from sophisticated medical care facilities. In addition, the racial and cultural backgrounds of the people are quite different from those in the United States, as are the risk factors they imply—all of which contribute to adverse pregnancy outcome. So results based on studies of such societies may not be useful in counseling in the United States or other developed countries.

Visiting at High Altitude:

The authors of the Colorado study mentioned above commented that it is possible that visiting in a high-altitude region may actually be more harmful to the unborn child than living there. This, they said, is because it takes time for the woman's body to adjust and insure that sufficient oxygen is transported to tissues throughout her body and to her unborn child. However, this is only a theory, not yet proven.

Visitors should also be aware of acute mountain sickness (AMS), which can appear within the first few days of arrival in a high altitude. Some of the symptoms of AMS include headache, listlessness, inability to sleep, loss of appetite, nausea, and insomnia.

AMS can develop in anyone, although some people are more susceptible than others. The pregnant woman who plans a strenuous exercise program immediately after arriving is at risk for developing AMS. In general, exercising at high altitudes during pregnancy probably increases the danger of hypoxia. This can be minimized by going easy for several days after arriving.

Nonstress tests to assure the well-being of the unborn child have been recommended for women in the third trimester of pregnancy on the following schedule: when they first arrive and for the next two days, then twice a week for the duration of their stay.[4] Please check with your own doctor regarding his or her own opinion on this matter.

References:

[1]P. Scholten, Pregnant stewardess—should she fly? *Aviation, Space and Environmental Medicine* 47 (1976): 77–81.

[2]R. Huch, H. Baumann, F. Fallenstein, K. T. M. Schneider, F. Holdener, and A. Huch, Physiologic changes in pregnant women and their fetuses during jet air travel, *American Journal of Obstetrics and Gynecology* 154 (1986): 996–1000.

[3]C. Ballew and J. D. Haas, Hematologic evidence of fetal hypoxia among newborn infants at high altitude. *American Journal of Obstetrics and Gynecology* 155 (1986): 166–69.

[4]D. W. Hershey and L. Vierira, Problems of pregnancy at high altitude, *Contemporary Ob/Gyn.* 23 (1984): 47–50.

[5]R. E. McCullough, J. T. Reeves, and R. L. Liljegren, Fetal growth retardation and increased infant mortality at high altitude, *Archives of Environmental Health* 32 (1977): 36–39.

MEDICATION CLASSIFICATION: **AMINOGLYCOSIDES**

GENERLIC NAMES: **AMIKACIN, GENTAMICIN, KANA-MYCIN, NEOMYCIN, PAROMOMYCIN, STREPTOMY-CIN** (separate entry), **TOBRAMYCIN**

Brand names: **(Amikin, Apogen, Bristagen, Garamycin, Humatin, Jenamicin, Kantrex, Klebcil, Mycifradin Sulfate, Nebcin, Neobiotic)**

FDA Pregnancy Category: —

ESTIMATED RISK SUMMARY:

Time of Exposure throughout pregnancy

Risk Risk assessment is not possible for amikacin, gentamicin, neomycin, paramomycin, and tobramycin, but *a possible risk may exist*

Pregnancy Outcome uncertain

Documentation insufficient

*above the 4% background risk

Time of Exposure can not be specified due to lack of specific information
Risk Suspected risk* for kanamycin
Pregnancy Outcome uncertain: favorable and adverse outcomes observed
Documentation inconclusive, based on minimal data

pre-conception	All or None		Organ Development – (in weeks)						Maturation – (in weeks)				
←	1	2	3	4	5	6	7	8	9	10	12	20-36	38

conception ←——Time of Greatest Risk——→ birth

Aminoglycosides are antibiotics reserved for the treatment of serious bacterial infections. Studies show that these drugs cross the placenta and enter fetal circulation, but this conveys nothing about their ability to affect the developing baby. There have been no reports of physical birth defects, but aminoglycosides have not yet been systematically evaluated during pregnancy by scientific investigations.

Complications from aminoglycosides in adults include damage to the kidney and to the eighth cranial nerve (responsible for hearing and balance). Eighth cranial nerve damage has also been observed in the children of mothers treated with both **streptomycin** (see streptomycin, page 302) and **kanamycin**, but no other aminoglycoside. A review of 391 women receiving kanamycin at various times during pregnancy found 9 children with hearing loss.[1] There is also a case report of a child with complete hearing loss born to a woman treated (for four and a half days) with kanamycin and another drug, ethacrynic acid during her twenty-eighth week of pregnancy.[2] Even though there is no evidence of eighth cranial nerve damage in the fetus from other aminoglycosides, this possibility must be considered.

Gentamicin given to prevent infection in women with premature rupture of birth membranes caused no recognizable birth defects in the newborns.[3]

References:

[1] H. Nishimura and T. Tanimura, *Clinical Aspects of the Teratogenicity of Drugs* (Amsterdam: Excerpta Medica, 1976), p. 131.

[2] H. C. Jones, Intrauterine ototoxicity. A case report and review of the literature, *Journal of the National Medical Association* 65 (1973): 201–3.

[3] D. Freeman, J. Matsen, and N. Arnold, Amniotic fluid and maternal and cord serum levels of gentamicin after intra-amniotic instillation in patients with premature rupture of the membranes, *American Journal of Obstetrics and Gynecology* 113 (1972): 1138–41.

MEDICATION CLASSIFICATION: **AMPHETAMINES**

GENERIC NAMES: **AMPHETAMINE SULFATE, DEXTROAMPHETAMINE, METHAMPHETAMINE**

Brand Names: **(Benzedrine, Biphetamine, Desoxyn, Dexampex, Dexedrine, Ferndex, Methampex, Obetrol-10, Obetrol-20, Oxydess II, Spancap No 1)**

FDA PREGNANCY CATEGORY: C

ESTIMATED RISK SUMMARY:

Time of Exposure throughout pregnancy
Risk No known risk* for birth defects
Pregnancy Outcome appears favorable
Documentation inconclusive

Time of Exposure in the latter part of pregnancy
Risk Possible risk* for poor pregnancy outcome and withdrawal symptoms with illicit use
Pregnancy Outcome appears favorable
Documentation inconclusive

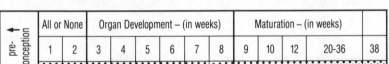

← pre-conception ←	All or None		Organ Development – (in weeks)						Maturation – (in weeks)				
	1	2	3	4	5	6	7	8	9	10	12	20-36	38

conception   ←— Time of Greatest Risk —→   birth

Amphetamines are stimulant drugs prescribed to treat a variety of conditions, including narcolepsy (an uncontrollable urge to sleep), appetite suppression for obesity or weight control, and hyperactivity (attention deficit disorder) in children. In addition to their prescribed uses, the illicit use of these drugs, and **methamphetamine** (or "crystal") in particular, is increasing dramatically among those of child-bearing age.

Isolated birth defects have been reported in a small number of children exposed to amphetamines before birth. But since the malformations have not followed a recognizable pattern, it is less likely that a single cause was responsible.

*above the 4% background risk

An association of amphetamines with heart defects[1] and biliary atresia[2] was found though relevant retrospective studies. However, the reliability of the conclusions drawn from the studies are questionable (see retrospective studies, page 43). This is because data collection depended on the mother's memory to record what drug was used and specifically when it was taken. Mothers of babies with birth defects recall the events during their pregnancy much differently than do mothers of normal children. The children with heart defects also had family histories of the problem, suggesting involvement of a genetic factor. Of the five children with biliary atresia whose mothers took amphetamines during pregnancy, one took them in the last two months of pregnancy, a time when they could not have caused the abnormality. Two others took other drugs, as well. A causal relationship between amphetamines and these two abnormalities cannot be inferred without confirmation by additional evidence.

A large prospective study investigated the effects of amphetamines and **phentermine** (another appetite supressant). It compared the rate of severe birth defects in two groups of children: 1,834 (354 first trimester exposures) five-year-olds born to white women who had prescriptions for these drugs during pregnancy and 8,989 otherwise similar children whose mothers did not.[3] No difference in the frequency of severe birth defects was observed. The greatest criticisms of this investigation are that only live born children were included and that subtle abnormalities and growth retardation, the most common teratogenic effects, were not even considered.

A prospective study examined the effect of **dextroamphetamine** prescribed during pregnancy on fetal growth. It discovered that decreased birth weight (by about 5 oz.) occurred only when the drug was taken after 28 weeks of pregnancy.[4]

A preliminary retrospective investigation of twenty-three children born to amphetamine-addicted mothers observed an increase in premature births.[5] This study served as a pilot for a larger prospective evaluation of 69 amphetamine-addicted women who delivered seventy-one infants.[6] Seventeen women stopped taking drugs once they were aware of their pregnancy. Fifty-two women continued using amphetamines. Women who continued using drugs and alcohol obtained less prenatal care, and as expected, their overall pregnancy outcome was poorer than those who stopped using amphetamines and received more care during their pregnancy. Overall, the study reported a high incidence of pregnancy and obstetric complications, including bleeding after delivery and premature births. A total of four babies had birth defects (no specific pattern was found) and two babies born to mothers who continued using drugs were stillborn. Breathing problems (respiratory distress) were found in 16% of the babies whose mothers remained on drugs and several infants were noted to have withdrawal-like symptoms, including drowsiness, poor feeding, and jitteriness. Sixty-six of the surviving children were evaluated at 1 and 4 years of age, their growth and development did not differ from that of other children. Some children whose parents continued to take drugs were disturbed emotionally.[7,8]

A recent investigation gathered information on the pregnancies of women using cocaine or methamphetamine or both.[9] Only women and infants who had evidence of these drugs in their system were studied. This study also found a higher incidence of pregnancy complications and prematurity. An increased frequency of fetal distress and poorer growth was also reported in these drug-exposed babies. A high rate of no prenatal care and the concomitant use of other drugs, cigarettes, and alcohol probably influenced some of these observed outcomes. Withdrawal symptoms were similar to previous observations and included irritability, tremors, drowsiness, and poor feeding.

References:

[1]J. J. Nora, T. A. Vargo, A. H. Nora, K. E. Love, D. G. McNamara. Dexamphetamine: A possible trigger in cardiovascular malformations. *Lancet* 1 (1970): 1290–91.

[2]J. N. Levin, Amphetamine ingestion with biliary atresia. *Journal of Pediatrics* 79 (1971): 130–31.

[3]L. Milkovich and B. J. Van den Berg, Effects of antenatal exposure to anorectic drugs. *American Journal of Obstetrical Gynecology* 129 (1977): 637–42.

[4]R. L. Naeye, Maternal use of dextroamphetamine and growth of the fetus, *Pharmacology* 26 (1983): 117–20.

[5]G. Larrson, The amphetamine-addicted mother and her child, *Acta Paediatrica Scandinavica* 278 (suppl) (1980): 8–24.

[6]M. Eriksson, G. Larrson, and R. Zetterström, Amphetamine addiction and pregnancy. II. Pregnancy, delivery, and the neonatal period. Socio-medical aspects. *Acta Obstetrica Gynecologica Scandinavica* 60 (1981): 253–59.

[7]L. Billing, M. Eriksson, G. Larrson, and R. Zetterström, Amphetamine addiction and pregnancy. III One year follow-up of the children. Psychosocial and pediatric aspects. *Acta Paediatrica Scandinavica* 69 (1980): 675–80.

[8]L. Billing, M. Eriksson, G. Steneroth, and R. Zetterström, Pre-school children of amphetamine-addicted mothers. I. Somatic and psychomotor development. *Acta Paediatrica Scandinavica* 74 (1985): 179–84.

[9]A. S. Oro and S. D. Dixon, Perinatal cocaine and methamphetamine exposure: Maternal and neonatal correlates. *Journal of Pediatrics* 111 (1987):571–78.

MEDICATION CLASSIFICATION: **ANDROGENS**

GENERIC NAMES: **FLUOXYMESTERONE, METHYLTESTOSTERONE, TESTOSTERONE**

Brand Names: **Android, Android-F, Android-T, Andro LA, Andryl 200, Anthatest, Delatestryl, Depo-Testosterone, Duratest, Everone, Halotestin, Metandren, Ora-Testryl, Oreton Methyl, Testate, Testone, Testred, Virilon**

FDA Pregnancy Category: —

ESTIMATED RISK SUMMARY:

Time of Exposure primarily from the 8th to the 12th week, although sensitivity to male hormones does continue beyond this time

Risk Known risk*

Pregnancy Outcome adverse

Documentation conclusive, based on current knowledge

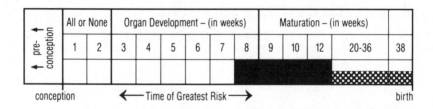

← pre-conception ←	All or None		Organ Development – (in weeks)						Maturation – (in weeks)				
	1	2	3	4	5	6	7	8	9	10	12	20-36	38

conception　　←— Time of Greatest Risk —→　　birth

Androgens are male sex hormones (see also danazol, page 133). These hormones have been prescribed for women for a variety of reasons, including antitumor therapy. Cases gathered from the 1950s and 1960s have associated their use during pregnancy with abnormal development of the external sex organs of female fetuses.[1] Approximately thirty-five cases of what is referred to as "female masculinization" have been reported.

Abnormalities in affected females include enlarged clitoris with or without partial to complete closure of the labia (skin folds on either side of the vaginal opening). The risk for this is highest during the "critical period" of development of the external sex organs, primarily from the eighth to the twelfth week after conception. However, sensitivity to male hormones does continue beyond this time.[2]

It is reassuring to know that these problems can be surgically corrected and that the internal reproductive organs do not appear to be affected by the drug.

There have been no reports of adverse effects in males.

Long-term studies on children whose mothers took these hormones have not yet been conducted. Of interest is a study that examined eleven adult women who were masculinized before birth by progestins (a female sex hormone that can be converted into androgens in the mother and unborn baby). There were no long-term effects, and the women looked and behaved like other females their age.[3]

References:

[1] J. L. Schardein, Congenital abnormalities and hormones during pregnancy: A critical review, *Teratology* 22 (1980): 251–70.

*above the 4% background risk

[2]P. Saenger, Abnormal sexual differentiation, *Journal of Pediatrics* 104 (1984): 1–17.
[3]J. Money and D. Mathews, Prenatal exposure to virilizing progestins: An adult follow-up study of twelve women, *Archives of Sexual Behavior* 11 (1982): 73–83.

MEDICATION CLASSIFICATION: **ANESTHETICS, INHALATION**

GENERIC NAMES: **ENFLURANE, HALOTHANE, METHOXYFLURANE, NITROUS OXIDE**

Brand Names: **(Ethrane, Fluothane, Penthrane)**

FDA Pregnancy Category: —

ESTIMATED RISK SUMMARY:

   Time of Exposure throughout pregnancy

   Risk No known risk* for birth defects

   Pregnancy Outcome appears favorable

   Documentation inconclusive, based on minimal data

Occupational Exposure

   Time of Exposure cannot specify, assumed to be early pregnancy

   Risk Possible risk* for miscarriage

   Pregnancy Outcome uncertain: favorable and adverse outcomes observed

   Documentation inconclusive, based on minimal data

Acute Exposure

   Time of Exposure possibly the first 6 months

   Risk Possible risk* for miscarriage

   Pregnancy Outcome uncertain: favorable and adverse outcomes observed

   Documentation inconclusive, based on minimal data

pre-conception	All or None		Organ Development – (in weeks)						Maturation – (in weeks)				
	1	2	3	4	5	6	7	8	9	10	12	20-36	38

conception   ←——Time of Greatest Risk——→   birth

*above the 4% background risk

Chronic or Occupational Exposure to Inhalation Anesthetics:

Data from the 1970s raised the question of possible increased frequency of miscarriages and birth defects in individuals exposed to inhalation anesthetics at work. Careful review of all the research leads to reappraisal of these concerns.[1] Some studies included only women, some included both sexes, and others included the wives of exposed males. All of the studies investigating this issue were retrospective, conducted after the known pregnancy outcome, and they suffer from the flaws of this approach (see retrospective studies, page 43). Most studies were surveys by mailed questionnaire, so their results reflected the outcome of only those who responded—possibly a large number of people with poor outcomes, making it difficult to collect accurate data on who was actually exposed, for how long, and how often. In all but one study no follow-up on the accuracy of the information was made. Furthermore, some studies required participants to recall events five to twenty years after the fact—presenting a large margin for error. Last, not all investigations controlled for other possible causes of poor pregnancy outcome.

In summary, the results from these investigations do suggest a possible increased risk for miscarriages in women who are themselves exposed to these gases *at work*. This risk might be more realistic for female dentists and chairside assistants, as exposure to trace amounts of anesthetics (primarily nitrous oxide) is thought to be higher for dental personnel than for those who work in operating rooms.[2] But there is no actual evidence of a higher risk. In fact, research not included in the above review found no increase rate of miscarriages among dental assistants.[3] These findings were from data collected in a prospective study that was flawed by using occupation as the only exposure criterion; actual exposures were determined by self-reporting.

Most of these studies failed to find either an increased frequency of miscarriages in the wives of men occupationally exposed to the anesthetics or more birth defects among the children of men and women who work with them.

Today operating rooms have scavenger systems that reduce trace levels of anesthetic gases, and the permissible level in hospitals is regulated in the United States. Clearly, new, well-controlled studies are needed to assess the risks from current exposure levels to inhalation anesthetics. It is hoped that the maintenance of low levels of inhalation anesthetics will make safer work environments for parents-to-be and their children.

Nonobstetric Surgery During Pregnancy and Acute Exposure to Inhalation Anesthetics:

An estimated 2 percent of all women who undergo surgery are pregnant. Data collected on the risks of surgery during pregnancy are scant, and they are complicated by the possibly greater risks from the indication for the surgery—for example, miscarriages have occurred in women who had surgical procedures for cervical incompetence. But these women were already at risk for losing the pregnancy because their cervix was not functioning properly.

For whatever reason—and again the underlying condition might be the strongest risk factor—an increased frequency of miscarriages has been reported after women have surgery and are given inhalation anesthetics in their first and second trimesters. For this reason, if you have the option, consider postponing the surgery until the latter part of pregnancy.[4]

Patients recovering from abdominal surgery, particularly when the uterus has been handled, have sometimes gone into premature labor. But this has not been linked to the anesthesia.

Of the few good studies of women who had either general or local anesthesia while pregnant, none has linked it to an increased risk of birth defects.[5]

Indirect effects from the surgery or anesthetic agent might influence the well-being of the mother and baby. These concerns are more related to the special medical considerations required for anesthetizing the pregnant woman, than to the specific teratogenic effect of the anesthetic agent itself. Such concerns are beyond the scope of this book.

Long-term follow-up studies of children exposed before birth have not been located.

References:

[1] T. N. Tannenbaum and R. J. Goldberg, Exposure to anesthetic gases and reproductive outcome, *Journal of Occupational Medicine* 27 (1985): 659–68.

[2] E. N. Cohen, B. W. Brown, M. L. Wu, C. E. Whitcher, J. B. Brodsky, H. C. Gift, W. Greenfield, T. W. Jones, and E. J. Driscoll, Occupational disease in dentistry and chronic exposure to trace anesthetic gases, *Journal of the American Dental Association* 101 (1980): 21–31.

[3] E. Z. Heidam, Spontaneous abortions among dental assistants, factory workers, painters and gardening workers: A follow up study, *Journal of Epidemiology and Community Health* 38 (1984): 149–55.

[4] J. B. Brodsky, Anesthesia and surgery during early pregnancy and fetal outcome, *Clinical Obstetrics and Gynecology* 26 (1983): 449–57.

[5] W. M. Barron, The pregnant surgical patient: Medical evaluation and management, *Annals of Internal Medicine* 101 (1984): 683–91.

MEDICATION CLASSIFICATION: **ANTACIDS**

GENERIC NAMES: **ALUMINUM-based, CALCIUM-based, MAGNESIUM-based, SODIUM BICARBONATE-based (and combination drugs)**

Brand Names: **Alagel, Algemol, Algenic, Alka, Alka-2, Alkets, Almacone, Alma-Mag, ALternaGEL, Aludrox, Alumid, Alumid**

Plus, Aluminum Hydroxide Gel, Alu-Cap, Alu-Tab, Amitone, Amphojel, Antagel, Basaljel, Bell/ans, Bisodol, Camalox, Calcilac, Calcium Carbonate, Calglycine, Chooz, Creamalin, Delcid, Dialume, Dicarbosil, Di-Gel, Duracid, Equilet, Escot, Estomul-M, Gaviscon, Gelamal, Gelusil, Gustalac, Kolantyl, Kudrox, Lo-Sal, Low Sium Plus, Maalox, Maalox Plus, Magmalin, Magnagel, Magnatril, Magnesium Carbonate, Magnesium Oxide, Magnesium Trisilicate, Mag-Ox 400, Mallamint, Maox, Marblen, Mi-Acid, Milk of Magnesia, Mintox, Mygel, Mylanta, Nephrox, Neutracomp, Noralac, Pama, Par-Mag, Phosphaljel, Ratio, Riopan, Riopan Plus, Rolaids, Rolox, Rulox, Silain Gel, Simaal, Simeco, Soda Mint, Sodium Bicarbonate, Spastosed, Titracid, Titralac, Tums, Tums E-X, Tralmag, Triconsil, Uro-Mag, WinGel

FDA Pregnancy Category:—

ESTIMATED RISK SUMMARY:
   Time of Exposure throughout pregnancy
   Risk No known risk*
   Pregnancy Outcome appears favorable
   Documentation inconclusive

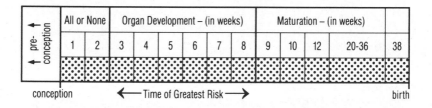

Antacids[1] provide relief of indigestion, heartburn, and conditions related to excessive stomach acid (ulcer, gastritis, hiatal hernia, esophagitis). There are a large number of anatacid products on the market, but there are only a few different kinds. Antacids are usually composed of calcium (Titralac, Tums), magnesium (Milk of Magnesia), aluminum (Amphojel) or a combination of these natural elements (Maalox, Mylanta). Sodium bicarbonate is another type of antacid, but one that

*above the 4% background risk

should be avoided in pregnancy because it could lead to problems in the mother and unborn child (fluid overload and a condition called metabolic alkalosis). Some antacids also contain an antigas ingredient (simethicone), as well as sodium (salt), which can cause you to retain excess water. Always evaluate the ingredients listed on the product. Choose one with the least amount of sodium and, as with all over-the-counter medications, look for the product with the fewest number of ingredients.

Even though 30–50 percent of pregnant women take antacids during the latter stages of their pregnancy, few studies have evaluated the effect they have on an unborn baby. One investigation compared drug consumption in pregnancies resulting in normal children and in malformed infants.[2] It found that mothers of children with major and minor abnormalities took antacids more often. But the researchers found no *individual* preparation was associated with an increase in birth defects. This study was conducted after the babies were born, a method in which mothers of malformed infants usually recall the events of pregnancy quite differently than those with normal children. This can affect the reliability of the conclusions drawn from the study. Also, the crucial issue of medication timing is extremely hard to determine in a study that relies on memory. The abnormalities cited among the children exposed to antacids were not similar. This means they probably were not the result of one specific cause, making it unlikely that antacids were responsible for the birth defects. In fact, most experts believe that antacids, in the normal therapeutic doses, can be safely used in pregnancy. The rather-safe-than-sorry approach would be to avoid these compounds in early pregnancy, and after the first trimester to take them as indicated and only when needed. Most importantly, please remember to check with your doctor before self-prescribing any drug during pregnancy.

Natural Remedies:*

Here are some safe alternatives[3] for dealing with the discomforts of heartburn or acid indigestion during pregnancy that don't rely on medications.

Avoidance. If you have an episode of heartburn, take note of the foods you have recently eaten. Then strike them from your menu. Likely candidates are fried foods, those with lots of seasonings, and coffee.

Frequency of eating. Rather than three ordinary meals, try eating several smaller ones.

Fluids. Drink adequate amounts of liquid, about eight glasses a day.

Clothing. Avoid garments that are tight around the waist.

---

*None of these commonsense remedies have been proven. They are listed here because I have found them useful.

Natural remedies. When heartburn strikes, try sipping small amounts of water, carbonated water, or milk.

Exercise. Sitting up, breathing exercises, and relaxation often lessen the discomfort of heartburn. Or sit cross-legged, hold your arms straight out to the sides, then bring them over the top of your head, touching the backs of your hands together. Repeating this exercise several times may bring relief.

References:

[1]J. H. Lewis and A. B. Weingold, The uses of gastrointestinal drugs during pregnancy and lactation. *American Journal of Gastroenterology* 80 (1985): 912–23.

[2]M. M. Nelson and J. O. Forfar, Associations between drugs administered during pregnancy and congenital abnormalities of the fetus. *British Medical Journal* 1 (1971): 523–27.

[3]The Over-the-Counter-Drug Committee of the Coalition for the Medical Rights of Women. *Safe and Natural Remedies for Discomforts of Pregnancy,* (San Francisco, Calif., January 1981; rev. 1982.)

MEDICATION CLASSIFICATION: **ANTIHISTAMINES**

GENERIC NAMES: **BROMPHENIRAMINE, CHLORPHENIRAMINE, DEXCHLORPHENIRAMINE, DIMENHYDRINATE, DIPHENHYDRAMINE, PHENIRAMINE, PYRILAMINE, TRIPELENNAMINE, TRIPROLIDINE**

Brand Names: **(see Table 5–1, page 86)**

FDA Pregnancy Category:
brompheniramine, dexchlorpheniramine triprolidine: B; all others—

ESTIMATED RISK SUMMARY:
Time of Exposure throughout pregnancy
Risk Risk assessment is not possible
Outcome uncertain
Documentation available information is insufficient

← pre-conception ←	All or None		Organ Development – (in weeks)						Maturation – (in weeks)				
	1	2	3	4	5	6	7	8	9	10	12	20-36	38

conception   ←——Time of Greatest Risk——→   birth

Antihistamines are most often used to help treat allergy symptoms—runny nose, watery eyes, or the "itchiness" of hives. Often they are combined with other drugs, such as decongestants and pain relievers, to relieve a variety of symptoms. Some antihistamines help alleviate nausea and are used for motion sickness. Most antihistamines make the user drowsy. So certain products have capitalized on this side effect to recommend antihistamines as a mild sleeping aid.

Runny or stuffy nose and other allergy or cold symptoms are common conditions for which there is no cure. Medicines, in this case antihistamines, will only help relieve the symptoms and make you feel more comfortable. While it's best to try to "tough it out" during pregnancy, the fact is that an extremely large number of pregnant women have been and continue to be treated with antihistamines for these symptoms. So considering their frequency of use during pregnancy, it is very surprising that antihistamines have not really been properly evaluated for their effect on the unborn baby. From the information we do have, I can tell you that there is no association of antihistamines as a class of medications with an increased risk for causing birth defects.

The Collaborative Perinatal Project, a large prospective study that evaluated pregnancy outcome in more than 50,000 mother-child pairs exposed to a wide variety of drugs, offers some of the only information available on antihistamines.[1]

Only sixteen mother-child exposures were reported with **tripolidine,** which is too small a sample size on which to base any conclusions.

Several drugs (**chlorpheniramine, dexchlorpheniramine, dimenhydrinate, diphenhydramine, pyrilamine, tripelennamine**) were *not* found to be associated with large categories of major or minor malformations. The use of some products (**chlorpheniramine, diphenhydramine, dimenhydrinate**, and **pheniramine**) during pregnancy did, however, result in several possible associations with individual birth defects. The statistical significance of these findings is not known. **Brompheniramine** was the *only* drug that was statistically more likely than other antihistamines to be associated with birth defects in the newborn. To my knowledge no other investigation has confirmed this finding.

Interpreting the meaning of all of these observations is difficult, because the value of the information from this study for use in teratogen risk counseling has been questioned for several reasons: There were few controls for other possible causes. The critical issue of medication timing was not specified. Because of frequent multiproduct use, of cold and allergy preparations in particular, it is hard to determine which drugs, if any, could cause birth defects. When several substances are examined together, as they were in this study, an association between any of the drugs and birth defects may simply be a chance occurrence. Last, even if there is an association, it does not prove that the substance actually caused the defect. So, further investigation is certainly required before the significance of the associations disclosed in this study can be determined.

Another investigation, which compared drug consumption in pregnancies resulting in normal children and in malformed infants, found that fewer mothers of infants with major and minor abnormalities took antihistamines in their first trimester.[2] In addition, no *individual* antihistamine compound was associated with an increase in birth defects. **Diphenhydramine** was the second most frequently used anithistamine and **chlorpheniramine** was the sixth. This study was conducted after the babies were born, so its findings are not entirely reliable. Gathered information was based on a mother's recall of events during pregnancy making it difficult to accurately document exactly what drugs were used and specifically when during pregnancy the drug was taken. Despite these shortcomings, this investigation does lend some support to antihistamines' apparent lack of obvious teratogenic effects.

A retrospective study compared drug consumption in pregnancies resulting in children with oral clefts (cleft lip and cleft palate) and in children without these defects.[3] It found that significantly more first trimester exposures to **diphenhydramine** occurred in children with cleft palate. This observation has not been confirmed by other investigations. Tremors and diarrhea observed in a 5-day-old newborn have been attributed to the use of diphenhydramine by the mother (150 mg per day, duration of drug was not specified).[4] These symptoms were interpreted as representing drug withdrawal.

Tripelennamine has been abused in conjunction with the drug pentazocine, a pain reliever. The combination is known as T's and Blues, and it first became popular during the 1970s as a heroin substitute. (*T's* comes from the *T* in Talwin, the brand name for pentazocine. *Blues* comes from the blue color of the tripelennamine tablet.) Although birth defects have not been reported from the combination used during pregnancy, withdrawal symptoms and low birth weight have been observed.[5,6] Withdrawal symptoms begin approximately twenty-four hours after birth and usually disappear within three to eleven days. Such symptoms usually result from *consistent* use of the drug in the latter part of pregnancy, particularly near the time of delivery. Withdrawal symptoms are characterized by jitteriness, irritability, hyperactivity, feeding difficulties (vomiting and weak suck), increased muscle tone, and a loud shrill cry. These problems are most likely attributed to pentazocine, although additional or additive effects from tripelennamine are certainly possible (see pentazocine, page 260).

Long-term follow-up studies of children exposed before birth to antihistamines have not been located.

Many physicians believe that judicious use of most antihistamines is relatively safe during pregnancy. These feelings are based on longtime clinical experience with their use during pregnancy without any obvious ill effects. Nevertheless, the rather-safe-than-sorry approach would be to try to avoid these medicines in early pregnancy. After the first trimester, take them only as indicated and when absolutely necessary. Most important, because many of these products are available without a prescription, please remember to check with your doctor before self-prescribing any drug during pregnancy.

Probably the best advice I can give you is to try to avoid whatever you are allergic to. This will reduce your need to treat allergy symptoms.

If you choose to take an antihistamine, avoid any product that might be linked to problems, choose one with the *lowest dose* (perhaps a children's preparation) and, as with all over-the-counter medications, look for the product with the *fewest* number of ingredients!

Natural Remedies:*

While antihistamines will provide a source of temporary relief from some allergy symptoms, a natural alternative[7] might provide a little peace of mind, while making you feel more comfortable.

- Breathing steam from a vaporizer, a hot shower, or even a pot of very hot water will help your stuffy nose.
- Normal saline nose drops can also provide some relief. These can be purchased at your drugstore or you can make your own by mixing one-fourth teaspoon of salt in one cup of warm water.
- Soothe your sore sinuses with a moistened warm towel across the nasal area.
- Sinus pressure may also be relieved with gentle finger pressure over the bones under your eyebrows, down the sides of your nose, and under your eyes.

References:

[1]O. P. Heinonen, D. Slone, and S. Shapiro, *Birth Defects and Drugs in Pregnancy* (Littleton, Mass: Publishing Sciences Group, 1977).

[2]M. M. Nelson and J. O. Forfar, Associations between drugs administered during pregnancy and congenital abnormalities of the fetus, *British Medical Journal* 1 (1971): 523–27.

[3]I. Saxen, Cleft palate and maternal diphenhydramine intake, *Lancet* 1 (1974): 407–8.

[4]D. E. Parkin, Probable Benydryl withdrawal manifestations in a newborn infant, *Journal of Pediatrics.* 85 (1984): 580.

[5]D. W. Dunn and J. Reynolds, Neonatal withdrawal symptoms associated with "T's and Blue's" (pentazocine and tripelennamine), *American Journal of Diseases of Children.* 136 (1982): 644–45.

*None of these commonsense remedies have been proven. They are listed here because I have found them useful.

[6] R. J. Wapner, R. D. Ross, J. M. Fitsdimmons et al. Fetal growth in drug dependent women: Quantitative assessments, abstracted, *Pediatric Research* 15 (1981): 1222.

[7] The Over-the-Counter-Drug Committee of the Coalition for the Medical Rights of Women, *Safe and Natural Remedies for Discomforts of Pregnancy* (San Francisco, Calif., January 1981; rev. 1982).

MEDICATION CLASSIFICATION: **ANTITHYROID HORMONES**

GENERIC NAMES: **METHIMAZOLE, PROPYLTHIOURICIL, SODIUM IODIDE I[131]**
(separate entry)

Brand Names: (**Propylthiouricil, Tapazole**)

FDA Pregnancy Category: D

ESTIMATED RISK SUMMARY:
> *Time of Exposure* after 10 weeks*
> *Risk* Known risk**
> *Pregnancy Outcome* adverse
> *Documentation* conclusive, based on current knowledge

← pre-conception	All or None		Organ Development – (in weeks)						Maturation – (in weeks)				
	1	2	3	4	5	6	7	8	9	10	12	20-36	38

conception   ←—Time of Greatest Risk—→   birth

Propylthiouracil (PTU) and methiamazole are ***anthithyroid hormones***[1,2] given to people who have hyperthyroidism (overactive thyroid glands). These drugs suppress thyroid activity. Mothers with significant but untreated hyperthyroidism have an increased frequency of pregnancy complications. These include toxemia, premature births, babies who are small for their age at birth, and an increased chance that the babies will die shortly before or after birth. For these reasons, drug therapy is usually warranted.

Ulcer-like scalp defects in nine infants have been linked to the mother's use of

*I do not know the time of exposure associated with the methimazole-related scalp defects
**above the 4% background risk

Table 5-1 ANTIHISTAMINES

BRAND NAMES	diphenhydramine	tripelennamine	chlorpheniramine	dexchlorpheniramine	brompheniramine	tripolidine	pheniramine	pyrilamine	aspirin	decongestant	acetaminophen	other*
Benadryl	•											
Benaphen	•											
PBZ		•										
Aller-Chlor			•									
Chlortab 4			•									
Chlor-Trimeton			•									
Phenetron			•									
Dexclor				•								
Poladex				•								
Polaramine				•								
Bromphen				•								
Dimetane				•								
Coricidin Tablets			•								•	
Rhinosyn Capsules			•							•		
Fedahist Gyrocaps			•							•		
Anafed Capsules			•							•		
Ornade Spansules			•							•		
Triaminic-12			•							•		
Allerest—12 hour			•							•		
Dristan—12 hour			•							•		
Bromfed					•					•		
Nasafed					•					•		
Dimetapp Extentabs					•					•		
Drixoral					•					•		
Nasahist			•						•			
Brometapp					•					•		
Bromphen Compound					•					•		
Histatapp					•					•		
A.R.M.			•							•		
Actifed						•				•		
Triafed						•				•		
Triacin						•				•		
Sine-off Extra Strength			•							•	•	
Sinarest			•							•	•	
Sinutab			•							•	•	
Dristan			•							•	•	
Naldecon			•							•		•1
Novahistine DH			•							•		•2

*Other: 1. phenyltoloxamine (an antihistamine) 2. alcohol and codeine

methimazole, or carbimazole in one case.[3] (Carbimazole, which is not available in the United States, is metabolized to methimazole.) Two of these infants also had umbilical defects, which might also be methimazole-related.

PTU is usually preferred for treatment during pregnancy because of the problems observed with methimazole. Occasionally, birth defects have coincided with a mother's use of **PTU**. But these problems have not occurred above the expected incidence of birth defects and have not been similar to each other. This means they probably were coincidental and not the result of one specific cause.

Early descriptions of goiter (enlarged thyroid gland) and other adverse effects on the fetus of **PTU** and **methimazole** may reflect the use of iodine in addition to *unnecessarily high doses* of antithyroid medication. (Iodine use during pregnancy is associated with causing goiter and underactive thyroid activity in the newborn; see iodine, page 203). Today, it is customary to closely monitor pregnant hyperthyroid patients and treat them with the minimum amount of antithyroid drugs required to maintain a normal thyroid functioning. Such conservative management may not completely eliminate the fetus's risk of goiter, but more likely the baby could develop hypothyroidism (underactive thyroid activity) and thyrotoxicosis (toxic activity of the thyroid gland) after birth. These problems usually disappear by themselves within a few days. For this reason, infants exposed to antithyroid medication should be followed after delivery, as these drugs can block the expression of thyrotoxicosis.

Antithyroid medications taken in early pregnancy do not adversely affect the fetus's thyroid function. Although the thyroid gland begins to develop between the second and seventh weeks, it does not really *begin* to *function* until about ten weeks of pregnancy. The risk for thyroid problems appears to be highest when antithyroid drugs are taken near term. In some instances, where the mother's thyroid state has remained normal for several weeks, antithyroid medication can be withdrawn four to six weeks before delivery. This will prevent hypothyroidism in the newborn.

Natural thyroid hormone does not cross the placenta (see page 317). For this reason, thyroid hormone given along with maternal antithyroid treatment is of no help to the fetus. In fact, the addition of thyroid hormone may require higher doses of antithyroid drugs before a normal functioning thyroid state is achieved.

Long-term follow-up studies of children exposed before birth have not been located.

References:

[1] J. H. Mestman, Thyroid disease in pregnancy, *Clinics in Perinatology* 12 (1985): 651–67.

[2] J. H. Mestman, Diagnosis and management of hyperthyroidism in pregnancy, *Current Problems in Obstetrics and Gynecology* 4 (1981): 1–51.

[3] S. Milham, Scalp defects in infants of mothers treated for hyperthyroidism with methimazole or carbimazole during pregnancy, *Teratology* 32 (1985): 321.

GENERIC NAME: **ASPARTAME**

Brand Name: **(Equal, NutraSweet)**

FDA Pregnancy Category:—

ESTIMATED RISK SUMMARY:
  Time of Exposure throughout pregnancy
  Risk No known risk* **(exception: women with phenylketonuria [PKU])**
  Pregnancy Outcome appears favorable
  Documentation inconclusive, based on minimal data

← pre-conception	All or None		Organ Development – (in weeks)						Maturation – (in weeks)				
	1	2	3	4	5	6	7	8	9	10	12	20-36	38

conception   ←—— Time of Greatest Risk ——→   birth

Aspartame is a low-calorie sweetener approved by the U.S. Food and Drug Administration for addition to some dry foods (1981) and carbonated drinks (1983). When ingested, aspartame is broken down into three parts: aspartic acid, phenylalanine, and methanol. Even though aspartame has not been evaluated for its potential effects on the unborn baby, knowing a little about its three parts provides some reassurance.

Aspartic acid is an amino acid and is present in many of the foods we eat every day. Aspartic acid does not readily pass from the mother's system to the unborn baby's system. In fact, one expert has said that it would be virtually impossible to take in enough aspartame to send significant amounts of aspartic acid to the unborn child.

In order to determine whether or not doses of *methanol* received from consuming aspartame could be dangerous, researchers gave a single dose of aspartame to a test group. This dose of aspartame equaled the amount in 50 twelve-ounce cans of aspartame-sweetened soda or 250 cans of aspartame-saccharin sweetened soda. The test subjects' blood levels of some methanol by-products rose briefly, but not enough to cause concern. Methanol appears to present no added risk, especially since the amount permitted in sweetened foods is lower than that found naturally in fruit juices.

Like aspartic acid, *phenylalanine* is also an amino acid and it, too, is in the foods

*above the 4% background risk

we eat (both spinach and chicken contain phenylalanine). Phenylalanine passes easily from the mother to the unborn child. For most individuals this naturally available substance poses no risk. But women who have the inherited disease phenylketonuria (PKU) need to restrict their intake of phenylalanine during pregnancy, because *sustained* high levels of phenylalanine can cause mental retardation in the unborn baby. Theoretically, if a pregnant woman who did not have PKU but who carried the gene for the disease, consumed extremely high doses of aspartame, her levels of phenylalanine might raise to levels that could threaten the health of her developing baby.

In various tests on people, the blood levels of phenylalanine were below that required to cause retardation. Even when eaten with a hamburger and a shake, the phenylalanine contributed by the aspartame, plus that in the meat, fell well below the danger limit. From these studies, added risk to a pregnancy from the phenylalanine in aspartame seems unlikely. Still, aspartame should be avoided by pregnant women who must consume a phenylalanine-free diet.

Long-term follow-up studies of children exposed before birth have not been located.

Reference:

[1] F. M. Sturtevant, Use of aspartame in pregnancy, *International Journal of Fertility* 30 (1985): 85–87.

GENERIC NAME: **ATENOLOL**

Brand Name: **(Tenormin)**

FDA Pregnancy Category: C

ESTIMATED RISK SUMMARY:

Time of Exposure first 3 months
Risk Risk assessment is not possible
Pregnancy Outcome uncertain
Documentation insufficient

Time of Exposure last 6 months of pregnancy
Risk No known risk*
Pregnancy Outcome appears favorable
Documentation inconclusive

*above the 4% background risk

Time of Exposure near the time of delivery

Risk Suspected risk* for slower than normal heartbeat (bradycardia)

Pregnancy Outcome uncertain: favorable and adverse outcomes observed

Documentation inconclusive, based on minimal data

pre-conception	All or None		Organ Development – (in weeks)						Maturation – (in weeks)				
	1	2	3	4	5	6	7	8	9	10	12	20-36	38

conception   ←—Time of Greatest Risk—→   birth

Atenolol belongs to a group of drugs that are classified as beta-adrenergic blocking agents (beta blockers). It is used to treat high blood pressure (hypertension.) This drug has been successfully used during pregnancy with no reported birth defects. However, information relative to the effects of its use during the first three months of pregnancy is lacking.

A decrease in average birth weights of atenolol-exposed infants has been reported by some studies,[1,2] and not by others.[3] The mother's illness along with other medications she might also be taking could have contributed to an observed effect on birth weight.

As with other antihypertensive drugs, there have been reports of infants with slower than normal heartbeat (bradycardia) and, in one case, low blood pressure, when their mothers received atenolol near the time of delivery. For this reason, babies born to women using this drug should be observed for a couple of days for any evidence of these symptoms.

No differences in either growth, or behavior were observed in 1-year-old infants born to women treated with atenolol some time during their last trimester of pregnancy.[4]

References:

[1]D. Dubois, J. Peticolas, B. Temperville, and A. Klepper, Treatment with atenolol of hypertension in pregnancy, *Drugs* 25 (suppl 2) (1983): 215–18.

[2]H. Lardoux, J. Gerard, G. Blazquez, F. Chouty, and B. Flouvat, Hypertension in pregnancy: Evaluation of two beta blockers atenolol and labetalol, *European Heart Journal* 4 (Suppl G) (1983): 35–40.

[3]P. C. Rubin, L. Butters, D. M. Clark, B. Reynolds, D. J. Sumner, D. Steedman, R. A. Low, and J. L. Reid, Placebo-controlled trial of atenolol in treatment of pregnancy-associated hypertension, *Lancet* 1 (1983): 431–34.

*above the 4% background risk

[4]B. Reynolds, L. Butters, J. Evans, T. Adams, and P.C. Rubin, First year of life after the use of atenolol in pregnancy associated hypertention, *Archives of Disease in Childhood* 59 (1984): 1061–63.

MEDICATION CLASSIFICATION: **BENZODIAZEPINES**

GENERIC NAMES: **ALPRAZOLAM, CHLORDIAZEPOXIDE** (separate entry), **CLONAZEPAM** (separate entry), **DIAZEPAM** (separate entry), **FLURAZEPAM, LORAZEPAM, MIDAZOLAM, OXAZEPAM, TEMAZEPAM, TRIAZOLAM**

Brand Names: **(Ativan, Dalmane, Halcion, Restoril, Serax, Versed, Xanax)**

FDA Pregnancy Category: midazolam D; all others—

ESTIMATED RISK SUMMARY:

Time of Exposure throughout most of pregnancy
Risk Risk assessment is not possible
Pregnancy Outcome uncertain
Documentation insufficient

Time of Exposure near term or during delivery
Risk Possible risk*
Pregnancy Outcome uncertain: favorable and adverse outcomes observed
Documentation inconclusive, based on minimal data

pre-conception	All or None		Organ Development – (in weeks)						Maturation – (in weeks)				38
	1	2	3	4	5	6	7	8	9	10	12	20-36	38
													▓

conception ←— Time of Greatest Risk —→ birth

Benzodiazepines are primarily used to treat anxiety disorders but are also prescribed for insomnia (difficulty in falling asleep). These drugs are among the most commonly prescribed drugs in the world. Prolonged use of benzodiazepines can lead to drug dependence in some patients.

I am not aware that the use of **alprazolam, flurazepam, lorazepam, midazolam, oxazepam, temazepam**, or **triazolam** has been associated with an increased frequency of birth defects, but you need to know that controlled studies of their use by pregnant women are lacking.

Birth defects have, however, been associated with other benzodiazepines, specifically, chlordiazepoxide and diazepam. But not all researchers have discovered adverse effects (see chlordiazepoxide, page 108, and diazepam, page 138). Unfortunately, most of the investigations have some shortcomings, so negative findings can not be interpreted as proof that these drugs are safe. Similarly, finding an association does not prove that they actually cause birth defects.

The American Academy of Pediatrics Committee on Drugs, in its review of psychotropic drugs in pregnancy and lactation, commented that the reports of abnormalities following benzodiazepine use during pregnancy have been inconsistent. The committee says that the drug's relationship to birth defects is not clear and that additional research is needed.[1] And it advised the conservative practice of a pregnant woman not taking drugs except to protect her health or that of her unborn child.

Various benzodiazepines have been linked to withdrawal symptoms, including tremors, irritability, increased muscle tone, vigorous sucking, vomiting, and diarrhea. Some of these drugs are also linked to the so-called floppy baby syndrome, characterized by poor muscle tone, lethargy, and sucking difficulties. Both of these complications are observed in newborns whose mothers received the drug near or during delivery. The possibility of these complications must be considered for all benzodiazepines used near or during delivery.

Long-term follow-up studies of children exposed before birth have not been located.

Reference:

[1]Committee on Drugs, Academy of Pediatrics, Psychotropic drugs in pregnancy and lactation, *Pediatrics* 69 (1982): 241–44.

GENERIC NAME: **BUCLIZINE**

Brand Names: **(Bucladin-S Softabs)**

FDA Pregnancy Category:—

ESTIMATED RISK SUMMARY:
   Time of Exposure throughout pregnancy
   Risk Risk assessment is not possible
   Pregnancy Outcome uncertain
   Documentation insufficient

		All or None	Organ Development – (in weeks)						Maturation – (in weeks)				
← pre-conception ←		1	2	3	4	5	6	7	8	9	10	12	20-36	38

conception   ←— Time of Greatest Risk —→   birth

Buclizine is used to treat and prevent nausea, vomiting, and the dizziness associated with motion sickness. This drug is similar to cyclizine (see page 130) and meclizine (see page 226).

The Collaborative Perinatal Project, which evaluated pregnancy outcome in more than 50,000 mother-child pairs exposed to a wide variety of drugs, offers the only information available on buclizine.[1] This drug was not associated with a pattern of malformation among forty-four children whose mothers took it during the first trimester. A total of sixty-two mothers took buclizine at various times during their pregnancy and three birth defects were reported in their children, but the significance of this finding is not known. More research is needed on buclizine before its true effects on a developing baby are understood.

Long-term follow-up studies of children exposed before birth have not been located.

Reference:

[1] O. P. Heinonen, D. Slone, and S. Shapiro, *Birth Defects and Drugs in Pregnancy* (Littleton, Mass.: Publishing Sciences Group, 1977).

COMMON NAME: **CAFFEINE**

Brand Names: **(There are too many to list individually.)**

FDA Pregnancy Category: C

ESTIMATED RISK SUMMARY:

Time of Exposure throughout pregnancy

Risk No known risk*, particularly in modest amounts

Pregnancy Outcome appears favorable

Documentation inconclusive, based on minimal data

*above the 4% background risk

pre-conception	All or None		Organ Development – (in weeks)						Maturation – (in weeks)				
	1	2	3	4	5	6	7	8	9	10	12	20-36	38

conception   ← Time of Greatest Risk →   birth

The stimulant drug *caffeine*[1] an ingredient in coffee, tea, chocolate, cocoa, and soft drinks, as well as other foods. Some of them are:

Food or beverage	Milligrams per serving
Coca-Cola	45.0
Dr Pepper (regular and sugar free)	39.6
Mountain Dew	54.0
Pepsi-Cola	38.4
Tab	46.5
Brewed tea	41.4
Instant tea	29.3
Brewed coffee	88.0
Instant coffee	70.7
Chocolate cake	13.8
Chocolate candy	7.7
Chocolate-covered candy	2.8
Chocolate ice cream	4.5
Chocolate milk	7.5
Instant chocolate pudding	5.5
Nut fudge brownie	7.7

More than 200 over-the-counter medications, including those used for weight control, pain relief, water loss, drowsiness, and colds and allergies also contain caffeine. Products containing caffeine specify this on the package. If you have any question about whether caffeine is an ingredient in a product you use, ask your pharmacist.

The topic of caffeine and pregnancy is truly a victim of media sensationalism, and the scientific facts are often difficult to sort out. Concern over caffeine's potential teratogenicity developed primarily from the results of laboratory animal studies. These reported an increase in lower birth weight, abnormalities of the skeleton, and other birth defects in the offspring of pregnant rats that were given caffeine. However, it is important to realize that these observations cannot be applied to humans. because (1) rats and humans metabolize caffeine very differently, (2) the doses used were extremely large (the caffeine equivalent of up to eighty cups of coffee) and were not comparable to human consumption, and (3) the caffeine was administered directly into the animal's gut, rather than being consumed by eating or drinking.

Although the FDA "has concluded that the data are insufficient to link caffeine with birth defects in humans,"[2] it issued a press statement in 1980 advising pregnant women to "be rather safe than sorry" and avoid caffeine-containing foods and drugs or to use them sparingly.

Caffeine does cross the human placenta, but it is not suspected of causing malformations in children exposed before birth.

Investigations have failed to agree on the possibility that caffeine consumption during pregnancy increases the risk of miscarriage, stillbirth, and premature birth. Studies reporting such outcomes link them to a minimum daily consumption of 400 to 600 mg during pregnancy. (Amounts of caffeine vary according to cup size and brewing style, but this is probably equal to four and a half to seven cups per day, assuming a six-ounce cup.) One study reported a very small reduction in birth weight when caffeine consumption during pregnancy exceeded 300 mg (three and a half cups) daily. Life-style and cigarette smoking may have contributed to these findings, since many studies have noticed a strong association betweeen caffeine use and cigarette smoking. The known adverse effects of cigarette smoking, which include low birth weight and an increase in miscarriages, makes it hard to evaluate caffeine's individual effect, if any.

In summary, pregnant women need to recognize caffeine as a drug. Like all drugs, it should be taken during pregnancy only if deemed necessary by your doctor. While there is no evidence to suggest that modest amounts of caffeine will harm your developing baby, thoughtful selection of caffeine substitutes is a safer and healthier option.

References:

[1]B. Watkinson and P. A. Fried, Maternal caffeine use before, during and after pregnancy and effects upon offspring, *Nuerobehavioral Toxicology and Teratology* 7 (1985): 9–17.

[2]Caffeine: Deletion of GRAS status, proposed declaration that no prior sanction exists, and use on an interim basis pending additional study: Proposed regulations, *Federal Register* 45 (Oct. 21, 1980): 69817–838.

GENERIC NAME: **CAPTOPRIL**

Brand Name: **(Capoten)**

FDA Pregnancy Category: C

ESTIMATED RISK SUMMARY:
　　Time of Exposure throughout pregnancy
　　Risk Risk assessment is not possible
　　Pregnancy Outcome uncertain
　　Documentation insufficient

← pre-conception ←	All or None		Organ Development – (in weeks)						Maturation – (in weeks)				
	1	2	3	4	5	6	7	8	9	10	12	20-36	38

conception　　　　←——Time of Greatest Risk——→　　　　birth

Captopril is used to treat hypertension (high blood pressure). Studies of high doses of the drug in pregnant rabbits and rats have revealed an increased incidence of the death of embryos and decreased newborn survival rates.[1] These results cannot be used to predict risks in humans. But they have made physicians cautious about prescribing captopril during pregnancy.

Controlled studies in pregnant humans have not yet been conducted. An isolated case report describes a limb abnormality (one leg ended at the midthigh) in the aborted fetus of a woman taking captopril, amiloride, and propranolol.[2] Since other drugs were involved and because one of the doctors could not rule out that the damage might have been caused by the elective abortion, cause and effect cannot be inferred.

Complications also occurred in two separate instances where newborns had been exposed to captopril before birth. Both infants had low blood pressure, which persisted for a number of days. One of the infants whose mother took captopril from the twenty-sixth to the twenty-eighth week of pregnancy had kidney failure and died; the kidneys were found to be structurally normal.[1] The other infant was exposed throughout the pregnancy; he was growth retarded, displayed low blood pressure for about ten days, and also had a heart defect (patent ductus arteriosis), which was surgically repaired.[3]

Again, while these reports reinforce the suspicion of adverse effects, together they do not prove that captopril was responsible for the observed problems. A total of three isolated case reports is not enough information to estimate risks. Clearly, further investigation into the potential teratogenicity of captopril is warranted.

Long-term follow-up studies of children exposed before birth have not been located.

References:

[1]W. F. Lubbe, Hypertension in pregnancy. Pathophysiology and management, *Drugs* 28 (1984): 170–88.

[2]P. C. Duminy and P. T. Burger, Fetal abnormality associated with the use of captopril during pregnancy, *South African Medical Journal* 60 (1981): 805.

[3]M. J. Boutroy, P. Vert, B. Hurault de Ligny and A. Milton, Captopril administrations in pregnancy impairs fetal angiotension converting enzyme activity and neonatal adaption, *Lancet* 2 (1984): 935–36.

GENERIC NAME: **CARBAMAZEPINE**

Brand Name: **(Tegretol)**

FDA Pregnancy Category: C

ESTIMATED RISK SUMMARY:
> *Time of Exposure* throughout pregnancy
> *Risk* Risk assessment is not possible
> *Pregnancy Outcome* uncertain
> *Documentation* insufficient; available information is insufficient

pre-conception	All or None		Organ Development – (in weeks)						Maturation – (in weeks)				
	1	2	3	4	5	6	7	8	9	10	12	20-36	38

conception　　　　←—— Time of Greatest Risk ——→　　　　birth

Carbamazepine is an anticonvulsant—a drug that inhibits recurrent seizures, or epilepsy.

Opinions differ about the specific risk of anticonvulsants. Many experts say there is two to three times the risk of major malformations in the children of epileptic women as in the general population. Some think the underlying disease is the cause. Others believe this statistic reflects a population of women who are exposed more often to anticonvulsant drugs, particularly hydantoins (see hydantoins, page 191), which are known teratogens.

To date, no increased risk has been reported in infants born to mothers receiving only carbamazepine during pregnancy. Researchers report one instance of a malformed fetus and a few cases of unrelated minor abnormalities, following exposure before birth to carbamazepine alone or with other anticonvulsants.[1,2,3] There is no characteristic pattern of malformation, and according to most studies, women on carbamazepine have normal children.[3,4,5,6]

Smaller than normal head size has been observed in a few children exposed before birth to carbamazepine alone or with another anticonvulsant.[3,7] In one study the difference was still evident at 18 months of age.[7] Unfortunately, developmental and intellectual functions were not assessed in these children.

Because there are so few reported cases, it is impossible to conclude whether or not carbamazepine used alone has a causal role in the production of birth defects. On the other hand, there is evidence that carbamazepine specifically combined with phenobarbitol and/or phenytoin, together with valproic acid can dramatically increase the frequency of birth defects.[8] This finding cannot be explained solely by an additive effect of the drugs. Apparently, the increase in teratogenic activity is the result of the metabolic interaction of this specific drug combination.[8]

Using carbamazepine might reduce your levels of one of the B-complex vitamins, folic acid, or folate. The need for folate increases greatly during pregnancy, as it is required for fetal growth and development. Some suggest that taking folic acid supplements during pregnancy might reduce the risk for having a baby with abnormalities.[9]

Some experts recommend carbamazepine as the drug of choice for women contemplating pregnancy and needing an anticonvulsant for the first time.[10,11] But there may be too little scientific evidence to support such a recommendation at this time. On the other hand, there is no support for changing or eliminating carbamazepine as anticonvulsant therapy.

Many women question how epilepsy or anticonvulsant medication in the father might affect their baby. Although not all scientists agree, most experts think this presents no increased risk. They believe that children fathered by men taking these drugs have the same chance of being normal and healthy as anyone else's, and well-conducted animal research confirms this belief.[12] (For more information on this, see Risks from Exposures in the Baby's Father, page 14.)

Most women continue taking anticonvulsant medication during pregnancy, unless they have been seizure free for many years. *Under no circumstances should you ever discontinue your anticonvulsant medication, unless under the direction and supervision of the prescribing physician.* Sudden withdrawal could cause a seizure. And while seizures are not known to cause malformations, they do present a possible risk to both you and your unborn baby.

References:

[1]E. P. Hicks, Carbamazepine in two pregnancies, *Clinical and Experimental Neurology* 16 (1979): 269–75.

[2]I. G. Robertson, D. Donnai, and S. D'souza, Cranial nerve agenesis in a fetus exposed to carbamazepine. *Developmental Medicine and Child Neurology* 25 (1983): 540–41.

[3]W. Kuhnz, E. Jager-Roman, D. Rating, A. Deichl, J. Kunze, H. Helge, and H. Nau, Carbamazepine and carbamazepine-10, 11-epoxide during pregnancy and postnatal period in epileptic mothers and their nursed infants: Pharmokinetics and clinical effects, *Pediatric Pharmacology* 3 (1983): 199–208.

[4]T. W. Bodendorfer, Fetal effects of anticonvulsant drugs and seizure disorders, *Drug Intelligence and Clinical Pharmocology* 12 (1978): 14–21.

[5]A. A. E. Starreveld-Zimmerman and W. J. Van der Kolk, Are anticonvulsants teratogenic? *Lancet* 2 (1973): 48–49.

[6]J. R. Niebyl, D. A. Blake, J. M. Freeman, and R. D. Luff, Carbamazepine levels in pregnancy and lactation, *Obstetrics and Gynecology* 53 (1979): 139–40.

[7]V. K. Hilesmaa, K. Teramo, M. L. Granström, and A. H. Bardy, Fetal head growth retardation associated with maternal antiepileptic drugs, *Lancet* July 25, 1981: 165–67.

[8]D. Lindhout, R. J. E. A. Höppener, and H. Meinardi, Teratogenicity of antiepileptic drug combinations with special emphasis on epoxidation (of carbamazepine), *Epilepsia* 25 (1984): 77–83.

[9]Y. Biale and H. Lewenthal, Effect of folic acid supplementation on congenital malformations due to anticonvulsive drugs, *European Journal of Obstetrics, Gynecology and Reproductive Biology* 18 (1984): 211–16.

[10]G. W. Paulson and R. B. Paulson, Teratogenic effects of anticonvulsants, *Archives of Neurology* 38 (1981): 140–43.

[11]C. D. Butler, Carbamazepine, seizure disorders and pregnancy, *Journal of the American Medical Association* 250 (1983): 3164.

[12]R. H. Finnell and J. F. Baer, Congenital defects among the offspring of epileptic fathers: Role of the genotype and phenytoin therapy in a mouse model, *Epilepsia* 25 (1986): 697–705.

MEDICATION CLASSIFICATION: CEPHALOSPORINS AND CEPHAMYCINS

GENERIC NAMES: CEPHALOSPORINS:

CEFACLOR, CEFADROXIL, CEFAMANDOLE NAFATE, CEFAZOLIN SODIUM, CEFONICID SODIUM, CEFOPERAZONE SODIUM, CEFORANIDE, CEFOTAXIME SODIUM, CEFTAZIDIME, CEFTIZOXIME SODIUM, CEFTRIAXONE SODIUM, CEFUROXIME SODIUM, CEPHALEXIN, CEPHALOTHIN SODIUM, CEPHAPIRIN SODIUM, CEPHARADINE

CEPHAMYCINS:

CEFOTETAN DISODIUM, CEFOXITIN SODIUM

Brand Names: CEPHALOSPORINS:

(Ancef, Anspor, Ceclor, Cefadyl, Cefizox, Cefobid, Claforan, Duricef, Fortaz, Keflex, Keflin Neutral, Kefzol, Mandol, Monocid, Precef, Rocephin, Seffin Neutral, Tazidime, Ultracef, Velosef, Zinacef)

CEPHAMYCINS: (Cefotan, Mefoxin)

FDA Pregnancy Category: B

ESTIMATED RISK SUMMARY:

Time of Exposure throughout pregnancy

Risk No known risk*

Pregnancy Outcome appears favorable

Documentation inconclusive, based on minimal data

pre-conception		All or None		Organ Development – (in weeks)						Maturation – (in weeks)				
		1	2	3	4	5	6	7	8	9	10	12	20-36	38

conception   ←——Time of Greatest Risk——→   birth

Cephalosporins and cephamycins[1] are antibiotics very similar to the penicillins. Like penicillins, these drugs destroy bacteria by weakening their cell walls. Human cells do not have walls, so the process affects only bacteria. These antibiotics are sometimes used to treat urinary tract infections during pregnancy. For more information about this type of infection, see page 331.

There is no evidence that cephalosporins and cephamycins cause birth defects when used during any stage of pregnancy. But you should know that while many of the first generation (older) cephalosporins have been examined for their effect on the developing baby, no single drug has been thoroughly investigated in controlled studies.

Cephalosporins and cephamycins are usually considered safe for use in pregnancy both because of the way they act on cells and because of the lack of evidence against them.

Long-term follow-up studies of children exposed before birth have not been located.

Reference:

[1]D. V. Landers, J. R. Green and R. L. Sweet, Antibiotic use during pregnancy and the postpartum period, *Clinics in Obstetrics and Gynecology* 26 (1983): 391–406.

*above the 4% background risk

COMMON NAME: **CHEMICALS**

Chemical Names: **(too many to list)**

FDA Pregnancy Category: not applicable

ESTIMATED RISK SUMMARY:

Time of Exposure throughout pregnancy
Risk Risk assessment is not possible for most home and work exposures
Pregnancy Outcome uncertain
Documentation insufficient

Time of Exposure throughout pregnancy
Risk Possible risk* for abusing solvents (high dose, prolonged use)
Pregnancy Outcome uncertain: favorable and adverse outcomes observed
Documentation inconclusive, based on minimal data

← pre-conception	All or None		Organ Development – (in weeks)						Maturation – (in weeks)				
	1	2	3	4	5	6	7	8	9	10	12	20-36	38

conception   ←——Time of Greatest Risk——→   birth

The majority of questions I receive on *chemical* exposures during pregnancy relate to occupational exposures in industry and in laboratory work. However, public awareness on potential environmental dangers continues to increase. As a result, prospective parents are more frequently questioning the effects of household cleaning products and the chemicals used in hobbies.

Well over 50,000 different chemicals are used in industry and in the home. Because researchers have just begun to address this area, very little information is available regarding their effects on pregnancy. One cannot predict pregnancy outcome after a particular exposure has occurred, unless there is published information on the pregnancy outcome and the well-being of children born to women with similar exposures. Unfortunately, there has been no systematic evaluation of the effect any one particular chemical agent has on the unborn baby. Even studies using pregnant animals are not always available.

*above the 4% background risk

Most of the information I encounter relates to laboratory experiments on the cancer-causing potential of chemicals, or research conducted on the toxicity of various compounds. Too often people mistakenly conclude that such research means these chemicals also cause birth defects. While it's certainly true that chemicals can be poisonous, cause cancer, and interfere with reproduction, we only know this for sure when studies focus on that particular possibility. But toxicity does not necessarily mean teratogenicity.

From the few available investigations,[1] animal studies suggest that, as is usually true, dosage and length of exposure are the most important factors. For humans, this also means contact with food, air, and skin.

Abuse of solvents for recreational use appears to cause a "fetal solvent syndrome," similar to the fetal alcohol syndrome. Babies born to women who have sniffed gasoline or abused toluene[2] and other solvents show altered facial appearance, abnormal muscle tone, growth deficiency, mental retardation, and developmental delay. With appropriate safety measures, occupational exposures should be substantially less than these intentional abusive exposures, as should casual contact, such as at the gas station.

Adverse pregnancy outcome, primarily miscarriages, but also some isolated cases of major malformations, have been reported for women working in chemical laboratories, the printing industry, as painters, and in the paper and pulp industry. But no single chemical was identified as the probable cause.

Retrospective surveys—one of central nervous system abnormalities and the other of cleft lip—have questioned the possible relationship between them and solvent exposure at work. These studies, together with the observations mentioned above, serve as a warning about the effects of solvents in the workplace. But because so many other variables also come into play here—multiple chemicals and differences in exposures—a definitive statement about the effects of these chemicals cannot yet be made.

Reliable and useful data on the teratogenicity of chemicals in humans will be a long time in coming. But it doesn't make sense to wait until adverse effects are either proven or disproven before being careful around these products. The most reasonable approach for you to take is to create a safer working environment, whether at work or in your home. Pregnant women and women considering pregnancy are advised to adopt a better-safe-than-sorry approach in reducing exposures to chemicals in the workplace. Some commonsense safety procedures include not smoking or eating at work, use of protective equipment, and good ventilation. The Occupational Safety and Health Administration (OSHA) may be consulted regarding the recommended safety precautions for working with chemicals, though not specifically during pregnancy.

Keep in mind that an extremely brief exposure—"just a 'smell' in passing"—is very unlikely to increase your risk of birth defects.

Long-term follow-up studies of children exposed before birth have not been located.

References:

[1]Is there a fetal solvent syndrome? Reproductive Toxicology, a medical letter on Environmental Hazards to Reproduction. (1983), Reproductive Toxicology Center, Washington, D.C. 2(5).
[2]J. H. Hersh, P. E., Podruch, G. Rogers, and B. Weisskopf, Toluene embryopathy, *Journal of Pediatrics* 106 (1985): 922–26.

MEDICATION CLASSIFICATION: **CHEMOTHERAPEUTIC DRUGS**

GENERIC NAMES (not all drugs are listed): **AMINOPTERIN, BUSULFAN, CHLORAMBUCIL, CYCLOPHOSPHAMIDE, CYTARABINE, DAUNORUBICIN HCL, FLUOROURA-CIL, METHOTREXATE, NITROGEN MUSTARD, THIO-GUANINE, VINBLASTINE, VINCRISTINE**

Brand Names: **(Adrucil, Cerubidine, Cytosara-U, Cytoxan, Folex, Leukeran, Mexate, Mustargen, Myleran, Neosar, Oncovin, Velban)**

FDA Pregnancy Category: cyclophosphamide, cytarabine: C; busulfan, methotrexate: D; all others:—

ESTIMATED RISK SUMMARY:

Women Who Receive Treatment
Time of Exposure before pregnancy
Risk No known risk* for birth defects
Pregnancy Outcome appears favorable
Documentation inconclusive, based on minimal data

Time of Exposure during pregnancy, specifically in the first trimester
Risk Suspected risk*
Pregnancy Outcome uncertain: favorable and adverse outcomes observed
Documentation inconclusive, based on minimal data

Time of Exposure during early pregnancy (particularly 4–9 weeks)
Risk Known risk* for **aminopterin** and **methotrexate**

*above the 4% background risk

Pregnancy Outcome adverse
Documentation conclusive, based on current knowledge

Women Who Work with These Drugs

Time of Exposure during early pregnancy
Risk Possible risk* for miscarriages
Pregnancy Outcome uncertain: favorable and adverse outcomes observed
Documentation inconclusive, based on minimal data

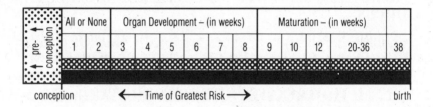

pre-conception	All or None		Organ Development – (in weeks)						Maturation – (in weeks)				
	1	2	3	4	5	6	7	8	9	10	12	20-36	38

conception   ←—— Time of Greatest Risk ——→   birth

This entry is only a general overview of the topic, because you should discuss this issue with the treating cancer specialist and your personal obstetrician.

There are several possible questions surrounding the effects of *chemotherapeutic drugs* in pregnant women and in women of childbearing age. First there is the woman who actually receives chemotherapy while she is pregnant. Then there is the woman who, in the past, had chemotherapy and is concerned about her ability even to become pregnant and then to have a normal, healthy baby. Last (but not least!), there is the pregnant health care worker who possibly is exposed to these drugs on the job.

Chemotherapy During Pregnancy

The information of the effects of these drugs in human pregnancy is not abundant.[1,2] Women usually avoid conceiving a child while on chemotherapy. And a large number of women who accidentally become pregnant during treatment terminate the pregnancy for fear of its damaging effect on the baby. Furthermore, the individual effects of these drugs on the developing baby are difficult to sort out because people often receive different combinations of drugs and dosages. The possibility that multiple drug combinations could be more teratogenic than any one drug used alone must also be considered.

As with all exposures to environmental agents, the effects of chemotherapy on the

---

*above the 4% background risk

developing baby are related to the time of the exposure, the dose used, and the individual susceptibility of the mother and fetus. Because these drugs are intended to interfere with rapidly dividing cells, by design their use in pregnancy, a time when the unborn baby is growing rapidly, carries a variety of theoretical risks and many well-founded concerns.

Beyond the theoretical concerns of chemotherapy during pregnancy are actual reports of birth defects caused by some of these drugs. The best-known offender is the drug **aminopterin.** Classified as a folic acid antagonist, aminopterin blocks the cell's use of folic acid, one of the B vitamins. Folic acid is needed for the cell to divide and multiply, and is also required for fetal growth, and development. In the past, high doses of aminopterin were used during the first trimester, primarily from four to nine weeks, for the specific purpose of terminating the pregnancy. Serious abnormalities were noted in aborted fetuses and in babies who survived and were born.

While there is little experience with most chemotherapeutic agents during the vital first three months of pregnancy, other drugs administered during this time have also caused malformations. These include: **cyclophosphamide** (Cytoxan), **busulfan, fluorouracil, methotrexate** (a derivative of aminopterin), **thioguanine** and **procarbazine.** In contrast, normal pregnancy outcomes after first trimester exposures to chemotherapeutic drugs have also been reported.[1,2,3] Various literature reviews have attempted to estimate the incidence of malformations from chemotherapy during the first trimester.[4] These estimates vary from around 10 percent to fewer than 8 percent. One report suggested that if aminopterin exposures were excluded, the risk would be 5 percent.

Several small studies and many case reports imply that the use of chemotherapeutic agents *after* the first three months of pregnancy results in normal babies in the majority of cases. An increased incidence of both premature birth and growth retardation, particularly low birth weight, has been observed.

If you are directly exposed to these drugs during pregnancy, your doctor should review with you all the potential risks of your specific treatment. References at the end of this entry provide a good starting place for a review of the available information.

Information gathered from surveyed parents has revealed normal development and intelligence in several children exposed to chemotherapeutic drugs before birth.[2] While reassuring, these observations need confirmation from larger, more formally designed studies.

Pregnancy After Chemotherapy

While treatment with chemotherapeutic drugs is associated with a risk for infertility, the great majority of women either retain or recover their reproductive potential. An increased frequency of miscarriage has been reported for some women who become pregnant subsequent to treatment. But there is no concrete evidence that receiving chemotherapy *prior* to becoming pregnant alters your chances of having a normal healthy child once you actually conceive.[5] This is true for both women and men.

Chemotherapeutic Drugs in the Work Place

Only limited information is available on occupational exposures to these drugs.[6,7] Retrospective studies conducted on nurses who work with chemotherapeutic drugs suggest that first trimester exposures might be associated with an increased risk for miscarriage and perhaps birth defects. Proof of this relationship does not yet exist. These results were based on information gathered by questionnaires and are subject to criticism because such studies require women to recall events that took place in the past. Actual exposures vary greatly among workers, and though accurate information is vital, it is very hard to gather this after the baby is born (see retrospective studies, page 43). Because such occupational exposures generate a considerable degree of concern in those who work with chemotherapeutic drugs, better studies are greatly needed. In the meantime, women working with these drugs should follow strict safety guidelines.

References:

[1]J. Gililland and L. Weinstein, The effects of cancer chemotherapeutic agents on the developing fetus, *Obstetrical and Gynecological Survey* 38 (1983): 6–13.

[2]J. Blatt, J. J. Mulvihill, J. L. Ziegler, R. C. Young, and D. G. Poplack, Pregnancy following cancer chemotherapy, *American Journal of Medicine* 69 (1980): 828–32.

[3]V. A. Catanzarite and J. E. Ferguson, Acute leukemia and pregnancy: A review of management and outcome, 1972–1982, *Obstetrical and Gynecological Survey* 39 (1984): 663–77.

[4]S. F. Williams and J. D. Bitran, Cancer in pregnancy, *Clinics in Perinatology* 12 (1985): 606–23.

[5]G. J. S. Rustin, M. Booth, J. Dent, S. Salt, F. Rustin, and K. D. Bagshawe, Pregnancy after cytoxic chemotherapy for gestational trophoblastic tumours, *British Medical Journal* 288 (1984): 103–6.

[6]S. G. Selevan, M. L. Lindbohm, R. W. Hornung, and K. Hemminki, A study of occupational exposure to antineoplastic drugs and fetal loss in nurses, *New England Journal of Medicine* 313 (1985): 1173–78.

[7]M. Sorsa, K. Hemminki, and H. Vainio, Occupational exposure to anticancer drugs: Potential and real hazards, *Mutation Research* 154 (1985): 135–49.

GENERIC NAME: **CHLORAMPHENICOL**

Brand Names: **(Chloramphenicol Sodium Succinate, Chloromycetin Kapseals, Chloromycetin Sodium Succinate)**

FDA Pregnancy Category:—

ESTIMATED RISK SUMMARY:

   Time of Exposure throughout most of pregnancy

Risk No known risk*
Pregnancy Outcome appears favorable
Documentation inconclusive, based on minimal data

Time of Exposure near the time of delivery
Risk Possible risk*
Pregnancy Outcome uncertain: favorable and adverse outcomes observed
Documentation inconclusive, based on minimal data

← pre-conception	All or None		Organ Development – (in weeks)						Maturation – (in weeks)				
	1	2	3	4	5	6	7	8	9	10	12	20-36	38

conception   ←—Time of Greatest Risk—→   birth

Chloramphenicol[1] is an antibiotic generally reserved for the treatment of serious infection, particularly when alternative drugs are unavailable. Various case reports and a few controlled studies have failed to detect an increased risk of birth defects in children exposed to this drug before birth. Although birth defects have not been found, chloramphenicol is usually avoided during late pregnancy because of the concern for "gray baby syndrome" (also called "gray syndrome").

Gray syndrome is a life-threatening complication caused by a toxic accumulation of chloramphenicol. This occurs when chloramphenicol is administered to newborns, particularly premature babies, who cannot metabolize and effectively excrete this drug from their system. While only one report has actually claimed that gray syndrome resulted from the use of chloramphenicol during late pregnancy, the theoretical risk calls for its avoidance or cautious use near the time of delivery.

Long-term follow-up studies of children exposed before birth have not been located.

Reference:

[1]D. V. Landers, J. R. Green, and R. L. Sweet, Antibiotic use during pregnancy and the postpartum period, *Clinics in Obstetrics and Gynecology* 26 (1983): 391–406.

*above the 4% background risk

GENERIC NAME: **CHLORDIAZEPOXIDE**

Brand Names: **(A-Poxide, Libritabs, Librium, Lipoxide, Sereen, SK-Lygen)**

FDA Pregnancy Category: D

ESTIMATED RISK SUMMARY:

Time of Exposure throughout most of pregnancy
Risk Risk assessment is not possible
Pregnancy Outcome uncertain
Documentation insufficient

Time of Exposure near term or during delivery
Risk Suspected risk*
Pregnancy Outcome uncertain: favorable and adverse outcomes observed
Documentation inconclusive, based on minimal data

← pre-conception	All or None	Organ Development – (in weeks)						Maturation – (in weeks)				
	1	2	3	4	5	6	7	8	9	10	12	20-36	38

conception   ←—Time of Greatest Risk—→   birth

Chlordiazepoxide belongs to a group of drugs known as benzodiazepines. These drugs are among the most commonly prescribed drugs in the world. Chlordiazepoxide is used to treat anxiety disorders and their symptoms. This drug is also useful in treating the symptoms of acute alcohol withdrawal. Prolonged use of benzodiazepines can lead to drug dependence in some patients.

Research into the effect of chlordiazepoxide on the developing baby has produced conflicting results. One investigation compared the prenatal drug exposure of children with congenital heart disease and normal infants. The rate of chlordiazepoxide exposure was higher in the children with defects.[1] Another retrospective study described an increase in serious birth defects when chlordiazepoxide was prescribed during the first forty-two days of gestation.[2] (The term *gestation* often is used to describe the time from the first day of the last menstrual period to birth, as opposed to the period from

---

*above the 4% background risk

conception to birth. Here the first forty-two days of gestation is equivalent to the first twenty-eight days of pregnancy.) None of the children born to the 172 women who took this drug had evidence of congenital heart disease. There were four children with birth defects, none of which was similar to another, meaning that they probably weren't the result of one specific cause. Also, other potential risk factors were not excluded, and the use of over-the-counter preparations was not assessed. Confirmation of the findings in both investigations is needed before their results can be fully interpreted.

In contrast, several other investigations have failed to find an association between chlordiazepoxide and birth defects.[3,4,5] Among these studies was a large prospective investigation finding no association between chlordiazepoxide use anytime during pregnancy and birth defects, death in childhood, or delayed mental development at 4 years of age.[3] All of these studies have some shortcomings, so such negative findings cannot be interpreted as proof that chlordiazpoxide is safe. Similarly, finding an association does not yet provide that chlordiazepoxide actually causes birth defects.

The Academy of Pediatrics Committee on Drugs, in its review of psychotropic drugs in pregnancy and lactation, has commented that the reports of abnormalities following benzodiazepine use during pregnancy have been inconsistent and that their relationship to birth defects is not clear. The academy concluded that additional research is needed and reaffirmed the prudent policy of taking drugs only if necessary for the health of the mother or unborn child.[6]

Like other benzodiazepines, chlordiazepoxide has been linked to withdrawal symptoms and depression in some newborns whose mothers received the drug near or during delivery (see also diazepam, page 138). Withdrawal symptoms have been characterized by irritability and severe tremors. Depressed newborns, referring to decreased functional activity and not to the emotional state, had poor muscle tone, were unresponsive and had some feeding difficulties.

References:

[1]K. J. Rothman, D. C. Flyer, A. Golblatt, and M. B. Kreidberg, Exogenous hormones and other drug exposures of children with congenital heart disease, *American Journal of Epidermiology* 109 (1979): 433–39.

[2]L. Milkovich and B. J. van den Berg, Effects of prenatal meprobamate and chlordiazepoxide hydrochloride on human embryonic and fetal development, *New England Journal of Medicine* 291 (1974): 1268–71.

[3]S. C. Hartz, O. P. Heinonen, S. Shapiro, V. Siskind, and D. Slone, Antenatal exposure to meprobamate and chlordiazepoxide in relation to malformations, mental development and childhood mortality, *New England Journal of Medicine* 292 (1975): 726–28.

[4]D. L. Crombie, R. J. Pinsent, D. M. Fleming, C. Rumeau-Rouguette, J. Goujard, and G. Huel, Fetal effects of tranquilizers in pregnancy, *New England Journal of Medicine* 293 (1975): 198–99.

[5]M. B. Braken and T. R. Holford, Exposure to prescribed drugs in pregnancy in association with congenital malformations, *Obstetrics and Gynecology* 58 (1981): 336–44.

[6]Committee on Drugs, Academcy of Pediatrics, Psychotropic drugs in pregnancy and lactation, *Pediatrics* 69 (1982): 241–44.

GENERIC NAMES: **CHLOROQUINE, HYDROXYCHLOROQUINE**

Brand Names: **(Aralen HCL, Aralen Phosphate, Cloroquine Phosphate, Plaquenil Sulfate)**

FDA Pregnancy Category:—

ESTIMATED RISK SUMMARY:

   Time of Exposure throughout pregnancy

   Risk No known risk,* when taken in the recommended preventive doses for malaria

   Pregnancy Outcome appears favorable

   Documentation inconclusive

pre-conception	All or None		Organ Development – (in weeks)						Maturation – (in weeks)				
	1	2	3	4	5	6	7	8	9	10	12	20-36	38

conception   ←— Time of Greatest Risk —→   birth

   Chloroquine and hydroxychloroquine are used to prevent and treat malaria. They are also used to treat "lupus" (systemic lupus erythematosis), some amebic infections and in certain circumstances, rheumataoid arthritis. Chlorquine is the drug of choice for people traveling to and living in malarious areas free of chloroquine resistance.

   Note to women who need information on hydroxychloroquine: Hydroxychloroquine acts similarly to chloroquine. Research studies have not addressed the potential teratogenicity of hydroxychloroquine but have focused on the use of chloroquine by pregnant women. For this reason it is necessary to use information on chloroquine to provide you with an idea on how hydroxychloroquine might affect a developing baby.

*above the 4% background risk

Concern about the potential teratogenicity of chloroquine was generated from a report of birth defects in three children whose mother took daily doses (200 mg–600 mg) of this drug throughout her pregnancy.[1] Damage to the inner ear was observed in each child. Of interest is that three other children born to this woman were normal; one was prenatally exposed to chloroquine and two were not.

A 1985 study that looked at the effects of normal preventive doses of this drug during pregnancy found more reassuring evidence.[2] The medical records of 169 infants exposed before birth to chloroquine showed an incidence of birth defects of 1 percent, which is lower than the 4 percent expected incidence in our population. I should mention that a study of this small size could not be expected to detect a very subtle increase in birth defects. The study is also flawed by collecting data only from medical records (see retrospective studies, page 43). Nevertheless, these results do support earlier research suggesting that chloroquine in the recommended preventive doses for malaria is not harmful.

There is no known increased risk to an unborn baby when cloroquine is used to prevent malaria, but only one dose per week is required and this is taken for only a short period of time. Based on the above information, we must consider the possibility that the effects of chloroquine on an unborn baby could be related to the duration of the treatment and dose used. If this is so, *pregnant women who require high daily doses of hydroxychloroquine or chloroquine on a continuing basis might face an increased risk for having a child with birth defects.* However, I am not aware of any studies that have fully investigated this relationship.

Malaria during pregnancy is associated with miscarriages, growth retardation before birth, and, rarely, congenital infection. The incidence of prematurity and stillbirth may also increase, but more studies must be performed to confirm this belief. It is important to realize that the risks from malaria infection to both the mother and unborn child are significantly greater than are any remote risks from preventive drug therapy. In addition, treatment for acute malaria during pregnancy requires higher drug doses than are needed to prevent it. Therefore, pregnant women who are not immune to malaria should not travel to areas with a high incidence of malaria without consulting a physician and beginning antimalarial drug therapy. Therapy usually begins one or two weeks before departure and is continued after returning for another six to eight weeks. Commonsense precautions to help avoid bites by infected insects include: sensible clothing, screens, nets, and insect repellents.

References:

[1] C. W. Hart and R. F. Naunton, The ototoxicity of chloroquine phosphate, *Archives of Otolaryngology* 80 (1964): 407–12.

M. S. Wolfe and J. F. Cordero, Safety of chloroquine in chemosuppression of malaria during pregnancy, *British Medical Journal* 290 (1985): 1466–67.

COMMON NAME: **CIGARETTE SMOKING**

Brand Name/Chemical Name: **not applicable**

FDA Pregnancy Category: not applicable

ESTIMATED RISK SUMMARY:
Time of Exposure primarily after the first 20 weeks of pregnancy
Risk Known risk*
Pregnancy Outcome adverse
Documentation conclusive, based on current knowledge

← pre-conception	All or None		Organ Development – (in weeks)						Maturation – (in weeks)				
	1	2	3	4	5	6	7	8	9	10	12	20-36	38
												■	■

conception   ← Time of Greatest Risk →   birth

Cigarette smoking[1,2] increases the risk for heart disease, lung disease, and cancer in adults. It also jeopardizes the health of the unborn children of pregnant women who smoke. The best-known consequence of cigarette smoking during pregnancy is the increased incidence of low birth weight. The more cigarettes the expectant mother smokes, the lower the birth weight of her child. Low birth weight makes an infant more likely to have medical complications and is the major contributor to infant death.

A reduction in weight is particularly hazardous to a premature infant, whose already small size impairs its survival. To complicate matters further, women who smoke have twice the rate of premature deliveries as do nonsmokers.

Placental complications and bleeding disorders often complicate the pregnancies of women who smoke. These conditions certainly contribute to the problems observed among pregnant smokers and their children.

The risk of miscarriage (spontaneous abortion) is 30–70 percent higher among

*above the 4% background risk

pregnant smokers than among nonsmokers. This, too, increases with the number of cigarettes smoked. Smoking also increases the frequency of stillbirths and infant deaths. Infant deaths are increased by 20 percent in women who smoke less than a pack a day and by 36 percent in women who smoke more.

The illness and death rate increases further in children up to the age of 5 years in women who continue to smoke after pregnancy. Children of smokers have more hospitalizations (primarly pneumonia and bronchitis) and make more visits to the doctor. Sudden infant death syndrome (SIDS) is also more frequent in children with smoking parents. Some researchers claim that smoking can affect child development, intellectual ability, and behavior, but an actual association has not yet been proven.

There is no convincing evidence that smoking during pregnancy causes physical abnormalities.[3]

Passive smokers are people who inhale someone else's cigarette smoke. Passive smoking by pregnant *non*smokers might affect the growth and birth weight of their unborn children. But more research is needed before definitive conclusions about the effect of "secondhand" smoke can be drawn. Until then women who don't smoke are encouraged to avoid long stays in smoke-filled places.

Other reproductive risks associated with cigarette smoking in women include difficulty in conceiving and earlier menopause. Studies show that male smokers have a lower sperm count than nonsmokers.

Smoking during pregnancy is gambling not only with your own health but also with the health of your unborn child. Smoking less or quitting altogether will make a big difference. In fact, research suggests that if you stop smoking by the twentieth week of your pregnancy, your risk will be close to that of a nonsmoker.[4]

If you are already pregnant, I urge you to stop smoking now! Help is available to meet your special quit-smoking needs, in the form of a highly successful program from the American Lung Association. In ten days you will be able to quit on your own. I encourage you to contact your local branch of the Amerian Lung Association to obtain further information about this fabulous self-help program.

References:

[1]H. Cole, Studying reproductive risks, smoking, *Journal of the American Medical Association* 255 (1986): 22–23.

[2]L. Longo, Some health consequences of maternal smoking: Issues without answers, *Birth Defects*, Original Article Series 18 (1982): 13–31.

[3]P. H. Shiono, M. A. Klebanoff, and H. W. Berendes, Congenital malformation and maternal smoking during pregnancy, *Teratology* 34 (1986): 65–71.

[4]N. R. Butler, H. Goldstein, and E. M. Ross, Cigarette smoking in pregnancy: Its influence on birth weight and perinatal mortality, *British Journal of Medicine* 2 (1972): 127–30.

GENERIC NAMES: **CIMETIDINE, RANITIDINE**

Brand Names: **(Tagamet, Zantac)**

FDA Pregnancy Category:—

ESTIMATED RISK SUMMARY:
Time of Exposure throughout pregnancy
Risk Risk assessment is not possible
Pregnancy Outcome uncertain
Documentation insufficient

← pre-conception	All or None		Organ Development – (in weeks)						Maturation – (in weeks)				
	1	2	3	4	5	6	7	8	9	10	12	20-36	38

conception   ←—Time of Greatest Risk—→   birth

Cimetidine[1] *and ranitidine* are drugs used to treat gastrointestinal ailments, primarily peptic ulcer disease.

To date, systematic studies evaluating the effects of these drugs in human pregnancy have not been conducted. Based on the widespread use of cimetidine and ranitidine, it is noteworthy that there is no anecdotal evidence associating these drugs with birth defects. Information from the manufacturer on fifty babies exposed before birth to cimetidine, also has not revealed an increased risk, but the time and duration of the exposures were not noted.[1]

There is an isolated incident, not confirmed by later reports, of one infant with short-term liver impairment. The baby was exposed to cimetidine and Titralac (a calcium antacid) during the last trimester.[2]

Cimetidine is sometimes used as a pre-anesthetic agent to prevent inhaling of acid gastric contents during labor.[3] No adverse effects on the course of delivery or in the newborn baby from such use have been reported.

Long-term follow-up studies of children exposed before birth have not been located.

References:

[1] J. H. Lewis, A. B. Weingold, and the committee on FDA-related matters, American College of Gastroenterology, *American Journal of Gastroenterology* 80 (1985): 912–23.

[2]G. Glade, C. L. Saccar, and G. R. Pereira, Cimetidine in pregnancy: Apparent transient liver impairment in the newborn, *American Journal of Diseases of Children* 134 (1980): 87–88.

[3]N. Qvist, K. Storm, and A. Holmskov, Cimetidine as pre-anesthetic agent for cesarean section: Perinatal effects on the infant, the placental transfer of cimetidine and its elimination in the infants, *Journal of Perinatal Medicine* 13 (1985): 179–83.

GENERIC NAME: **CLINDAMYCIN**

Brand Name: **(Cleocin)**

FDA Pregnancy Category:—

ESTIMATED RISK SUMMARY:

Time of Exposure throughout pregnancy
Risk Risk assessment is not possible
Pregnancy Outcome uncertain
Documentation unavailable

pre-conception →	All or None		Organ Development – (in weeks)						Maturation – (in weeks)				
	1	2	3	4	5	6	7	8	9	10	12	20-36	38

conception   ←— Time of Greatest Risk —→   birth

Clindamycin is an antibiotic usually reserved for serious infections. To date, there is no evidence that this drug used during pregnancy causes birth defects. But there has not been a systematic evaluation of its potential teratogenicity.

Rarely, clindamycin causes a severe, or even fatal, form of colitis in adults. Pregnant women are at no greater risk for this complication.

GENERIC NAME: **CLOMIPHENE CITRATE**

Brand Names: **(Clomid, Serophene)**

FDA Pregnancy Category:—

ESTIMATED RISK SUMMARY:

Time of Exposure immediately before pregnancy
Risk Known risk*
Pregnancy Outcome multiple pregnancies
Documentation conclusive, based on current knowledge

Time of Exposure immediately before or during pregnancy
Risk Suspected risk* for miscarriage, ectopic pregnancies, and molar pregnancies
Pregnancy Outcome uncertain: favorable and adverse outcomes observed
Documentation inconclusive

Time of Exposure immediately before or during pregnancy
Risk No known risk* for birth defects
Pregnancy Outcome appears favorable
Documentation inconclusive

pre-conception	All or None		Organ Development – (in weeks)						Maturation – (in weeks)				
	1	2	3	4	5	6	7	8	9	10	12	20-36	38

conception   ←— Time of Greatest Risk —→   birth

Clomiphene is a "fertility drug" used to stimulate ovulation.

Ovulation induction with clomiphene has been reported to cause an increase in ectopic pregnancies (those occurring outside of the uterus),[1] molar pregnancies (those that do not develop but result in a mass of cysts),[2] twin or other multiple pregnancies,[3,4,5,6] and miscarriages.[4] Clomiphene-related multiple pregnancies, primarily twins, occur ten times more often than expected. These pregnancies are at risk for premature births as well as a number of other complications. The incidence of molar pregnancy is suspected to be 1 in 659. Published reports suggest that there is a twofold relative risk for ecotpic pregnancy.[2]

In considering these possible increased risks, keep in mind that clomiphene is prescribed for women with fertility problems. Women with fertility problems more often have miscarriages. In fact, regardless of whether or not they are taking clomiphene, their rate of miscarriage is similar (22.3%[7] without drugs and 25.5%[3] after using clomiphene). It is also important to understand that women taking clomiphene are

*above the 4% background risk

watched more closely than others and this provides a greater opportunity to document any problems. So their miscarriage rate, for example, may only appear higher.

The reported incidence of miscarriage varies greatly, from 11 percent to 30 percent, and it is thus hard to define clomiphene's true role in causing it. One large prospective study found no differences in miscarriages between women who spontaneously conceived and women receiving either clomiphene or another fertility drug (gonadotropins).[8] Another study found that miscarriages were higher than expected after the first and after the seventh cycle of clomiphene treatment.[9] And yet another study observed that miscarriages were nearly twice as high in women who conceived while taking clomiphene than in those who conceived after clomiphene therapy.

After miscarriages, some of the embryos and fetuses were found to have abnormal chromosomes. The chromosomal defects are primarily those that preclude survival of the fetus. It is important to realize that this increases the incidence of miscarriages, rather than the number of children born live with abnormalities.[10]

One exception was a study that found a twofold increase in Down syndrome (formally referred to as mongolism) in women taking fertility drugs (clomiphene or another type, gonodotropins).[11,12,13] This increase over the expected incidence in the general population is similar to the increased risk for Down syndrome in women 35 years and older. Since no other evidence supports this observation, further studies are needed before a cause-and-effect relationship between clomiphene and Down syndrome can be made. Prenatal diagnosis can detect Down syndrome (see "Diagnosing and Treating Problem Pregnancies," page 21). But these procedures carry certain risks and are not ordinarily recommended after clomiphene treatment.

Several investigations have failed to detect an increase in birth defects among children born to women using clomiphene to conceive.[3,4,5,8] One study of 1034 clomiphene-related pregnancies found the incidence of minor and major malformations comparable to a group of children born to women who conceived without drug treatment.[5] Several years ago, individual case reports raised the suspicion that clomiphene caused defects of the brain and spinal cord (the neural tube defects spina bifida and anencephaly).[14,15,16,17,18] To date, these concerns remain unfounded; a causal relationship is not suspected.

Infants born from clomiphene-induced pregnancies showed normal development at 6 and 12 months.[5] However, there have been no long-term follow-up studies.

As with many drugs that are necessary or cannot be avoided during pregnancy, a possible increased risk resulting from the reason for the mother's drug treatment must be considered.

References:

[1]P. A. Marchbanks, C. B. Coulam, and J. F. Annegers, An association between clomiphene citrate and ectopic pregnancy: A preliminary report, *Fertility and Sterility* 22 (1985): 268–70.

[2]S. Mor-Joseph, S. O. Antebury, M. Grant, A. Brzezinsky, and S. Evron, Recurrent molar pregnancies associated with clomiphene citrate and human gonadotropins, *American Journal of Obstetrics and Gynecology* 151 (1985): 1085–86.

[3]E. Y. Adashi, J. A. Rock, K. C. Sapp, E. J. Martin, A. C. Wentz, and G. S. Jones, Gestational outcome of clomiphene-related conceptions, *Fertility and Sterility* 31 (1979): 620–26.

[4]R. H. Asch and R. B. Greenblatt, Update on the safety of clomiphene citrate as a therapeutic agent, *Journal of Reproductive Medicine* 17 (1976): 175–80.

[5]M. Hack, M. Brish, D. M. Serr, M. Insler, M. Salomy, and B. Lunenfeld, Outcome of pregnancy after induced ovulation, *Journal of the American Medical Association* 220 (1972): 1329–33.

[6]A. F. Goldfarb, A. Morales, A. E. Rakoff, and P. Protos, Critical review of 160 clomiphene-related pregnancies, *Obstetrics and Gynecology* 31 (1968): 342–45.

[7]C. L. Buxton and A. L. Southam in *Human Infertility* (New York: Hoeber, 1958), p. 18.

[8]K. Kurachi, T. Aono, J. Minagawa, and A. Miyake, Congenital malformations of newborn infants after clomiphene-inducted ovulation, *Fertility and Sterility* 40 (1983): 187–89.

[9]T. Toshinobu, F. Seiichiro, S. Noriaki, I. Kihyoe. Correlation between dosage or duration of clomid therapy and abortion rate, *International Journal of Fertility* 1979; 24: 193–7.

[10]J. Boué, A. Boué, and P. Lazar, Retrospective and prospective epidemiological studies of 1,500 karyotyped spontaneous human abortions, *Teratology* 12 (1975): 11–26.

[11]G. P. Oakley and J. W. Flynt. Jr. Increased prevalence of Down's syndrome among offspring treated with ovulation-inducing agents, *Teratology* 5 (1972): 264.

[12]S. Harlap, Ovulation induction and congenital malformation, *Lancet* 2 (1976): 961.

[13]M. Ahlgren, B. Källén, and G. Rannevik, Outcome of pregnancy after clomiphene therapy, *Acta Obstetrica et Gynecologica Scandinavica* 55 (1976): 371–75,.

[14]Y. Biale, L. M. Altaras, and N. Ben-Aderet, Anencephaly and clomiphene-induced pregnancy, *Acta Obstetrica et Gynecologica Scandinavica* 57 (1978): 483–84.

[15]B. Field and C. Kerr, Ovulation stimulation and defects of neural tube closure, *Lancet* 2 (1974): 1511.

[16]B. Sandler, Anencephaly and ovulation stimulation, *Lancet* 2 (1973): 379.

[17]C. Barrett and C. Hakim, Anencephaly, ovulation stimulation, subfertility and illegitimacy, *Lancet* 2 (1973): 916–17.

[18]J. L. Dyson and H. G. Kohler, Anencephaly and ovulation stimulation, *Lancet* 1 (1973): 1256–57.

GENERIC NAME: **CLOTRIMAZOLE**

Brand Names: **(Gyne-Lotrimin, Lotrimin, Mycelex)**

FDA Pregnancy Category: B

ESTIMATED RISK SUMMARY:

Time of Exposure throughout pregnancy

Risk No known risk*

Pregnancy Outcome appears favorable

Documentation inconclusive, based on minimal data

*above the 4% background risk

← pre-conception ←	All or None	Organ Development – (in weeks)						Maturation – (in weeks)				
	1	2	3	4	5	6	7	8	9	10	12	20-36	38

conception   ←—Time of Greatest Risk—→   birth

Clotrimazole is an antibiotic used to treat moniliasis, a fungal or "yeast" infection of the vagina. The infection is sometimes called candida, after the fungus *Candida albicans.*

Several studies monitoring the topical use of this drug by pregnant women, have not observed any birth defects caused by it.[1,2]

Long-term follow-up studies of children exposed before birth have not been located.

References:

[1]K. Haram and A. Digranes, Vulvovaginal candidiasis in pregnancy treated with clotrimazole, *Acta Obstetrica et Gynecologica Scandinavica* 57 (1978): 453–55.

[2]E. Svendsen, S. Lie, T. H. Gunderson, I. Lyngstad-Vik, and J. Skuland, Comparative evaluation of miconazole, clotrimazole and nystatin in the treatment of candidal vulvo-vaginitis, *Current Therapeutic Research* 23 (1978): 666–72.

GENERIC NAME: **COCAINE**

Brand Name/Chemical name: **not applicable**

FDA Pregnancy Category: not applicable

ESTIMATED RISK SUMMARY:

Time of Exposure throughout pregnancy

Risk Risk assessment for birth defects is not possible

Pregnancy Outcome uncertain

Documentation insufficient

Time of Exposure difficult to be specific, possibly throughout pregnancy

Risk Highly suspected risk* for pregnancy complications and behavioral disturbances in exposed infants

Pregnancy Outcome uncertain: favorable and adverse outcomes observed

Documentation inconclusive, based on minimal data

*above the 4% background risk

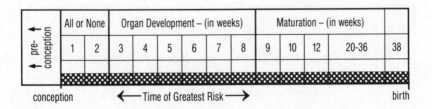

← pre-conception ←	All or None	Organ Development – (in weeks)						Maturation – (in weeks)				
	1	2	3	4	5	6	7	8	9	10	12	20-36	38

conception   ← Time of Greatest Risk →   birth

Cocaine is a stimulant drug that produces an intense euphoric high. Today, cocaine is one of the most widely abused drugs in the United States, with an estimated 30 million Americans having used it at least once. Contributing to the popularity of this drug is the less expensive and more potent form called rock cocaine, or "crack." Named for the crackling sound it makes when smoked, the availability of crack has removed the price barrier from cocaine, whose high price once prohibited experimentation. Paralleling the rise in the use of this drug by the general population, is the alarming increase in cocaine use reported among pregnant women.

Currently only preliminary information on the effects of this drug on the unborn have been published. Many of the cocaine-using women in the studies were also smoking cigarettes and using other drugs, including alcohol. Even though most researchers tried to take these variables into account, it is likely that the polydrug use and the bad health habits of some mothers adversely influenced their pregnancy outcomes. It is too early to know whether or not the various methods of using this drug (inhaling, smoking, and injecting) could have different effects on the developing baby. Also most of the reports on cocaine use during pregnancy have focused more on regular use of the drug (although not necessarily throughout pregnancy) or on large single doses. For this reason, it is difficult to determine the risks involved with very small amounts of cocaine. Nevertheless, the possibility that some of the observed complications could occur with lesser doses cannot be excluded.

At the time of this writing, there is no strong evidence to suggest that cocaine causes malformations in the developing baby. There is, however, a report of a child with a kidney defect and testes which failed to descend into the scrotum. His mother took 4–5 grams of cocaine in a single day.[1] Cause and effect cannot be deduced from this isolated instance.

Several researchers have reported a number of complications other than birth defects in both the pregnancies and infants of cocaine-using women. Some of the adverse effects include an increased frequency of: early miscarriages,[1] premature labor and delivery,[2,3] spontaneous labor with premature detachment of the placenta (abruptio placentae),[1,2,4] intrauterine growth retardation,[2] fetal distress,[2] risk factors associated with sudden infant death syndrome,[5] and a variety of behavioral disturbances.[1,2,6] Many of these problems could be explained by cocaine's physiologic effects: it constricts the blood vessels, it increases the heart rate, and it causes an acute rise in blood pressure (hypertension).

A case report described a baby born to a cocaine-using woman who had a rapid heart rate (tachycardia) and mild decreased muscle tone on his upper right side but otherwise appeared normal at birth.[7] Soon afterward, the baby developed seizures, his blood pressure and heart rate were elevated, and at 24 hours of age he was diagnosed as having suffered a "stroke." The exact timing of the "stroke" is not known. Although the doctors suspect it occurred before birth, there is no way to know for certain. The baby's mother used cocaine intranasally during her first five weeks of pregnancy, then stopped, but took another 5 grams in the 3 days immediately preceding delivery. Recently, another case of "stroke" in a cocaine-exposed baby was reported.[2] Unfortunately, the details of the exposure were not provided.

The investigators who have reported behavioral disturbances in babies born to cocaine-using women are not certain whether they are drug withdrawal symptoms or represent direct effects of the drug. The disturbances are characterized by tremulousness, irritability, irregular sleeping patterns, muscular rigidity, and poor feeding. One study found that on the average, such symptoms appeared when the baby was two days of age.[8]

Although long-term follow-up of infants born to cocaine-using mothers has not been conducted, one research group has tested early infant behavior by using the Brazelton Neonatal Behavioral Assessment Scale.[1] These investigators discovered that some of the babies did not respond appropriately. They believe that their behavior could potentially interfere with the process of bonding, which normally occurs in healthy mother/infant relationships. To help address possible problems, parents or caregivers of affected babies should first know what to expect. Beyond this, normal infant development can be enhanced through various handling techniques, which are discussed in detail in a recent publication.[6]

In conclusion, it is important to realize first that there are too few studies to conclude that cocaine actually causes all of the problems that have been reported. Second, not all investigations have associated cocaine with adverse effects.[9] Last, other factors such as little or no prenatal care, poor nutrition, and the concomitant use of cigarettes and other drugs (including marijuana, heroin, methadone, amphetamines, and alcohol) also contribute to poor pregnancy outcome in drug-using women. Nevertheless, the emerging findings are alarming and they should serve as a strong warning about the potential risks of using cocaine during pregnancy.

Andrea's Story:

I've been using coke for a few years now. I don't use it all the time, but it just seems to be around a lot. Since I found out I was pregnant I have tried not to use any. At first it was easy, because I wanted to do everything just right for my baby. But after awhile, the temptation overwhelmed me. I justified in my own mind that doing a little wouldn't hurt. I'll tell ya, that was a big mistake! After I did some, I worried about it a lot! I wish I had thought about how I would feel *beforehand.* My doctor told me that there wasn't enough research on cocaine yet to know whether the little I did could harm my unborn baby. We talked about taking chances, and my doctor explained that using cocaine during pregnancy was definitely taking a chance. I decided to ask my boyfriend and all of our friends not to do any cocaine in my presence and not even to have it around. Fortunately for me, everyone was extremely supportive. Now every time I think about doing just a little, I remember how I felt last time—it just wouldn't be worth it!

References:

[1] I. J. Chasnoff, W. J. Burns, S. H. Schnoll, and K. A. Burns. Cocaine use in pregnancy. *New England Journal of Medicine* 313 (1985): 666–69.

[2] A. S. Oro and S. D. Dixon, Perinatal cocaine and methamphetamine exposure: Maternal and neonatal correlates. *Journal of Pediatrics* 111 (1987): 571–78

[3] S. N. MacGregor, L. G. Keith, I. J. Chasnoff, M. A. Rosner, G. M. Chisum. P. Shaw, and J. P. Minogue, Cocaine use during pregnancy: Adverse perinatal outcome, *American Journal of Obstetrics and Gynecology* 157 (1987): 686–90.

[4] D. Acker, B. P. Sachs, K. J. Tracey, W. E. Wisw, Abruptio placentae associated with cocaine use. *American Journal of Obstetrics and Gynecology* 146 (1983): 220–21.

[5] Ward S. L. Davidson, S. Scheutz, V. Krishna, X. Bean, W. Wingert, L. Wachsman, and T. G. Keens. Abnormal sleeping ventilatory pattern in infants of substance-abusing mothers, *American Journal of Diseases of Children* 140 (1986): 1015–

[6] J. W. Schneider and I. J. Chasnoff. Cocaine abuse during pregnancy: Its effects on infant motor development—a clinical perspective. *Top Acute Care Trauma Rehabilitation* 2 (1987): 59–69.

[7] I. J. Chasnoff, M. E. Bussey, R. Savich, and C. M. Stack, Clinical and laboratory observations. Perinatal cerebral infarction and maternal cocaine use. *Journal of Pediatrics* 108 (1986): 456–59.

[8] P. E. LeBlanc, A. J. Parekh, B. Naso, L. Glass, Effects of intrauterine exposure to alkaloidal cocaine ("crack"), *American Journal of Diseases of Children* 141 (1987): 937–38.

[9] J. D. Madden, T. F. Payne, and S. Miller, Maternal cocaine abuse and effect on the newborn. *Pediatrics* 77 (1986): 209–11.

GENERIC NAME: **CODEINE**

Brand Names: **(available only in generic form; medicines that contain codeine must say so)**

FDA Pregnancy Category: C

ESTIMATED RISK SUMMARY:

Time of Exposure throughout pregnancy
Risk No known risk* for birth defects
Pregnancy Outcome appears favorable
Documentation inconclusive, based on minimal data

Time of Exposure particularly near delivery or during labor
Risk Known risk* (related to dose and duration)
Pregnancy Outcome adverse
Documentation conclusive, based on current knowledge

pre-conception	All or None		Organ Development – (in weeks)						Maturation – (in weeks)				
	1	2	3	4	5	6	7	8	9	10	12	20-36	38

conception   ←—Time of Greatest Risk—→   birth

Codeine is a narcotic analgesic, used to relieve moderate pain. It is popularly used as a suppressive in cough syrups. Although codeine is a weak narcotic, it can become habit-forming if used for prolonged periods, and the potential for its abuse does exist. Abuse of any narcotic during pregnancy always carries with it the risk for addiction not only in the mother but in the unborn baby as well.

There are three relevant retrospective studies, two of which focused on children with specific birth defects, the other looking at newborns with various abnormalities. They investigated the relationship of narcotic analgesics, opiates or codeine in particular, with an increased frequency of congenital heart disease,[1] cleft lip and cleft palate,[2] and malformations in general.[3] Basically these studies concluded that the mothers of children with abnormalities took codeine more often than did mothers of normal babies.

None of these investigations demonstrates that codeine caused any of the birth defects. It is important to realize that collecting the data depended on the mother's remembering what drug she took and specifically when during pregnancy she took it (see retrospective studies, page 43). Mothers of babies with birth defects recall the events during their pregnancies much differently than do mothers of normal children. Therefore, relying on mothers' memories can affect the reliability of the study's conclusions. Also it's important to realize that when several substances are examined

*above the 4% background risk

together, an association between any of the drugs and birth defects may simply be a chance occurrence. Last, all known teratogens display a recognizable pattern of malformation, but no such pattern has been described in codeine-exposed children.

The Collaborative Perinatal Project, which evaluated pregnancy outcome in more than 50,000 mother-child pairs, reported on birth defects after prenatal exposure to a wide variety of drugs.[4] Here, too, the combinations of drugs examined risked the possibility that the defects were chance occurrences. This study has other weaknesses: Other possible causes were not excluded, and the critical issue of medication timing was not specified. Even so, the use of codeine during pregnancy (there were 563 first trimester exposures) was not associated with large categories of major or minor birth defects.

Current research does not implicate codeine as a teratogen. Well-controlled studies are needed before the relationship between codeine and birth defects can be accurately defined.

Withdrawal symptoms have been reported in the newborns of *non*addicted women using codeine near term.[5] Symptoms were similar to those reported with heroin and methadone and disappeared either spontaneously or when treated with phenobarbital. Other risks affecting infant well-being, such as poor maternal health and nutritional habits, lack of prenatal care, additional drug use during pregnancy, and poor care-taking environment, are not expected from the nonaddicted mother.

Breathing difficulty (respiratory depression) is a reported risk with all narcotic analgesics when given during labor. Among these drugs, effects are similar in degree and are related to the dose used and the duration of the exposure.

Long-term follow-up studies of children exposed before birth have not been located.

References:

[1]K. J. Rothman, D. C. Flyer, A. Goldblatt, and M. B. Kreidberg, Exogenous hormones and other drug exposures of children with congenital heart disease, *American Journal of Epidemiology* 109 (1979): 433–39.
[2]I. Saxen, Associations between oral clefts and drugs taken during pregnancy, *International Journal of Epidemiology* 4 (1975): 37–44.
[3]M. B. Bracken, and T. R. Holford, Exposure to prescribed drugs in pregnancy and association with congenital malformations, *Obstetrics and Gynecology* 58 (1981): 336–44.
[4]O. P. Heinonen, D. Slone, and S. Shapiro, *Birth Defects and Drugs in Pregnancy* (Littleton, Mass.: Publishing Sciences Group, 1977).
[5]H. H. Mangurten, and R. Benawra, Neonatal codeine withdrawal in infants of nonaddicted mother, *Pediatrics* 65 (1980): 159–60.

COMMON NAME: **COPY MACHINES**

Brand Name/Chemical Name: **not applicable**

FDA Pregnancy Category: not applicable

ESTIMATED RISK SUMMARY:

Time of Exposure throughout pregnancy
Risk No known risk*
Pregnancy Outcome appears favorable
Documentation inconclusive

pre-conception	All or None		Organ Development – (in weeks)						Maturation – (in weeks)				
	1	2	3	4	5	6	7	8	9	10	12	20-36	38

conception   ←—— Time of Greatest Risk ——→   birth

Copy machines do not emit ionizing radiation (the kind produced by X-ray machines) or any harmful form of radiation.

The flash that you see is produced by an intense light. I am not aware of any investigation that has evaluated the pregnancy outcome in women who work around copy machines. While it might not be wise to stare at the light flash, I know of no information that would indicate avoidance of this exposure during pregnancy.

The specific chemicals used in the machines have also not been evaluated for their use during pregnancy. Nothing is really known about the effects of these chemicals in pregnancy, so if you come in actual contact with them, handle them especially carefully (see chemicals, page 101).

MEDICATION CLASSIFICATION: **CORTICOSTEROIDS**

GENERIC NAMES: BECLOMETHASONE, BETAMETHASONE, CORTISONE, DEXAMETHASONE, HYDROCORTISONE, METHYLPREDNISOLONE, PREDNISONE, PREDNISOLONE

Brand Names: **(Alphatrex, Baycadron, Beclovent, Beconase Nasal Inhaler, Benisone, Beta-Val, Celestone, Cortalone, Cortan, Cortef, Cortone, Decadron, Delta-Cortef, Deltasone, Dexone, Diprolene, Diprosone Dipropionate, Fernisolone Betatrex, Hexadrol, Hydrocortone, Liquid Pred, Medrol,**

*above the 4% background risk

Meticorten, Orasaone, Prednicen-M, SK-Dexamethasone, SK-Prednisone, Sterane, Sterapred, Uticort, Valisone, Valnac, Vancenase Nasal Inhaler, Vanceril)

FDA Pregnancy Category: topical corticosteroids; C; intranasal steroids: C; all others:—

ESTIMATED RISK SUMMARY:
   Time of Exposure before conception and throughout pregnancy
   Risk No known risk*
   Pregnancy Outcome appears favorable
   Documentation inconclusive

pre-conception	All or None		Organ Development – (in weeks)						Maturation – (in weeks)				
	1	2	3	4	5	6	7	8	9	10	12	20-36	38

conception   ←——Time of Greatest Risk——→   birth

Corticosteroids[1,2] are hormones produced by the adrenal gland, or synthetic versions that act just like those naturally produced. Corticosteroids (also referred to as steroids) are available in a variety of forms to treat many different conditions, including: allergies, asthma, certain skin ailments, eye problems, lupus erythematosis, rheumatoid arthritis, inflammatory bowel disease, endocrine disorders, and particular types of cancer. Corticosteroid creams and oral and nasal inhalers have a local action, working directly on the inflamed or irritated tissue. Used in these forms, little of the drug is absorbed into the bloodstream, making fetal exposure less likely.

Corticosteroids are well-established teratogens in laboratory animals, best known for causing cleft palate. In fact, these agents are often given to pregnant animals for the specific purpose of studying cleft palate. Some sources have inappropriately used such animal research as the basis for warnings of a similar effect in humans. (Cleft lip and cleft palate are among the most common birth defects in our population, occurring in 1/1000 births.) This is unfortunate, as such inaccurate information has caused many pregnant women to worry needlessly.

Numerous studies have consistently failed to reveal an increased incidence of

*above the 4% background risk

miscarriages, cleft palate, or any other birth defects in infants exposed to corticosteroids before birth. These include large studies that followed women on corticosteroids through their pregnancies.[3] Also included are hundreds of cases of pregnant patients with inflammatory bowel disease, rheumatoid arthritis, and asthma who take these drugs in various doses and for various lengths of time.

This is not to say that a birth defect has never been observed in a child whose mother used a corticosteroid during pregnancy. There have been isolated instances. But as you know, there is a risk of birth defects with every pregnancy, and corticosteroids are frequently used products. For these reasons, such isolated instances are most likely just chance occurrences. Some of these case reports probably originate in an increased awareness of possible dangers generated by the animal studies. As a result, more adverse effects are reported.

In adults on longtime steroid therapy, the adrenal gland may lose the ability to produce these hormones itself. Corticosteroids cross the placenta, so a mother's long-term therapy theoretically could reduce the ability of the baby's adrenal gland to function. This risk, however, appears negligible, as the majority of these infants show no such signs.

Steroids, **betamethasone** and **dexamethasone** in particular, are commonly administered to fetuses likely to be born prematurely. The procedure is a way to prevent a serious complication called respiratory distress syndrome—a life-threatening condition characterized by lung immaturity. Steroids can accelerate fetal lung maturity, increasing the chances of survival for the premature newborn. Although certain circumstances prohibit the use of steroids for this purpose, under the appropriate circumstances there are no known significant risks to the mother, fetus, or newborn. In fact, evaluation of 4- and 6-year-old children whose mothers received **betamethasone** revealed no adverse development effects.[4] Long-term follow-up of children prenatally exposed to **dexamethasone** has also failed to reveal adverse effects.[5]

In one study, thirty-four pregnant women receiving **prednisolone** showed an increased incidence of difficult deliveries and stillbirths over that for pregnant women with similar conditions not receiving steroids.[6] Subsequent investigations have not confirmed these observations.

A study of 119 women being treated for infertility with **prednisone** revealed no birth defects among their infants but did find an increased frequency of low birth weight. Only long-term follow-up studies can reveal the significance of these findings. Nevertheless, it is reassuring that other studies have not indicated that prednisone causes low birth weight.

References:

[1]J. H. Lewis, A. B. Weingold, and the committee on FDA-related matters, American College of Gastroenterology, *American Journal of Gastroenterology* 80 (1985): 912–23.

[2]R. J. Vender and H. M. Spiro, Inflammatory bowel disease and pregnancy. *Journal of Clinical Gastroenterology* 4 (1982): 231–82.

[3]A. M. Bongiovanni and A. J. McPadden, Steroids during pregnancy and possible fetal complications, *Fertility and Sterility* 11 (1960): 181–86.

[4]B. A. MacArthur, R. N. Howie, J. A. Dezote, et al., School progress and cognitive development of 6-year-old children whose mothers were treated antenatally with betamethasone, *Pediatrics* 70 (1982): 99–105.

[5]Collaborative Group on Antenatal Steroid Therapy, Effects of antenatal dexamethasone administration in the infant: Long-term follow-up, *Journal of Pediatrics* 104 (1984): 259–67.

[6]D. Warrell and R. Taylor, Outcome for the fetus of mothers receiving prednisolone during pregnancy, *Lancet* 1 (1968): 117.

MEDICATION CLASSIFICATION: **COUMARIN DERIVATIVES**

GENERIC NAMES: **DICUMAROL, PHENOPROCOUMON, WARFARIN**

Brand Names: **(Coumadin, Dicumarol, Liquamar, Panwarfin)**

FDA Pregnancy Category:—

ESTIMATED RISK SUMMARY:

Time of Exposure throughout most of pregnancy, 6–9 weeks for the fetal warfarin syndrome

Risk Known risk*

Pregnancy Outcome adverse

Documentation conclusive, based on current knowledge

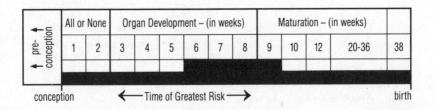

← pre-conception	All or None		Organ Development – (in weeks)						Maturation – (in weeks)				
	1	2	3	4	5	6	7	8	9	10	12	20-36	38

conception   ←— Time of Greatest Risk —→   birth

Coumarin derivatives are anticoagulants—drugs that thin the blood by interfering with clotting (coagulation.) Of the group, **warfarin** is the most commonly used.

*above the 4% background risk

Anticoagulants are used to treat and prevent blood clots (thrombophlebitis, pulmonary emboli), certain types of heart conditions, and stroke.

One study of 437 pregnant women exposed to coumarin derivatives showed that 67 percent delivered normal babies.[1] Of the others, half miscarried or produced stillbirths. The rest of the children exhibited birth defects.

Abnormalities associated with prenatal exposure to coumarin derivatives are referred to as the warfarin embryopathy or the fetal warfarin syndrome. The most characteristic feature of the fetal warfarin syndrome is underdeveloped nasal cartilage, occurring in all reported cases.[1,2,3,4,5] This defect causes breathing problems in about one-half of the newborns. Cartilage defects seen by X rays in most of the children with the syndrome may no longer be evident after the first year. About 20 percent have eye abnormalities— blindness, abnormally small eyes, and degeneration of the nerves of the eye.

Some experts think there are other defects, as well: In 3 percent of exposed infants there are brain abnormalities, abnormally small heads (microcephaly), mental retardation, deafness, seizures, and spasticity.[1] Low birth weight and growth failure have also been observed.

Keep in mind that these studies were all retrospective (see retrospective studies, page 43). They may show only the most severe defects, and under-report more subtle problems of the central nervous system and other organs.

The critical period for the fetal warfarin syndrome is six to nine weeks. The critical period for central nervous system defects has not been determined, but the greatest risk probably occurs in the second and third trimesters. Developmental retardation can result from exposures throughout pregnancy.

Fetal and placental bleeding are additional risks associated with coumarin derivatives. Use of heparin, although not a completely safe alternative, would eliminate these and other risks posed by coumarin derivatives (see heparin, page 176).

References:

[1]J. G. Hall, R. M. Pauli, and K. M. Wilson, Maternal and fetal sequelae of anticoagulation during pregnancy, *American Journal of Medicine* 68 (1980): 122–40.

[2]J. M. Lamontagne, J. E. Leclerc, C. Carrier, and M. Bureau, Warfarin embryopathy—A case report, *Journal of Otolaryngology* 13 (1984): 127–29.

[3]M. F. Whitfield, Chrondrodysplasia punctata after warfarin in early pregnancy: Case report and summary of the literature, *Archives of Diseases in Childhood* 55 (1980): 139–42.

[4]M. J. E. Harrod and P. S. Sherrod, Warfarin embryopathy in siblings, *Obstetrics and Gynecology* 57 (1981): 673–76.

[5]M. Baillie, E. D. Alenm, and A. R. Elkington, The congenital warfarin syndrome: A case report, *British Journal of Ophthalmology* 64 (1980): 633–5.

GENERIC NAME: **CYCLIZINE**

Brand Name: **(Marezine)**

FDA Pregnancy Category: B

ESTIMATED RISK SUMMARY:
   Time of Exposure throughout pregnancy
   Risk No known risk*
   Pregnancy Outcome appears favorable
   Documentation inconclusive

← pre-conception	All or None	Organ Development – (in weeks)						Maturation – (in weeks)				
	1	2	3	4	5	6	7	8	9	10	12	20-36	38

conception   ← Time of Greatest Risk →   birth

Cyclizine is used to treat and prevent nausea, vomiting, and the dizziness associated with motion sickness. This drug is similar to buclizine (see page 92) and meclizine (see page 226).

Cyclizine has been evaluated in three studies (two prospective and one retrospective) that have failed to associate its use with an increase in birth defects.[1,2,3] The Collaborative Perinatal Project, which evaluted pregnancy outcome in over 50,000 mother-child pairs exposed to a wide variety of drugs, found no association between the use of cyclizine during the first three months of pregnancy and congenital malformations.[1] But only fifteen exposures were included, making the finding less meaningful.

Another prospective study that examined the pregnancy outcomes of 111 women who took cyclizine as an antinauseant also found no adverse effects from its use.[2] The retrospective investigation compared drug consumption in pregnancies resulting in normal children and in malformed infants.[3] It found that significantly fewer mothers of children with major malformations took antinausea drugs during their first three months of pregnancy. Cyclizine was the fifth most commonly consumed antinausea agent. While each of these studies suffers from some shortcomings, together their similar conclusions have more meaning.

*above the 4% background risk

Long-term follow-up studies of children exposed before birth have not been located.

References:

[1]O. P. Heinonen, D. Slone, and S. Shapiro, *Birth Defects and Drugs in Pregnancy* (Littleton, Mass.: Publishing Sciences Group, 1977).

[2]L. Milkovich and B. J. Van den Berg, An evaluation of the teratogenicity of certain antinauseant drugs, *American Journal of Obstetrics and Gynecology* 125 (1976): 244–48.

[3]M. M. Nelson and J. O. Forfar, Associations between drugs administered during pregnancy and congenital abnormalities of the fetus, *British Medical Journal* 1 (1971): 523–27.

COMMON NAME: **CYTOMEGALOVIRUS (CMV)**

Brand Name/Chemical Name: **not applicable**

FDA Pregnancy Category: not applicable

ESTIMATED RISK SUMMARY:

Time of Exposure difficult to determine, possibly 4 to 24 weeks

Risk Suspected risk* from a reactivated infection

Pregnancy Outcome uncertain: favorable and adverse outcomes observed

Documentation inconclusive, based on minimal data

Time of Exposure difficult to determine, possibly 4 to 24 weeks

Risk Known risk* from a primary infection

Pregnancy Outcome adverse

Documentation conclusive, based on current knowledge

pre-conception	All or None		Organ Development – (in weeks)						Maturation – (in weeks)				
	1	2	3	4	5	6	7	8	9	10	12	20-36	38

conception   ←——Time of Greatest Risk——→   birth

Cytomegalovirus (CMV)[1,2] is one of the herpesviruses and it is an extremely common infection that is nearly always "silent" (without symptoms). (Other herpesviruses include: Epstein-Barr virus [mononucleosis]; varicella-zoster virus [chickenpox and

*above the 4% background risk

herpes zoster or "shingles"]; and herpes simplex virus 1 and 2 [oral and genital herpes]). Transmission of CMV, which occurs from person to person, does appear to require close physical contact.

By the time of puberty 30–80 percent of girls have acquired CMV and the vast majority of our population has acquired it by the age of 40. But having had the infection once does not prevent it from reactivating or recurring again. Unlike other viral infections such as the "German measles" (rubella) or the mumps, CMV tends to persist within your body for an indefinite period of time, resulting in later reactivation of the disease.

During pregnancy, the greatest risk from CMV is when you contract it for the very first time (primary infection). But even a reactivated infection can increase the risk that CMV will be passed from the mother to her developing baby.[2] However, infection under these circumstances is much less likely to produce complications than is a primary CMV infection.

CMV is the most common virus known to be transmitted before birth. Each year in the United States, an estimated 33,000 (1%) babies are born with this infection. Most of these infants (90%) have no symptoms at birth. A study following normal-appearing children born with silent CMV infection into their fifth year, showed that one-third of them developed some type of neurologic abnormality, including mental retardation, learning disabilities, and hearing loss.

Very severely affected infants with symptoms of the disease probably account for less than 5 percent of all infected newborns. As many as 20–30 percent of these children may die from disease complications. Features typical of congenital CMV infection include: enlargement of the liver and spleen, jaundice (yellowing of the skin due to high levels of bilirubin in the blood), purpura (a specific type of skin rash), microcephaly (abnormally small head size), mental retardation (ranging from severe retardation to mild to moderate developmental deficits[3]), eye abnormalities, hearing loss and, less commonly, pneumonia, and a type of anemia (hemolytic anemia). Heart defects, gastrointestinal abnormalities, and defects involving the muscles and skeleton have been observed in infected children. But it is not clear whether these other birth defects are coincidental or are truly the result of CMV.

For the most part, the time of CMV infection during pregnancy has little influence on how often the virus is passed to the developing baby. However, there is some evidence that the risk of complications is higher when the infection occurs during weeks four to twenty-four, although the most severely affected child reported in one study was born to a woman with CMV infection early in her third trimester of pregnancy.[4]

Several researchers have concluded that routine screening of pregnant women for

CMV would be of limited value. The primary reason is that as yet there are no practical ways to determine if the unborn baby has actually acquired the infection or to assess the severity of the disease.

In addition to CMV's being transmitted across the placenta, the baby can also acquire it through contact with an infected cervix during birth or through the mother's milk when breast-feeding.

Large amounts of the virus appear in the saliva and urine of affected infants. As a result, child-care personnel who are in contact with these children may face a risk of infection. However, evidence from one study suggests that pediatric health care workers are at no greater risk for contracting CMV than are women in the general population.[5] Until more information becomes available, women who are pregnant or who plan to be, need to be aware that children infected with CMV could be present in any child-care setting.[6] As a result, prevention of CMV is best accomplished by observing good personal hygiene (washing your hands) and careful handling and disposal of all items contaminated by potentially infectious secretions (urine and respiratory tract secretions).

References:

[1]J. S. Remington and J. O. Klein (eds.), *Infectious Diseases of the Fetus and Newborn Infant,* 2d ed. (Philadelphia: W. B. Saunders 1983), pp. 104–42.

[2]S. Stagno and R. J. Whitley, Herpesvirus infections of pregnancy. Part 1: Cytomegalovirus and Epstein-Barr virus infections, *New England Journal of Medicine* 313 (1985): 1270–74.

[3]T. J. Conboy, R. F. Poiss, S. Stagno, C. A. Alford, G. J. Myers, W. J. Britt, F. P. McCollister, M. N. Summers, and C. E. McFarland, Early clinical manifestations and intellectual outcome in children with symptomatic congenital cytomegalovirus infection, *Journal of Pediatrics* 111 (1987): 343–48.

[4]P. D. Griffiths and C. Baboonian, A prospective study of primary cytomegalovirus infection during pregnancy: Final report, *British Journal of Obstetrics and Gynecology* 91 (1984): 307–15.

[5]M. E. Dworsky, K. Welch, G. Cassady, and S. Stagno, Occupational risk for primary cytomegalovirus infection among pediatric health workers, *New England Journal of Medicine* 309 (1983): 950–53.

[6]Prevalence of cytomegalovirus excretion from children in five day-care centers, Alabama, *Morbidity and Mortality Weekly Report* 34 (1985): 49–51.

GENERIC NAME: **DANAZOL**

Brand Name: **Danocrine**

FDA Pregnancy Category:—

ESTIMATED RISK SUMMARY:

> *Time of Exposure* primarily from the 8th to the 12th week, although sensitivity to male hormones does continue beyond this time.
>
> *Risk* Known risk*

*above the 4% background risk

Pregnancy Outcome adverse
Documentation conclusive, based on current knowledge

← pre-conception ←	All or None		Organ Development – (in weeks)						Maturation – (in weeks)				
	1	2	3	4	5	6	7	8	9	10	12	20-36	38

conception   ←—Time of Greatest Risk—→   birth

Danazol is a synthetic androgen, a male hormone (see also: androgens, page 74). This drug is used to treat endometriosis, a condition that makes it very difficult for a woman to conceive a child. In endometriosis, cells from the lining of the uterus (the endometrium) migrate to the ovaries or other locations in the pelvis. By treating this condition, danazol can improve a woman's chances of becoming pregnant. But conception should not be attempted until *after* danazol therapy has been completed because its use during pregnancy has been associated with abnormal development of the unborn female's external sex organs. For this reason, women are advised to use a nonhormonal method of birth control while taking this drug.

I have located eleven instances, primarily case reports, where female fetuses have been affected by their mothers' use of danazol during the first three months of pregnancy.[1] Exactly how often this occurs is not clear. Miscarriages during danazol therapy have also been reported, but whether these were actually caused by the drug is not clear.[1] Abnormalities in affected females include enlarged clitoris with or without partial to complete closure of the labia (skin folds on either side of the vaginal opening). The risk for this occurring is highest during the "critical period" of development of the external sex organs, primarily from the eighth to the twelfth week after conception; however, sensitivity to male hormones does continue beyond this time.[2] It is reassuring to know that these problems can be surgically corrected and that the internal reproductive organs do not appear to be affected by the drug.

There are no reports of ill effects in males.

Normal infant[3,4] and early childhood[5] growth and development have been observed, but long-term studies of children exposed before birth have not yet been conducted. There is a study that examined eleven adult women who were masculinized before birth by progestins (a female sex hormone that can be converted into androgens in the mother and unborn baby). There were no long-term effects, and the women looked and behaved like other females their age.[6]

References:

[1] F. W. Rosa, Virilization of the female fetus with maternal danazol exposure, *American Journal of Obstetrics and Gynecology* 149 (1984): 99–100.

[2] P. Saenger, Abnormal sexual differentiation, *Journal of Pediatrics* 104 (1984): 1–17.

[3] M. R. Peress, A. K. Kreutner, R. S. Mathur, and H. O. Williamson, Female pseudohermaphroditism with somatic chromosomal anomaly in association with in utero exposure to danazol, *American Journal of Obstetrics and Gynecology* 142 (1982): 708–9.

[4] R. W. Shaw, Female pseudohermaphroditism associated with danazol exposure in utero case report, *British Journal of Obstetrics and Gynecology* 91 (1984): 386–89.

[5] S. C. Duck and K. P. Katayama, Danazol may cause female pseudohermaphroditism, *Fertility and Sterility* 35 (1981): 230–31.

[6] J. Money and D. Mathews, Prenatal exposure to virilizing progestins: An adult follow-up study of twelve women, *Archives of Sexual Behavior* 11 (1982): 73–83.

MEDICATION CLASSIFICATION: **DECONGESTANTS**

GENERIC NAMES: **EPHEDRINE, EPINEPHRINE, PHENYLEPHRINE, PHENYLPROPANOLAMINE, PSEUDOEPHEDRINE**

Brand Names: **(see Table 5–2, page 139)**

FDA Pregnancy Category: epinephrine: C; all others:—

ESTIMATED RISK SUMMARY:

Time of Exposure throughout pregnancy

Risk Risk assessment is not possible

Outcome uncertain

Documentation available information is insufficient

← pre-conception →	All or None		Organ Development – (in weeks)						Maturation – (in weeks)				
	1	2	3	4	5	6	7	8	9	10	12	20-36	38

conception   ← Time of Greatest Risk →   birth

Decongestants[1,2] are widely used to relieve symptoms of the common cold and various allergies. They are available as tablets, liquids, and nose drops and sprays. Nose drops and nasal sprays produce almost immediate relief, whereas tablets work more slowly but produce longer-lasting relief.

Decongestants are commonly combined with a variety of medicines, including antihistamines, cough suppressants, expectorants (used to thin out mucus secretions), and pain relievers. Some of these drugs are also used to treat other conditions. Phenylpropanolamine acts as an appetite suppressant and is contained in many over-the-counter diet pills. Epinephrine and phenylephrine are used to treat shock; epinephrine is also used for glaucoma. Ephedrine and epinephrine are used to treat bronchial asthma; as bronchodilators, they cause constricted air passages to become wider.

Stuffy or runny nose and other cold or allergy symptoms are common ailments for which there is no cure. Medicines will only help relieve the symptoms and make you feel more comfortable. While it's best to try to "tough out" a cold or minor allergies during pregnancy, the fact is that an extremely large number of pregnant women have been and continue to be treated for their symptoms. In addition, it is not always advisable to let asthma and severe allergies go untreated during pregnancy, since both can pose a threat to the mother and her unborn baby. In such cases, pregnant women are often advised to continue on their customary medications. Based on the frequency of their use during pregnancy, it is very surprising that decongestants have not really been properly evaluated for their effect on the developing baby.

Ephedrine, epinephrine, phenylephrine, phenylpropanolamine and pseudoephedrine belong to a class of drugs called sympathomimetics. The Collaborative Perinatal Project, a prospective study that evaluated pregnancy outcome in more than 50,000 mother-child pairs exposed to a wide variety of drugs, offers some of the only information available on these medicines. This study found an association between first trimester exposure to the sympathomimetic class of drugs and minor (cosmetic, non-life-threatening) birth defects.[3] *No* relationship appeared between **ephedrine** exposures and large categories of major or minor malfunctions. The use of **epinephrine, phenylephrine**, and **phenylpropanolamine** during the first trimester was associated with a greater frequency of major anad minor malfunctions. Minor malformations were greater for both **phenylephrine** and **phenylpropanolamine.** The use of **phenylephrine** and **phenylpropanolamine** also resulted in several possible associations with individual birth defects, the majority of which were not statistically significant. Too few exposures were recorded with **pseudoephedrine** to allow any conclusions.

Interpreting the meaning of these observations is difficult, in part because the value of the study's information for use in teratogen risk counseling has been questioned, for several reasons: There were few controls for other possible causes; in some cases it is possible that the condition for which the drug was prescribed might have caused the birth defects. For example, ephedrine is often used in emergency treatment for acute asthma or anaphylaxis (a very severe allergic reaction). And decongestants were given to women who might have viral infections. These conditions might of themselves pose a risk for birth defects.

The critical issue of medication timing was also not specified in the Collaborative Perinatal Project study, making it difficult to link an exposure to a specific defect. Because of frequent multiproduct use of cold and allergy preparations, in particular, it is hard to determine which drugs, if any, could cause birth defects. When several substances are examined together, as they were in this study, an association between any of the drugs and birth defects may simply be a chance occurrence. Last, even if there is an association, it does not prove that the substance actually caused the defect. So, further investigation is certainly required before the significance of the associations disclosed in this study can be determined.

Finally, there is some concern that the use of **epinephrine, phenylephrine,** and **phenylpropanolamine** could constrict the blood vessels in the placenta and uterus, thus affecting blood flow that could reduce the oxygen supply to the fetus.

Long-term follow-up studies of children exposed before birth to decongestants have not been located.

Many physicians believe that judicious use of certain decongestants is relatively safe during pregnancy. These feelings are based on long-time clinical experience with their use during pregnancy without any obvious ill effects. The Collaborative Perinatal Project doesn't clearly implicate these drugs as teratogenic. But it does serve as a warning against their indiscriminate use during pregnancy. Many believe that during pregnancy a topical nasal decongestant is safer than an oral one, because it exerts its effect directly on swollen nasal vessels and tissues. Still, small amounts of even these products can be absorbed into your system.

Certainly the rather-safe-than-sorry approach would be to try to avoid these medicines in early pregnancy. After the first trimester, take them only as indicated and when absolutely necessary. (Of course, use them if your physician has determined that you need the medication.) Most important, because many of these products are available without a prescription, please remember to check with your doctor before self-prescribing any drug during pregnancy. If you use a prescribed medication for asthma or allergies, be certain to inform your doctor before or as soon as you become pregnant.

When choosing a decongestant, avoid any product that might be linked to problems, choose one with the *lowest dose* (perhaps a children's preparation), and, as with all over-the-counter medications, look for the product with the *fewest* number of ingredients!

Natural remedies:*

While decongestants will provide a source of temporary relief from some cold and allergy symptoms, a commonsense alternative[4] might provide a little peace of mind, as well as help you to feel more comfortable.

- Breathing steam from a vaporizer, a hot shower, or even a pot of very hot water will help your stuffy nose.
- Normal saline nose drops can also provide some relief. These can be purchased at your drugstore or you can make your own by mixing a quarter-teaspoon of salt in one cup of warm water.
- Soothe your sore sinuses with a moistened warm towel across the nasal area.
- Gently finger-massage the sinus area, down the sides of your nose, under your eyebrow bones, and under your eyes.

References:

[1]E. S. Turner, P. A. Greenberber, and R. Patteson, Management of the pregnant asthmatic patient, *Annals of Internal Medicine* 6 (1980): 905–18.

[2]P. A. Greenberber and R. Patteson, Safety of therapy for allergic symptoms during pregnancy, *Annals of Internal Medicine* 89 (1978): 234–37.

[3]O. P. Heinonen, D. Slone, and S. Shapiro, *Birth Defects and Drugs in Pregnancy* (Littleton, Mass.: Publishing Sciences Group, 1977).

[4]The Over-the-Counter-Drug Committee of the Coalition for the Medical Rights of Women, *Safe and Natural Remedies for Discomforts of Pregnancy* (San Francisco, Calif., January 1981; rev. 1982).

GENERIC NAME: **DIAZEPAM**

Brand Names: **Valium, Valrelease**

FDA Pregnancy Category: D

ESTIMATED RISK SUMMARY:

Time of Exposure first trimester
Risk Possible risk**
Pregnancy Outcome uncertain: favorable and adverse outcomes observed
Documentation inconclusive

Time of Exposure near term or during delivery
Risk Known risk**

---

*None of these commonsense remedies have been medically proven. They are listed here for you because I have found them useful.
**above the 4% background risk

Table 5–2 DECONGESTANTS

BRAND NAMES	GENERIC NAMES*							
	ephedrine	epinephrin	phenylephedrine	phenylpropanolamine	pseudoephedrine	acetaminophen	antihistamine	other*
Anafed Capsules					•		•	
Chlor-Trimeton Decongestant Repetabs					•		•	
Triaminic-12 Tablets				•			•	
Allerest-12 Hour Capsules				•			•	
Cold Factor 12 Capsules				•			•	
Contac Capsules				•			•	
Dristan 12-Hour Capsules			•				•	
Nasafed Capsules			•				•	
Dimetapp Extentabs				•			•	
Drixoral Tablets					•		•	
Nasahist Capsules			•	•			•	
Bromatapp Tablets			•	•			•	
Fedahist Tablets					•		•	
Sudafed Plus Tablets					•		•	
Chlor-Trimeton Decongestant Tablets					•		•	
A.R.M. Tablets				•			•	
Triaminic Allergy Tablets				•			•	
Dimetane Decongestant Tablets			•				•	
Benadryl Decongestant Capsules					•		•	
Triafed Tablets					•		•	
Decohist Syrup			•				•	•
Sine-Off Extra Strength Tablets				•		•	•	
Allerest Sinus Pain Formula Tablets				•		•	•	
Sinarest Extra Strength Tablets				•		•	•	
Coricidin "D" Decongestant Tablets				•		•	•	
Sinutab Tablets					•	•	•	
Bronitin Mist		•						
Bronkaid Mist Supension		•						
Medihaler-Epi		•						
Primatene Mist Suspension		•						
Efed II	•							
Ephedrine Sulfate	•							

*Other: alcohol

Pregnancy Outcome adverse
Documentation conclusive, based on current knowledge

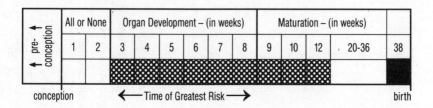

pre-conception	All or None		Organ Development – (in weeks)						Maturation – (in weeks)				
	1	2	3	4	5	6	7	8	9	10	12	20-36	38

conception   ←—Time of Greatest Risk—→   birth

Diazepam belongs to a group of drugs known as benzodiazepines. These drugs are among the most commonly prescribed drugs in the world. Benzodiazepines have a variety of uses as antianxiety drugs, hypnotics, anticonvulsants, and as muscle relaxants. Prolonged use of these drugs can lead to drug dependence in some individuals.

A casual relationship between the use of diazepam during pregnancy and an increased frequency of birth defects (specifically cleft lip and cleft palate) has not been proven. Both positive and negative evidence exists—leading to much debate and some speculation regarding the safety of its use.[1,2]

Before discussing any studies, I want you to understand a couple of things about cleft lip and cleft palate. First, these defects occur at very specific times during pregnancy. The lip is formed by thirty-five days after conception and the palate begins to develop at the end of the fifth week and is complete, for the most part, by seven weeks. Therefore, exposures to drugs beyond the first trimester cannot cause oral clefts (cleft lip with or without cleft palate or cleft palate alone). Second, the normal incidence of cleft lip and cleft palate in our population is approximately one in every thousand births. Because these defects are fairly common, a very slight increase in their frequency could be difficult to detect, requiring very large studies to do so.

Three retrospective studies,[3,4,5] all with inherent flaws in study design, have shown an association between oral clefts and the use of diazepam in pregnancy. Two retrospective studies[6,7] and one large prospective survey[8] do not support such an association.

One case report has described a child with facial abnormalities, including cleft lip and cleft palate, born to a woman whose single dose of diazepam (580 mg) was forty-three days after her last menstrual period (twenty-nine days after conception).[9]

In the retrospective studies, mothers of children with selected malformations were either interviewed or sent a questionnaire in an effort to investigate a possible relationship between diazepam and oral clefts. Therefore, these mothers were questioned *after*, and in some cases many years after, giving birth to a baby with an abnormality. The most significant problem with this approach is the difficulty of accurately documenting what drug was used and when during pregnancy it was taken (see retrospective studies, page 43). Only exposures occurring during cleft lip and cleft palate development could be linked to their cause. So it is critical that the issue of medication timing be closely determined. Further complicating the matter, mothers of babies with birth defects recall the events during their pregnancy much differently than do mothers of normal children. This can affect the reliability of a study's conclusions.

One of the retrospective studies not finding an association between diazepam use and oral clefts did find a slight increased frequency of inguinal hernia (hernia in the groin area).[7] Additional studies are needed to explore the significance of this observation.

The results of a prospective study are more dependable, because recall is not affected by time lapsed or influenced by pregnancy outcome (see prospective studies, page 42). In such a study, 33,249 women were questioned during their pregnancy about first trimester diazepam use.[8] The results revealed that oral clefts did not occur significantly more often in babies born to diazepam users.

But failing to show an association does not prove that diazepam is safe; just as finding an association does not prove that diazepam actually causes oral clefts.

Most of the studies did not look at a sufficient number of cases to allow meaningful conclusions about the use of diazepam during the first trimester as the cause of oral clefts.[5] From lack of supporting data, the possibility of chance occurrence cannot be dismissed. However, if a causal relationship does in fact exist, according to one study oral clefts might be four times more frequent in women taking diazepam during their first trimester.[4] This translates to: 996 of every 1000 babies would still be expected to be born *without* such a defect.

Certainly more studies are needed to resolve this issue. In the meantime, it would be safest to avoid the use of diazepam during the first trimester of pregnancy.

While diazepam associated malformations are questionable, there is little doubt that the use of this drug near term or during delivery causes withdrawal symptoms and listlessness in the newborn, referred to as "floppy baby syndrome." The floppy baby syndrome is characterized by poor muscle tone, lethargy, and sucking difficulties. The withdrawal symptoms have lasted from ten days to two weeks and include tremors, irritability, increased muscle tone, and vigorous sucking. Diazepam levels in newborns have reportedly been twice as high as that of their mothers. The apparent limited ability of newborns to metabolize and excrete this drug is thought to be responsible for the prolonged effects.

Long-term follow-up studies in children exposed before birth have not been located.

References:

[1]M. J. Safra and G. P. Oakley, Valium: An oral cleft teratogen? *Cleft Palate Journal* 13 (1976): 198–200.

[2]L. W. D. Weber, Benzodiazepines in pregnancy—academical debate or teratogenic risk? *Biological Research in Pregnancy* 6 (1985): 151–67.

[3]D. Aarskog, Association between maternal intake of diazepam and oral clefts. *Lancet* 2 (1975): 921.

[4]J. M. Safra and G. P. Oakley, Association between cleft lip with or without cleft palate and neonatal exposure to diazepam, *Lancet* 2 (1975): 478–80.

[5]I. Saxen and L. Saxen, Association between maternal intake of diazepam and oral clefts, *Lancet* 2 (1975): 498.

[6]A. Czeizel, Diazepam, phenytoin, and etiology of cleft lip and/or cleft palate, *Lancet* 1 (1976): 810.

[7]L. Rosenberg and A. A. Mitchell. Lack of relationship of oral clefts to diazepam use in pregnancy, *New England Journal of Medicine* 310 (1984): 1122.

[8]P. H. Shiono and J. L. Mills. Oral clefts and diazepam use during pregnancy. *New England Journal of Medicine* 311 (1984): 919–20.

[9]F. Rivas, Z. Hernandez, and J. M. Cantu, Acentric craniofacial cleft in a newborn female prenatally exposed to a high dose of diazepam, *Teratology* 30 (1984): 179–80.

GENERIC NAME: **DIAZOXIDE**

Brand Names: **(Hyperstate IV, Proglycem)**

FDA Pregnancy Category: C

ESTIMATED RISK SUMMARY:

Time of Exposure throughout most of pregnancy
Risk No known risk*
Pregnancy Outcome appears favorable
Documentation inconclusive, based on minimal data

Time of Exposure near the time of delivery
Risk Suspected risk*
Pregnancy Outcome uncertain: favorable and adverse outcomes observed
Documentation inconclusive, based on minimal data

*above the 4% background risk

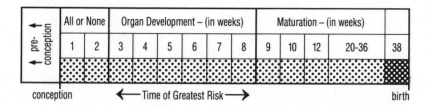

← pre-conception	All or None		Organ Development – (in weeks)						Maturation – (in weeks)				
	1	2	3	4	5	6	7	8	9	10	12	20-36	38

conception   ← Time of Greatest Risk →   birth

Diazoxide,[1] administered intravenously (IV), is used for the emergency treatment of severe hypertension (high blood pressure). Oral diazoxide is used to raise blood sugar levels in hyperinsulinism (when the pancreas secretes excessive amounts of insulin).

Studies have reported both normal and abnormal pregnancy outcomes from short- and long-term exposures to diazoxide. However, there have been no reports of birth defects after the use of this drug during pregnancy.

A newborn whose mother received IV diazoxide right before delivery had hyperglycemia (abnormally high blood sugar), which persisted for a few days. Decreased bone age, absence of hair, or excessive amounts of the fine hair that covers the body of the fetus have been observed with oral use of diazoxide in the last nineteen to sixty-nine days of pregnancy.

When IV diazoxide is administered too rapidly, it can cause an excessive drop in the mother's blood pressure. This has been associated with fetal distress. Fetal complications have been avoided by slow IV infusion of diazoxide, which reduces maternal blood pressure in a more controlled manner.

Diazoxide can interefere with spontaneous uterine contractions. To accomplish delivery, oxytocin, which promotes uterine contractions, might be required when diazoxide is taken near term.

Long-term follow-up studies of children exposed before birth have not been located.

Reference:

[1]R. P. Naden and C. W. Redman, Antihypertensive drugs in pregnancy, *Clinics in Perinatolgy* 12 (1985): 521–38.

GENERIC NAME: **DIETHYLSTILBESTROL (DES)**

Brand Name: **Diethylstilbestrol**

FDA Pregnancy Category: X

ESTIMATED RISK SUMMARY:

Time of Exposure weeks 11–20 might be the most important for structural abnormalities of the cervix and vagina, weeks 7– 12 might be important for noncancerous changes in the vagina and cervix, and the risk of cancer is higher when DES is given in the first 10 weeks.

Risk Known risk*

Pregnancy Outcome adverse

Documentation conclusive, based on current knowledge

pre-conception	All or None		Organ Development – (in weeks)						Maturation – (in weeks)				
	1	2	3	4	5	6	7	8	9	10	12	20-36	38

conception   ←—Time of Greatest Risk—→   birth

Diethylstilbestrol (DES)[1,2,3,4] is a synthetic estrogen (a female sex hormone, see page 161). One of DES's numerous uses as an estrogen substitute was to prevent and treat threatened abortions and reduce complications of late pregnancy. As it turned out, the therapy with DES was unsuccessful.

The most widespread use of DES occurred between 1946 and 1960, and an estimated 2–3 million pregnant women received it from 1940 to 1971. Despite its popularity, it was not until 1971 when the use of DES during pregnanacy was linked to cervical and vaginal cancer in a number of exposed female children—referred to as the "DES daughters"—later in life. Other harmful effects have since been discovered.

It was the recognition of cancer in young women (usually between 19 and 25 years of age) whose mothers took DES that alerted the medical community to the dangers of the drug. But the actual incidence of the cancer (clear cell adenocarcinoma) is rare. For every 10,000 women exposed to DES, somewhere between 1.4 and 14 will actually develop the cancer. More common are noncancerous changes in the vagina or cervix of the DES daughters: structural defects of the cervix (22–58% of those exposed), vagina (22–58%), uterus (66%), and fallopian tubes, as well as reproductive complications.

Adverse reproductive effects include infertility, miscarriages (18–47% of those exposed), pregnancies occurring outside of the uterus ("ectopic pregnancy," 2.6–6.5%),

*above the 4% background risk

and premature deliveries (10–30%). Finally, there may be an increased frequency of late pregnancy loss or death in the newborn.

Apparently DES exposure does not alter a DES daughter's chances of becoming pregnant, but it impairs her chances of giving birth to a full-term baby. Overall, approximately 82 percent of DES daughters who become pregnant give birth to healthy newborns.

There is conflicting information about men exposed to DES before birth. Some studies suggest they may have an increased risk for infertility, various urogenital abnormalities, and, less probably, testicular cancer. But not all studies confirm these findings, some investigations finding no increased risk of reported complications.[4] The differences in results are probably due to the way the studies are conducted, the amount of drug taken by the mother, and when during her pregnancy she took the drug.

The children of DES exposed sons and daughters are no more likely than those of unexposed parents to have birth defects.

Psychosexual development was evaluated in a two small groups of boys (twenty 6-year-olds and twenty 16-year-olds) whose diabetic mothers took female hormones (either DES or hydroxyprogesterone) in order to prevent pregnancy complications.[5] These boys were then compared to boys the same age whose mothers had not received such treatment. Hormone-exposed boys were rated as less assertive, less aggressive, and less athletic. The significance and meaning of these findings are very difficult to interpret.

If you don't already know if you are a DES daughter or son, your mother's medical records are the ideal way to find out. But these might not be available or it might be impractical to review them. If this is the case, you should ask your mother the obvious question: "Did you take DES?" You might also want to ask her particularly if she doesn't remember, "Did you have problems carrying a pregnancy to term?" "Did you bleed during pregnancy?" "Did you have miscarriages or pregnancies that threatened to miscarry?"

If your mother took DES, the best thing you can do is educate yourself. There are DES Action centers throughout the country (check your phone book) that are great sources of information. They will help you to find out about your exposure and the care you need. If there is no DES Action center in your community, contact the headquarters in San Francisco for more information: DES Action, 2845 24th Street, San Francisco, CA 94110, (415) 826–5060.

Alix Ann's Story:
Maybe you'll remember me as a panicky DES daughter who called you for help. My mother took DES when she was pregnant with me, and she and I have both been

worried about my own second pregnancy. I thought you'd like to know that after a normal pregnancy I had my second daughter, eight days early, in five hours of labor. It was a vaginal delivery, no instruments, and I took no medications at all. All of us are so happy, including my mother, who tends to worry a lot about me. Thanks again for all the help you gave me in learning about DES.

References:

[1] E. Eisenberg, Fertility problems of DES daughters, *Contemporary OB/GYN* August 1983: 197–99.

[2] J. A. Jefferies, S. J. Robby, P. C. O'Brien, E. J. Bergstralh, D. R. Labarthe, A. B. Barnes, K. L. Noller, P. A. Hatab, R. H. Kaufman, and D. E. Townsend, Structural anomalies of the cervix and vagina in women enrolled in the Diethylstilbestrol Adenosis (DESAD) Project, *American Journal of Obstetrics and Gynecology* 149 (1984): 59–66.

[3] NCI DES Summary, Prenatal Diethylstilbestrol (DES) exposure, *Clinical Pediatrics* 22 (1983)): 139–43.

[4] F. J. Leary, L. J. Resseguie, L. T. Kurland, P. C. O'Brien, R. F. Emslander, and K. L. Noller, Males exposed in utero to diethylstilbestrol, *Journal of the American Medical Association* 252 (1984): 2984–89.

[5] I. D. Yalom, R. Green, and N. Fisk, Prenatal exposure to female hormones: Effect on psychosocial development in boys, *Archives of General Psychiatry* 28 (1973): 554–61.

GENERIC NAME: **DIGITALIS**

RELATED GENERIC COMPOUNDS: **DIGITOXIN, DIGOXIN, GITALIN, LANATOSIDE C**

Brand Names: **(Cedilanid-D, Crystodigin, Digifortis, Kapseals, Digiglusin, Digitalis Pulvules, Gitaligin, Lanoxicaps, Lanoxin, Purodigin)**

FDA Pregnancy Category: digitalis: C; digitoxin: C; digoxin: A; gitalin: C; lanatoside C:—

ESTIMATED RISK SUMMARY:
   Time of Exposure throughout pregnancy
   Risk Risk assessment is not possible
   Pregnancy Outcome uncertain
   Documentation insufficient

pre-conception	All or None		Organ Development – (in weeks)						Maturation – (in weeks)				
	1	2	3	4	5	6	7	8	9	10	12	20-36	38

conception   ←—Time of Greatest Risk—→   birth

Digitalis[1] (whose use dates from the eighteenth century) and its related compounds are used to treat congestive heart failure and abnormal heart rate and rhythm. To date there is no evidence that these drugs cause birth defects. Only occasionally have low birth weight and shorter gestation periods (a difference of only one week) been reported in infants born to women using digitalis.

There have been two reported instances of digitalis causing fetal poisoning. One case was caused by drug overdose in the mother: the baby died at 3 days of age. In the other case, electrocardiographic (a graphic record of heart muscle action) changes were observed in the newborn. These observations are by no means routinely expected because digitalis concentrations in the blood of pregnant women are closely monitored.

Congestive heart failure in an unborn child has been treated with digoxin administered to the mother during pregnancy.

Long-term follow-up studies of children exposed before birth have not been located.

Reference:

[1] H. H. Rotmensch, U. Elkayam, and W. Frishman, Antiarrhythmic drug therapy during pregnancy. *Annals of Internal Medicine* 98 (1983): 487–97.

GENERIC NAME: **DISOPYRAMIDE**

Brand Name: **(Norpace)**

FDA Pregnancy Category:—

ESTIMATED RISK SUMMARY:

   Time of Exposure throughout pregnancy
   Risk Risk assessment is not possible
   Pregnancy Outcome uncertain
   Documentation insufficient

← pre-conception	All or None		Organ Development – (in weeks)						Maturation – (in weeks)				
	1	2	3	4	5	6	7	8	9	10	12	20-36	38

conception   ←—Time of Greatest Risk—→   birth

*above the 4% background risk

Disopyramide[1] is used to treat cardiac arrythmias (abnormal heartbeat rhythms). The use of this drug during pregnancy has not been associated with any adverse effects on the unborn baby. However, there is only limited obstetric experience with disopyramide, so the evidence is by no means conclusive.

Uterine contractions have been associated with the use of disopyramide in one woman. The contractions appeared to be drug-related, since they coincided with administration of the drug and subsided when therapy stopped. This effect was not observed in another woman who took disopyramide during her eighteenth and nineteenth week of pregnancy.

Long-term follow-up studies of children exposed before birth have not been located.

Reference:

[1] H. H. Rotmensch, U. Elkayam, and W. Frishman, Antiarrhythmic drug therapy during pregnancy, *Annals of Internal Medicine* 98 (1983): 487–97.

GENERIC NAME: **DOXYLAMINE**

Brand Names: **(Bendectin or Debendox** [no longer available], **Compōz*, Nervine Nighttime Sleep Aid*, Nytol with DPH*, Sleep-Eze 3,* Sominex 2,* Twilite, Unisom Nighttime Sleep Aid)**

FDA Pregnancy Category:—

ESTIMATED RISK SUMMARY:
   Time of exposure throughout pregnancy
   Risk No measurable risk**
   Pregnancy Outcome favorable
   Documentation conclusive, based on current knowledge

← pre-conception	All or None		Organ Development – (in weeks)						Maturation – (in weeks)				
	1	2	3	4	5	6	7	8	9	10	12	20-36	38
	o o	o o	o o	o o	o o	o o	o o	o o	o o	o o	o o	o o o o o o	o o
	o o	o o	o o	o o	o o	o o	o o	o o	o o	o o	o o	o o o o o o	o o
	o o	o o	o o	o o	o o	o o	o o	o o	o o	o o	o o	o o o o o o	o o

conception   ←——Time of Greatest Risk——→   birth

*also contains diphenhydramine (see antihistamines, page 81).
**above the 4% background risk

Doxylamine[1,2] is an antihistamine which because of its sedative effects is used as a sleeping aid.

At one time doxylamine was used to treat morning sickness associated with pregnancy. In the United States the drug was called **Bendectin**; elsewhere it was named **Debendox**. Bendectin is the only drug which was ever approved by the U.S. Food and Drug Administration for the specific use of treating nausea and vomiting during pregnancy. Its use during pregnancy has been more extensively evaluated than any other drug in history. During its twenty-seven years on the market, an estimated 33 million worldwide prescriptions of this drug were filled. Bendectin was removed from the market in 1983, because of the costs of legal actions brought against the manufacturer.

What is the Bendectin story?

Its sudden removal from the market led some people to assume it had been found to be teratogenic. On the contrary, thirty years of investigations showed it to be "safe" for the unborn child, as well as the mother. This position is also held by the FDA. The same conclusion was reached by a panel of independent experts, the Fertility and Maternal Health Drugs Advisory Committee, in a public hearing in September 1980.

After 1977, Bendectin contained only doxylamine and vitamin B_6 (pyridoxine). Prior to that time, it had also contained the antispasmodic, dicyclomine, that was later found to be ineffective.

Instances of Bendectin-associated birth defects have been described in case reports. Though provocative, case reports do not prove or disprove teratogenicity.

Prospective studies including 12,795 pregnancies have failed to demonstrate that the use of Benedectin is associated with a statistically significant increase in birth defects. One of these studies questioned the possible link between Bendectin and genital tract malformations, but other investigations failed to confirm this. A concern for an increase in the frequency of diaphragmatic hernias was raised by another study. The authors of this study made a point of stating that because so many comparisons were made, an association between the drug and birth defects may simply be a chance occurrence. The authors also called for confirming evidence before drawing conclusions.

The great majority of retrospective studies have also failed to reveal that Bendectin has a causal role in the production of birth defects, but some focusing on a particular birth defect have found a positive association. The relationship between Bendectin and congenital heart defects has been raised by some studies. But a 1985 investigation provided evidence against Bendectin's causing heart defects and concluded that the data presented in their study along with previously published research suggest a very small association, if any.[3]

Cleft lip ("harelip") or cleft palate was suspected in one study that questioned doctors about what they had prescribed for mothers of babies with such defects. The author of the study believed that her investigation introduced bias in the way she ascertained Bendectin use. She also thought that the findings offered no proof that Bendectin actually caused the clefts. Subsequent research has not found an increase in these birth defects.

Limb defects are another type of birth defect that retrospective investigations have only *weakly* linked to Bendectin. The authors who reported this finding concluded that a causal relationship between the drug and the observed birth defects could *not* be established. An increased frequency of pyloric stenosis (a constriction in the stomach's outlet) was observed, but again no causal relationship has been established. Other studies have not confirmed an increased risk for either of these defects.

Among the studies that have observed an increased frequency of some type of birth defect, the malformations have been different, suggesting that a single environmental cause was not responsible. All known teratogens display a recognizable pattern of malformation that has not been described in Bendectin-exposed children.

Given its longtime and widespread use, if Bendectin had been a teratogen, clinical evidence would have been abundant. This never occurred.

The large number of pregnant women using Bendectin—perhaps 25 percent in the United States at the height of its popularity—means that chance alone would be responsible for many birth defects among its users. From this numerical association, it was easy for many people to conclude that Bendectin was responsible for the defects.

Legal actions against the manufacturer followed. Proof in court of an association between the drug and the defect is much less rigorous than that required in science. As one expert has said, courts require only a 51 percent certainty, while scientists require 95 percent. Further, courts hear such cases out of the larger scientific context. As a result, judgments were based on other than the best scientific evidence. The final conclusion was that Bendectin was taken off the market for economic, not scientific, reasons.

Long-term follow-up studies of children exposed before birth have not been located.

Laura's Story:

I have four children. In all of my pregnancies I suffered from terrible morning sickness. Under normal circumstances I'm the type who doesn't even take an aspirin. But my daily responsibilities made it too difficult for me to just suffer through months of nausea and vomiting—so my doctor prescribed Bendectin.

My third child, Billy, was born with multiple birth defects. At the time, we were all so shocked and so unprepared. There was no evidence in my family or my husband's of anything like this ever happening. The doctors explained that they, too, were mystified as to the cause of Billy's problems. We were told that despite all the medical advances, there was still much to be learned about the specific causes of many birth defects. They couldn't give any reason for Billy's birth defects, but they thought it wouldn't happen if I got pregnant again.

The more I thought about Billy's problems, the more I wondered if they were the result of something I did, or perhaps didn't do. It wasn't until after my next baby, Niki, was born that I read about the possibility that Bendectin might cause birth defects. When I thought about it, I realized that Bendectin was the only drug I remembered taking during my pregnancy with Billy. But then, I had taken it with my two children born before him and again with my most recent pregnancy. Perhaps I was just lucky with them, I told myself. I read an ad in the local paper from a lawyer who was trying a case in federal court involving Bendectin and a child with birth defects. The ad said he needed help for epidemiological and statistical purposes and encouraged people with information to call or write. I thought that they had given me the answer to the cause of Billy's misfortune. It angered me that it could be the result of something that could have been prevented. I immediately went to my doctor and the experts who had come to know Billy, and presented them with my new found "evidence."

I was not the first mother who had asked them if Bendectin had been responsible for an ill-fated pregnancy. They explained that no drug had been researched more during pregnancy than Bendectin, the scientific evidence failing to find it teratogenic. And that its popularity resulted in literally millions and millions of prescriptions worldwide. The large numbers of pregnant women who took this drug, together with a certain expected number of malformations resulted in some unfortunate coincidences—a drug taken during pregnancy and a child born with a birth defect.

The logical part of me accepted the unfortunate coincidence. But the emotional part of me still battles with it. I wish the lawyers who advertised about Bendectin in my town paper knew the amount of unnecessary confusion, anxiety, guilt, and, yes, even misguided hope they brought to mothers like me.

References:

[1] L. J. Sheffield and R. Batagol, The creation of therapeutic orphans—or, what have we learnt from the Debendox fiasco? *Medical Journal of Australia* 143 (1985): 143–47.

[2] L. B. Holmes, Teratogen update: Bendectin, *Teratology* 27 (1983): 277–81.

[3]S. Zierler and K. J. Rothman, Congenital heart disease in relataion to maternal use of Bendectin and other drugs in early pregnancy, *New England Journal of Medicine* 313 (1985): 347–52.

GENERIC NAME/COMMON NAME: **not applicable**

Brand Name: **(Emetrol)**

FDA Pregnancy Category:—

ESTIMATED RISK SUMMARY:

Time of Exposure throughout pregnancy
Risk No known risk*
Pregnancy Outcome appears favorable
Documentation inconclusive

pre-conception	All or None		Organ Development – (in weeks)						Maturation – (in weeks)				
	1	2	3	4	5	6	7	8	9	10	12	20-36	38

conception   ←—— Time of Greatest Risk ——→   birth

Emetrol is a pleasantly mint flavored liquid containing balanced amounts of the sugars levulose (fructose) and dextrose (glucose), and orthophosphoric acid. Because of its local action, Emetrol works very quickly to relieve nausea and vomiting. For morning sickness, the recommended dose is one to two tablespoonfuls first thing in the morning, and again every three hours, or on feeling nauseated.

The use of this product by pregnant women has not been studied. But based on its safe ingredients, there is no indication that Emetrol would be harmful to an unborn baby.

Emetrol is available without a prescription. As with all over-the-counter products, please remember to check with your doctor before self-prescribing any drug during pregnancy.

*Natural remedies:***

"Morning sickness" is the popular name for pregnancy-related nausea that actually can occur at any hour. Not all pregnant women experience morning sickness. For

*above the 4% background risk
**None of these commonsense remedies have been medically proven. They are listed here for you because I have found them useful.

those who do, it usually disappears by the third month. If you experience nausea, you may wish to try some of the safe, nonmedicinal remedies[1] that many women have found to be effective:

• Eat nutritious foods frequently and in small amounts.
• Dry high-carbohydrate foods like crackers, cereal, and toast are stomach settlers.
• Drink lots of fluids, including soup and carbonated water.
• If you wake up feeling nauseated, lie still until your stomach feels more settled; then sit up slowly.
• At night, sleep with a window open for fresh air; during the day, take a walk outdoors.

Reference:

[1]The Over-the-Counter-Drug Committee of the Coalition for the Medical Rights of Women, *Safe and Natural Remedies for Discomforts of Pregnancy* (San Francisco, Calif., January 1981; rev. 1982).

COMMON NAME: **EPSTEIN-BARR VIRUS (MONONUCLEOSIS)**

Brand Name/Chemical Name: **not applicable**

FDA Pregnancy Category: not applicable

ESTIMATED RISK SUMMARY:
　Time of Exposure throughout pregnancy
　Risk Risk assessment is not possible
　Pregnancy Outcome uncertain
　Documentation insufficient

← pre- conception ←	All or None	Organ Development – (in weeks)						Maturation – (in weeks)				
	1	2	3	4	5	6	7	8	9	10	12	20-36	38

conception　　　←—Time of Greatest Risk—→　　　　　birth

　　Infectious mononucleosis (the "kissing disease") is caused by the *Epstein-Barr virus.*[1,2] Epstein-Barr virus is a very common infection, one which almost all women of childbearing age have had. In fact, studies following more than 12,000 pregnant women in the United States, Canada, and France indicate that only 1.1 percent to 4.2 percent had never had the disease. Unlike other viral infections, such as the German measles (rubella) or the mumps, after you first contract Epstein-Barr virus, it tends to persist within your body for an indefinite period, resulting in reactivation of the disease at a later time.

Controversy surrounds the effect of the virus on the unborn child. Theoretically, the greatest risk from having this infection during pregnancy would be for the unborn babies of women having it for the very first time. Several reports have claimed that this infection during the first trimester causes heart defects, cataracts, or multiple birth defects, but their conclusions are questionable. There was a lack of laboratory evidence confirming the presence of Epstein-Barr virus in all but three of these cases. In the three cases where the virus was confirmed by laboratory test, the children had multiple birth defects. In two cases, however, there was also evidence of cytomegalovirus, a known viral teratogen (see cytomegalovirus, page 131). Most of the complications in these two infants were characteristic of those found in babies born with cytomegalovirus infection.

In summary, at this time there is no evidence that Epstein-Barr virus causes birth defects. More precise studies are needed before this can be conclusively determined.

References:

[1] J. S. Remington and J. D. Klein (eds.), *Infectious Diseases of the Fetus and Newborn Infant*, 2d ed. (Philadelphia: W. B. Saunders, 1983), pp. 545–47.

[2] S. Stagno and R. J. Whitley, Herpesvirus infections of pregnancy. Part 1: Cytomegalovirus and Epstein-Barr virus infections, *New England Journal of Medicine* 313 (1985): 1270–74.

GENERIC NAMES: **ERYTHROMYCIN, ERYTHROMYCIN ESTOLATE, ERYTHROMYCIN STERATE**

Brand Names: **(Bristamycin, E-Mycin, Eramycin, ERYC, Erypar, Erythromycin Sterate, Ery-Tab, Ethril, Ilotycin, Ilosone, Pfizer-E, Robimycin Robitabs, RP-Mycin, Wyamycin)**

FDA Pregnancy Category:—

ESTIMATED RISK SUMMARY:

Time of Exposure throughout pregnancy
Risk No known risk*

---

*above the 4% background risk

Pregnancy Outcome appears favorable
Documentation inconclusive, based on minimal data

pre-conception	All or None		Organ Development – (in weeks)						Maturation – (in weeks)				
	1	2	3	4	5	6	7	8	9	10	12	20-36	38

conception   ⟵ Time of Greatest Risk ⟶   birth

Erythromycin[1] is an antibiotic often given to patients who are allergic to penicillins. There is no evidence that erythromycin is a teratogen when used during any stage of pregnancy.

If a pregnant woman has gonorrhea or syphilis, she should receive antibiotic treatment, so that both she and her unborn child will benefit from it (see gonorrhea, page 169, and syphilis, page 308). Erythromycin crosses the placenta. But since the levels that reach the fetus are low and unpredictable, erythromycin is not the ideal drug for treatment of these infections during pregnancy.

Erythromycin estolate should be avoided during pregnancy based on a study linking the drug to abnormal liver functioning in 10 percent of pregnant patients tested.[2] However, once the treatment ended, patients' livers functioned normally once again.

Long-term follow-up studies of children exposed before birth have not been located.

References:

[1]D. V. Landers, J. R. Green, and R. L. Sweet, Antibiotic use during pregnancy and the postpartum period, *Clinical Obstetrics and Gynecology* 26 (1983): 391–406.

[2]W. M. McCormick, H. George, A. Donner, L. F. Kodgis, S. Albert, E. W. Lowe, and E. H. Kass, Hepatotoxicity of erythromycine estolate during pregnancy, *Antimicrobial Agents Chemotherapy* 12 (1977): 630–35.

GENERIC NAME: **ETHACRYNIC ACID**

Brand Names: **(Edecrin, Sodium Edecrin)**

FDA Pregnancy Category:—

ESTIMATED RISK SUMMARY:

Time of Exposure throughout pregnancy

Risk Risk assessment is not possible
Pregnancy Outcome uncertain
Documentation insufficient

← pre-conception ←		All or None		Organ Development – (in weeks)						Maturation – (in weeks)				
		1	2	3	4	5	6	7	8	9	10	12	20-36	38

conception   ← Time of Greatest Risk →   birth

Ethacrynic acid is a very potent diuretic—a drug used to promote urine excretion. There has been only limited experience with the use of this drug in pregnant women, so it must be studied further to determine whether it can be safely used during pregnancy. Use of ethacrynic acid and kanamycin (an aminoglycoside antibiotic drug) during the third trimester was linked to deafness in one case report. This is not enough evidence for determining a cause-and-effect relationship, particularly since prenatal exposure to kanamycin has, in several instances, been associated with deafness (see aminoglycosides, page 70).

Long-term follow-up studies of children exposed before birth have not been located.

Refer to thiazides for a brief discussion on the use of diuretics during pregnancy and a natural remedy for discomfort relief, page 315.

Reference:

[1]A. L. Wilson and G. R. Matzke, The treatment of hypertension in pregnancy, *Drug Intelligence and Clinical Pharmacy* 15 (1981): 21–26.

GENERIC NAME: **ETHAMBUTOL**

Brand Name: **(Myambutol)**

FDA Pregnancy Category:—

ESTIMATED RISK SUMMARY:
Time of Exposure throughout pregnancy
Risk No known risk*

*above the 4% background risk

Pregnancy Outcome appears favorable

Documentation inconclusive, based on minimal data

← pre-conception	All or None		Organ Development – (in weeks)						Maturation – (in weeks)				
	1	2	3	4	5	6	7	8	9	10	12	20-36	38

conception ←——Time of Greatest Risk——→ birth

Ethambutol[1] is used to treat tuberculosis. An extensive review of the medical literature on pregnant women treated with various antitubercular medications was conducted in an effort to discover the effect of these drugs on the developing baby. The investigators located information on the pregnancies of 2,787 women and found that 94 percent of them had full-term infants who appeared normal at birth. Approximately 3 percent of the pregnancies resulted in miscarriages, stillbirths, or premature births, while 2.89 percent resulted in birth defects. The reported frequency of problems is within the expected range for the general population. As abnormalities are likely to be overrepresented in the literature, the small incidence of adverse pregnancy outcomes is particularly reassuring.

In this literature review, ethambutol was not identified as a teratogen. Many pregnant women exposed to ethambutol were also treated with additional antituberculins, usually isoniazid. From a total of 655 exposed to ethambutol, there were 592 normal term infants (90.3%), 1 miscarriage (0.15%), 5 stillbirths (0.76%), 26 premature births (3.9%), and 14 birth defects (2.1%), of which most were minor.

Long-term follow-up studies of children exposed before birth have not been located.

Reference:

[1]D. E. Snider, P. M. Layde, M. W. Johnson, and M. A. Lyle, Treatment of tuberculosis during pregnancy, *American Review of Respiratory Diseases* 122 (1980): 65–79.

GENERIC NAME: **ETRETINATE**

Brand Name: **(Tegison)**

FDA Pregnancy Category: X

ESTIMATED RISK SUMMARY:

Time of Exposure undetermined

Risk Known risk*
Pregnancy Outcome adverse
Documentation conclusive, based on current knowledge

pre-conception	All or None		Organ Development – (in weeks)						Maturation – (in weeks)				
	1	2	3	4	5	6	7	8	9	10	12	20-36	38

conception   ←—Time of Greatest Risk—→   birth

Etretinate[1,2] is a vitamin A derivative used to treat severe psoriasis that is unresponsive to other treatments. This drug has been marketed in other countries but was not available for use in the United States until December 1986. Like isotretinoin, another vitamin A derivative, etretinate is teratogenic in both animals and in humans.

At this writing I am aware of seven children with birth defects and ten apparently normal children all born to women who used this drug after a missed menstrual period. Three of the abnormalities involved birth defects arising from an error in the prenatal development of the brain and spinal cord (two cases of spina bifida and one case of encephalocele). Three babies had abnormalities of the skeleton and face, and another child had a severe brain defect. An eighth case involved a mother who discontinued etretinate four months before conceiving a baby with a leg malformation. This abnormality is considered uncharacteristic and is thought to have occurred by chance. Six other apparently normal pregnancy outcomes have been reported in women who discontinued the drug within one to four months before becoming pregnant.

Unlike isotretinoin, etretinate remains in the body for a very long period of time, as much as three years after discontinuance (see isotretinoin, page 206). For this reason, pregnant women or those who plan to become pregnant sometime in the future should not take this drug. And women who have been taking etretinate should postpone pregnancy for "an indefinite period of time."[2] A pregnancy test two weeks before beginning eretinate therapy is strongly recommended.

Long-term follow-up studies of children exposed before birth have not been located.

The possible effect of this drug on a man's sperm is not known and is under current investigation.

*above the 4% background risk

Referencnes:

[1]F. W. Rosa, A. L. Wilk, and F. O. Kelsey, Teratogen update: Vitamin A congeners, *Teratology* 33 (1986): 335–64.
[3]Etretinate approved, *FDA Drug Bulletin* 16 (1986): 16–17.

COMMON NAME: **EXERCISE**

Brand Name/Chemical Name: **not applicable**

FDA Pregnancy Category: not applicable

ESTIMATED RISK SUMMARY:

Time of Exposure throughout pregnancy
Risk No known risk* for regular exercise (if you have no pregnancy complications)
Pregnancy Outcome appears favorable
Documentation inconclusive, based on minimal data

Time of Exposure throughout pregnancy
Risk Risk assessment is not possible for extremely strenuous exercise
Pregnancy Outcome uncertain
Documentation insufficient

pre-conception	All or None		Organ Development – (in weeks)						Maturation – (in weeks)				
	1	2	3	4	5	6	7	8	9	10	12	20-36	38

conception ←—Time of Greatest Risk—→ birth

In recent times, the importance and benefits of regular *exercise*[1] have become widely recognized. Aerobic exercise has gained popularity becuase of its potential to increase cardiovascular health and minimize body fat. Most recently, exercise has been advocated for women as one preventive measure against osteoporosis, a thinning and weakening of the bones. It is not surprising, therefore, that you may question the risks and benefits of exercise during pregnancy.

Exercise places certain demands on the body: Oxygen consumption increases, the heart rate is increased, and body temperature rises. What impact does all of this have

*above the 4% background risk

on you and your developing baby? Although only limited information is available to answer this question, the evidence that does exist is very reassuring. Let's take a closer look.

During exercise the body distributes blood and its oxygen supply in favor of the heart and the muscles at work. When a pregnant woman exercises, her muscles compete with her uterus for blood supply, decreasing blood flow to the uterus. Since the fetus receives its oxygen and nutrients from uterine blood, then a potential risk for the unborn baby is hypoxia (reduced oxygen supply). Other complications such as fetal distress, growth retardation (particularly low birth weight), and possibly premature birth could also occur.

But the fact of the matter is that during exercise the mother's body helps protect the unborn baby through certain mechanisms that compensate for the decreased blood supply to the uterus. One way is that the pregnant uterus can extract higher amounts of oxygen from the blood it receives. Additionally, the blood is actually more concentrated, it contains more oxygen and more nutrients, including glucose, which supplies the body with energy. So it seems that even though the volume of blood that reaches the uterus during exercise is decreased, its high quality helps maintain normal oxygen uptake by both the uterus and the fetus.

Changes in fetal heart rates could reduce the amount of oxygen available to the baby's tissues and cause distress. Only a limited number of studies have investigated this issue. While some have observed *temporary* increases or decreases in the fetal heart rate, very little overall change during exercise has been reported. Fortunately, these changes in fetal heart rate patterns have not been associated with signs of hypoxia and/or distress.

The effects of elevated body temperature during exercise is another potential concern for the developing baby. But the effects of exercise-induced hyperthermia (abnormally high body temperature) on the unborn have not yet been studied. The primary concerns about hyperthermia during pregnancy are related to those incidents when the body temperature is elevated above 102, F. for a "prolonged period of time" in the early part of pregnancy (see hyperthermia, page 197). Regular moderate exercise would certainly not be associated with these circumstances. However, during some strenuous athletic activities, body temperature can reach the "high fever" range. For this reason, pregnant women and women contemplating pregnancy should discuss the safety of their physical activity level with their doctor.

Studies that focus on the general effects of exercise on pregnancy outcome most often conclude that strenuous activity during pregnancy does not adversely affect the infants of healthy women. However, not all studies concur. Consistent "intense" exercise during pregnancy has been linked to a small reduction in birth weight in some animal studies and in some human investigations. Whether this effect is truly related to exercise or due to some other factor can only be determined by large and well-designed human studies. As yet, no such study has been conducted.

Since exercise has a variety of psychological as well as physical benefits, experts recommend that women ideally begin conditioning programs before becoming pregnant and then continue them as long as possible during pregnancy—always in consultation with qualified health and exercise professionals. If you are healthy and *have no pregnancy complications*, regular moderate exercise such as walking, bicycling, swimming, or light jogging is usually considered safe. Exercise classes specifically designed for pregnant women are an alternative to these activities. In fact, most prenatal exercise classes will focus on strengthening muscles in the back, abdomen and pelvis—those which are especially needed during pregnancy and delivery.

Experts suggest that it's safest to avoid extremely strenuous exercise, such as intense aerobic dance, and activities that carry a high risk for injury, such as surfing, scuba diving, basketball, hockey, and horseback activities.[2] Certainly, some women are very skilled and are accustomed to particular sport activities. The risk of injury or overexertion might be less for them, and within reason, continued participation in their chosen activity could be safe. Still, the safety of exercise during pregnancy must be evaluated on an individual basis by a physician, who will take into consideration your medical history, your exercise experience, and the well-being of your pregnancy.

Probably the best advice anyone can give you about exercise during pregnancy, or anytime, for that matter, is: Pay attention to what your body is telling you. And don't overdo it!

References:

[1] F. K. Loterging, R. D. Gilbert, and L. D. Longo, The interactions of exercise and pregnancy: A review, *American Journal of Obstetrics and Gynecology* 149 (1984): 560–68.

[2] T. Jopke, Pregnancy: A time to exercise judgement, *The Physician and Sportsmedicine* 11 (1983): 139–48.

MEDICATION CLASSIFICATION: **FEMALE HORMONES (PROGESTINS and ESTROGENS, including ORAL CONTRACEPTIVES)**

GENERIC NAMES: **CONJUGATED ESTROGENS, ESTRADIOL, ESTRONE, ETHINYL, ETHISTERONE,**

ETHONODIOL, HYDROXYPROGESTERONE, MEDROXYPROGESTERONE, NORETHINDRONE, NORGESTREL, NORTHYNODREL, PROGESTERONE

Brand Names: **(Amen, Aygestin, Bestrone, Curretab Delautin, Duralutin, Estinyl, Estrocon, Feminone, Gerterol LA 250, Hy-Gesterone, Hylutin, Hyprogest 250, Hyproval PA, Hyroxon, Kestrone, Micronor, Norlutin, Norlutate, Nor-QD, Ovrette, Premarin, Pro-Depo, Progens, Provera, Theelin)** **To conserve space, brand names for oral contraceptives are not included.**

FDA Pregnancy Category: X

ESTIMATED RISK SUMMARY:

Time of Exposure before conception
Risk No known risk*
Pregnancy Outcome appears favorable
Documentation inconclusive

Time of Exposure early pregnancy, primarily 8–12 weeks, although some sensitivity to hormones does continue beyond this time
Risk Suspected risk* for genital defects only
Pregnancy Outcome uncertain: favorable and adverse outcomes observed
Documentation inconclusive

pre-conception	All or None		Organ Development – (in weeks)						Maturation – (in weeks)				
	1	2	3	4	5	6	7	8	9	10	12	20-36	38

conception   ←—— Time of Greatest Risk ——→   birth

Progestins and estrogens are *female hormones*[1,2] available in the natural and synthetic form, and are used individually and in combination.

Exposures to female hormones during pregnancy are from a variety of sources

*above the 4% background risk

including birth control pills (oral contraceptives), hormonal pregnancy tests, and hormone therapy used to induce late periods or treat a "threatened miscarriage." Although some of these procedures are no longer practiced, many of the studies identifying sex hormones as teratogens included women with such exposures. Today the most likely hormone exposures during pregnancy come from women who either take natural progestin (progesterone) to prevent miscarriage or else continue taking oral contraceptives, not realizing they are already pregnant. Oral contraceptives usually contain a combination of synthetic progestin and estrogen compounds, although the minipill contains only progestin.

There have been several hundred scientific papers considering the subject of female hormones as teratogens, with no consensus. It is reassuring to note that most investigations on the effects of female hormones, among them large-scale prospective studies, have *failed* to reveal an increased frequency of birth defects in children exposed before birth.[2] (see prospective studies, page 42). However, female hormones, *particularly* **progestins**, have been variously regarded as causing VACTERL* syndrome,[3] heart defects,[4] limb abnormalities,[5] defects of the external sex organs,[6,7] and an increased overall risk for malformations,[8] or of having no effect on the unborn baby.[9] Reevaluation of the research linking these hormones to an increased risk for heart defects failed to support the original findings.[10]

Many investigations finding a positive association between birth defects and exposure to female hormones in early pregnancy have been retrospective studies with small sample sizes (see retrospective studies, page 43). They often fail to specify the types and combinations of medications used. Collectively these studies have not revealed a consistent type or pattern of abnormalities, which is usually present if there is one specific cause. Some studies researched the relationship between birth defects and hormonal pregnancy tests.[11] The results of such investigations have minimal implications since the U.S. Food and Drug Administration eliminated pregnancy testing as an indication for hormone treatment in 1973. In addition, the subjects of some of the investigations reporting increased birth defects were women with first trimester bleeding. These women received progestin therapy for threatened miscarriage. It is a well-known fact, though, that serious bleeding during this time is associated with a slight increase in birth defects. For this reason, the cause of some detected birth defects might actually be related more to the threatened miscarriage than to the drug

---

*A group of abnormalities charaterized by the acronym VACTERL: Vertebral (bones of the spinal column), Anal, Cardiac (heart), Tracheal (windpipe), Esophageal (link from throat to stomach), Renal (kidneys), and Limb defects.

treatment. Last, with one exception, studies reporting an increased frequency of malformations have failed to correlate the time of exposure with the reported defects.

The exception is the relationship of synthetic progestins, and in some cases estrogens, with genital malformations.

A review of all the research on the topic leaves little doubt that these hormones can alter the normal development of the external sex organs, that is, *if* taken by a susceptible individual, *if* the dose is large enough, and *if* taken during the critical period of development (primarily eight to twelve weeks after conception). Individual susceptibility cannot yet be determined (see The Principles of Teratology, page 33). Fortunately, today's birth control pills are of low dosage and the time of highest risk is toward the end of the first trimester, by which time pregnancy is often recognized.

The observed modifications in the reproductive organs appear to be limited to the external sex organs, resulting in enlargement of the clitoris and labia (sometimes called "masculinization") in affected females and abnormally placed urethral opening on the penis (hypospadias) in affected males. It may be comforting to know that these birth defects can be corrected surgically. Internal reproductive organs are unaffected, so actual fertility is not impaired.

Practically all of the reported cases of affected *males* have involved use of **progestin** by their mothers—six cases were from natural progestin (progesterone) and thirty-nine from synthetic progestin. Hypospadias normally occurs in our population between 5 per 10,000 and 30 per 10,000 births. The occurrence is twice that rate in males whose mothers took progestins.

Some cases of clitoral and labial enlargement in *females* have occurred when natural progestin (**progesterone**) is taken during pregnancy. But most are attributed to the use of synthetic progestins (primarily **ethisterone** and **norethindrone**). Interestingly, progestins can be converted into androgens, male hormones, in the mother and unborn baby.

Excluding DES (diethylstilbestrol, see page 143), only rarely have **estrogens** been said to cause birth defects in females. This is curious, given the once widespread use of this hormone during pregnancy. Overall, these abnormalities do not occur frequently, and the incidence of affected females is particularly small.

Psychosexual development was evaluated in two small groups of boys (twenty 6-year-olds and twenty 16-year-olds) whose diabetic mothers took either **hydroxy-progesterone** or a synthetic estrogen (diethylstilbestrol) in order to prevent pregnancy complications.[12] These boys were then compared to boys the same age whose mothers had not received such treatment. Hormone-exposed boys were rated as less assertive, less aggressive, and less athletic. The significance and meaning of these findings are very difficult to interpret.

A study of eleven adult women "masculinized" by progestins before birth, later showed feminine physical characteristics appropriate to their age and what is considered normal social behavior.[13]

Careful consideration of the available data leads me to agree with the conclusions from the review of Drs. Wilson and Brent that female hormones have *not* been *proven* to cause malformations in the body other than in sex organs. If, however, some as yet unrecognized risk does exist, it is small enough to be below the expected 4 percent background risk.

In sum: Because of the variety of birth defects that have, at one time or another, been attributed to female hormones, women may still encounter outdated warnings of serious consequences from their use during pregnancy.

References:

[1]J. L. Schardein, Congenial abnormalities and hormones during pregnancy: A critical review, *Teratology* 22 (1980): 251–70.

[2]J. G. Wilson and R. L. Brent, Are female sex hormones teratogenic? *American Journal of Obstetrics and Gynecology* 141 (1981): 567–80.

[3]A. H. Nora and J. J. Nora, A syndrome of multiple congenital anomalies associated with teratogenic exposure, *Archives of Environmental Health* 30 (1975): 17–21.

[4]O. P. Heinonen, D. Slone, R. R. Monson, et al. Cardiovascular birth defects and antenatal exposure to female sex hormones, *New England Journal of Medicine* 296 (1977): 67–70.

[5]D. T. Janerich, J. M. Piper, and D. M. Glebatis, Oral contraceptives and congenital limb-reduction defects, *New England Journal of Medicine* 291 (1974): 697–700.

[6]A. M. Bongiovanni and A. J. McFadden, Steroids during pregnancy and possible fetal consequences, *Fertility and Sterility* 11 (1960): 181–86.

[7]D. Aarskog, Maternal progestins as a possible cause of hypospadias, *New England Journal of Medicine* 300 (1979): 75–78.

[8]D. Harlap, R. Prywes, and A. M. Davies, Birth defects and oestrogens and progesterones in pregnancy, *Lancet* 1 (1975): 682–83.

[9]Z. Katz, M. Lancet, J. Skornik, J. Chemke, B. M. Mogliner, and M. Klinberg, Teratogenicity of progestogens given during the frist trimester, *Obstetrics and Gynecology* 65 (1985): 775–80.

[10]R. A. Wiseman and I. C. Dodds-Smith, Cardiovascular birth defects and antenatal exposure to female sex hormones: A reevaluation of some base data, *Teratology* 30 (1984): 359–70.

[11]E. J. Lammer, and J. F. Cordero, Exogenous sex hormone exposure and the risk for major malformations, *Journal of the American Medical Association* 255 (1986): 3138–32.

[12]I. D. Yalom, R. Green, and N. Fisk, Prenatal exposure to female hormones: Effect on psychosocial development in boys, *Archives of General Psychiatry* 28 (1973): 544–61.

[13]J. Money and D. Mathews, Prenatal exposure to virilizing progestins: An adult follow-up study of twelve women, *Archives of Sexual Behavior* 11 (1982): 73–83.

GENERIC NAME/COMMON NAME: **not applicable**

Chemical Names: (**FORMALDEHYDE [formalin]**)

FDA Pregnancy Category: not applicable

ESTIMATED RISK SUMMARY:
  Time of Exposure throughout pregnancy
  Risk Risk assessment is not possible.
  Pregnancy Outcome uncertain
  Documentation insufficient

pre-conception	All or None		Organ Development – (in weeks)						Maturation – (in weeks)				
	1	2	3	4	5	6	7	8	9	10	12	20-36	38

conception   ⟵ Time of Greatest Risk ⟶   birth

Formaldehyde is a powerful disinfectant gas. When mixed with water (producing **formalin**) it is used as a preservative or as a fixing solution for laboratory specimens. Formaldehyde is also the major chemical in the home insulation, urea-formaldehyde foam, which was banned for use in 1982.

Contact with formaldehyde can be irritating to your system. In large doses it can be poisonous, causing itchy, watery eyes, headache, some difficulty in breathing, coughing and wheezing. Levels of insulation in homes are usually too low to cause such symptoms. But some people may be especially sensitive to it.

As discussed in a comprehensive review on urea-formaldehyde foam insulation, studies have not clearly linked exposures to this chemical with adverse health effects.[1]

In animals, formaldehyde may be carcinogenic (cancer-causing) in very high concentrations, but studies in humans have not shown consistent findings of this effect.

Investigations into the potential teratogenicity of formaldehyde in humans have been too few to draw any definitive conclusions from. One study compared menstrual and reproductive function in women exposed to formaldehyde in the manufacturing process of fabric with women who sold such fabrics. Of the women who came into direct contact with the chemical, 48 percent has menstrual disorders, whereas the relatively unexposed women had a rate of 19 percent. Another study reported an increased frequency of miscarriage in Russian women working with formaldehyde. Full-term babies born to these workers were 27 percent smaller than normal.[2]

Long-term follow-up studies of children exposed before birth have not been located.

Pregnant women who have a one-time or limited exposure to this chemical should remember that studies have evaluated the effects of *chronic* exposures, so the circumstances are not comparable.

There is not enough evidence to show whether exposure to formaldehyde presents a risk of birth defects. But it doesn't make sense to wait until adverse effects are proven before being careful around formaldehyde or any other chemical. As with any occupational hazard, pregnant women should attempt to minimize their exposure. Good safety procedures include working in a well-ventilated area.

References:

[1]K. A. L'Abbé and J. R. Hoey, Review of the health effects of Urea-Formaldehyde Foam Insulation, *Environmental Research* 35 (1984): 246–63.

[2]A. V. Shumilina, Menstrual'naia i detorodnaia funktsii rabontnits imeiushchikh po usloviiam proizvodstva kontakt s formal'degidom, *Gigiena Truda I Profossionalnye Zabolevaniia* 12 (1975): 18– 21.

GENERIC NAME: **FUROSEMIDE**

Brand Name: **(Lasix)**

FDA Pregnancy Category:—

ESTIMATED RISK SUMMARY:

Time of Exposure approximately during the first 12 weeks
Risk Risk assessment is not possible.
Pregnancy Outcome uncertain
Documentation insufficient; no information available

Time of Exposure after approximately 12 weeks
Risk No known risk*
Pregnancy Outcome appears favorable
Documentation inconclusive, based on minimal data

pre-conception	All or None		Organ Development – (in weeks)						Maturation – (in weeks)				
	1	2	3	4	5	6	7	8	9	10	12	20-36	38
												▓	▓

conception   ◄——Time of Greatest Risk——►   birth

*above the expected 4% background risk

Furosemide[1,2] is a very potent diuretic. Diuretics are substances that cause fluid loss through urination. Although there have been no evaluations of furosemide as a possible cause of birth defects, it is reassuring to note that none have been reported in children exposed to it before birth.

Unlike other diuretics, furosemide taken near the time of delivery has not been associated with a decrease in the newborn's blood platelets (thrombocytopenia), which are essential for blood coagulation.

Furosemide freely crosses the placenta and increases the fetus's urine production. For this reason, it is administered intravenously to the mother for ultrasound imaging of the unborn baby's bladder, in order to evaluate urinary tract function when a problem is suspected.

Long-term follow-up studies of children exposed before birth have not been located.

(Refer to thiazides for a brief discussion on the use of diuretics during pregnancy and a natural remedy for discomfort relief, page 315.)

References:

[1] A. L. Wilson and G. R. Matzke, The treatment of hypertension in pregnancy, *Drug Intelligence and Clinical Pharmacy* 15 (1981): 21–26.

[2] B. M. Sibai, R. A. Grossman, and H. G. Grossman, Effects of diuretics on plasma volume in pregnancies with long-term hypertension, *American Journal of Obstetrics and Gynecology* 150 (1984): 831– 35.

MEDICATION CLASSIFICATION: **GOLD COMPOUNDS**

GENERIC NAMES: **AURANOFIN, AUROTHIOGLUCOSE, GOLD SODIUM THIOMALATE**

Brand Names: **(Myochrysine, Ridaura, Solganal)**

FDA Pregnancy Category: C

ESTIMATED RISK SUMMARY:

Time of Exposure throughout pregnancy

Risk Risk assessment is not possible

Pregnancy Outcome uncertain

Documentation insufficient.

pre-conception ← ← conception	All or None		Organ Development – (in weeks)						Maturation – (in weeks)				
	1	2	3	4	5	6	7	8	9	10	12	20-36	38

conception   ← Time of Greatest Risk →   birth

Gold compounds are used in the treatment of selected cases of rheumatoid arthritis. Since gold does cross the placenta, most sources recommend avoiding the use of these compounds during pregnancy.

Laboratory animals receiving extremely high doses of gold during pregnancy have produced abnormal offspring. No scientific studies have been conducted on the use of gold in humans. Available information is limited to case reports. More than seventy cases of *normal* babies born to mothers receiving gold compounds during pregnancy have appeared in the medical literature.[1] Only one abnormal infant has been reported,[2] described as having facial peculiarities, cleft lip (harelip), cleft palate, and brain abnormalities. This isolated incident cannot prove cause-and-effect, though some of the reported defects were similar to those observed in laboratory animals.

Long-term follow-up studies of children exposed before birth have not been located.

References:

[1]D. L. Cohen, J. Orzel, and A. Taylor, Infants of mothers receiving gold therapy, *Arthritis and Rheumatism* 24 (1981): 104–5.

[2]J. G. Rogers, R. McD. Anderson, C. W. Chow, G. L. Gillam, and L. Markman, Possible teratogenic effect of gold, *Australian Paediatric Journal* 16 (1980): 194–95.

COMMON NAME: **GONORRHEA**

Brand Name/Chemical Name: **not applicable**

FDA Pregnancy Category: not applicable

ESTIMATED RISK SUMMARY:

    Time of Exposure throughout pregnancy
    Risk No measurable risk* for birth defects
    Pregnancy Outcome favorable
    Documentation conclusive, based on current knowledge

*above the 4% background risk

Time of Exposure during birth
Risk Known risk for infection*
Pregnancy Outcome adverse
Documentation conclusive, based on current knowledge

pre-conception	All or None		Organ Development – (in weeks)						Maturation – (in weeks)				
	1	2	3	4	5	6	7	8	9	10	12	20-36	38

conception   ←— Time of Greatest Risk —→   birth

Gonorrhea[1] is caused by the bacterium *Neisseria gonorrhoeae*. In the United States it is the most frequently reported communicable disease. The high incidence of this infection, together with the known risks during pregnancy, has caused many prenatal care providers to screen routinely for gonorrhea in pregnant women.

In the early stages of the disease, gonorrhea often appears without symptoms, particularly in women. The usual infection site is the cervix. Some women might detect a discharge from the vagina together with uncomfortable and frequent urination. Left untreated, the infection will move into the uterus and Fallopian tubes, where it can cause a severe pelvic infection referred to as pelvic inflammatory disease (PID). Severe abdominal pain and fever are symptoms associated with PID. If the gonorrhea continues beyond this acute stage it will eventually affect the large joints, resulting in gonococcal arthritis. Skin rashes can also appear anywhere on the body.

Gonorrhea can also be acquired through oral/genital contact, infecting the mouth and throat (pharyngeal gonorrhea).

Adverse Effects

During pregnancy. Gonorrhea is associated with an increased frequency of pregnancy occurring outside of the womb (ectopic pregnancy), a greater incidence of prematurely ruptured membranes that surround the fetus, which are more often inflamed (chorioamnionitis), and a higher occurrence of premature birth.

In the newborn: During birth, the baby can come into contact with gonorrhea through the infected birth canal or the prematurely ruptured membranes. This can result in an extremely contagious eye infection called opthalmia neonatorum. Unless

*above the 4% background risk

this infection is promptly treated, it can cause partial or complete blindness. Gonococcal arthritis has also been reported in newborns exposed to gonorrhea.

Treatment

Pregnant women can be safely treated for gonorrhea with antibiotic therapy. Penicillin, or a penicillin derivative, are the drugs of choice, but many strains of gonorrhea are now resistant to these drugs (see penicillins, page 257). Alternative drugs include spectinomycin and cefoxitin (a cephalosporin) (see spectinomycin, page 298 and cephalosporins, page 99).

Newborns born to mothers with gonorrhea receive penicillin immediately to protect against infection. Additional treatment with penicillin is given to babies with gonococcal arthritis and other complications of gonorrhea. Ophthalmia neonatorum is managed with silver nitrate drops to both eyes after birth. In addition, the baby's eyes are irrigated with saline or buffered ophthalmic solutions.

Reference:

[1] J. S. Remington and J. O. Klein (eds.), *Infectious Diseases of the Fetus and Newborn Infant,* 2d ed. (Philadelphia: W. B. Saunders, 1983), pp. 619–35.

GENERIC NAME: **GRISEOFULVIN**

Brand Names: **(Fulvicin-P/G, Fulvicin-U/F, Grisactin, Grisactin Ultra, Grisfulvin, Gris-PEG)**

FDA Pregnancy Category:—

ESTIMATED RISK SUMMARY:

Time of Exposure throughout pregnancy

Risk Risk assessment is not possible

Pregnancy Outcome uncertain

Documentation insufficient

← pre-conception →	All or None		Organ Development – (in weeks)						Maturation – (in weeks)				
	1	2	3	4	5	6	7	8	9	10	12	20-36	38

| conception | ←—Time of Greatest Risk—→ | birth |

Griseofulvin is an antifungal antibiotic used in the treatment of severe fungus infections of the skin, hair, and nails.

Data on the use of this drug by pregnant women is very limited. Clinical experience of 134 dermatologists who prescribed griseofulvin during pregnancy did not reveal an increase of adverse pregnancy outcome.[1] Fifty-five of these doctors withheld treatment until after the fourth month of pregnancy. Complications were however reported by other dermatologists, who observed four miscarriages, one genetic defect (Down syndrome), and one abnormality (unspecified). The author of the study comments that the incidence of the problems "makes it improbable that they could have been due to griseofulvin."[1] This information was collected by a questionnaire and is therefore subject to the criticisms of data collected in that manner (see retrospective studies, page 43).

Recently the U.S. Food and Drug Administration described two cases of conjoined (Siamese) twins, both born to mothers who used griseofulvin in early pregnancy.[2] If a drug were to cause conjoined twinning, it would probably do so earlier than twenty days after ovulation.[2] Specific exposure information was available for only one case: The mother took one tablet three times a day for her first two months of pregnancy. These types of twins are extremely rare and the use of griseofulvin during pregnancy is not common. For these reasons, the experts at the FDA do not believe the birth defects are just a coincidence.

In this same report the FDA presented additional, previously unpublished information on the effects of griseofulvin during the first trimester of pregnancy. Retrospectively collected data revealed other birth defects and a significant increase in the frequency of miscarriages. The birth defects included two babies with heart defects (one died) and two children with cleft palate. They did not speculate on the relationship between the malformations and the mother's use of griseofulvin.

Various malformations and impaired survival have been reported in the offspring in some animal species given very high doses of griseofulvin during pregnancy. No conjoined twins have been produced. Still, results from animal studies cannot be directly applied to human risk counseling.

Long-term follow-up studies of children exposed before birth have not been located.

References:

[1]H. Gotz, The side effects of griseofulvin therapy after 12 years of experience, *Archiv für Dermatologische Forschung* 244 (1972): 391–95.

[2]F. W. Rosa, C. Hernandez, and W. A. Carlo, Griseofulvin teratology, including two thoracopagus conjoined twins, *Lancet* 1 (1987): 171.

GENERIC NAME: **GUAIFENESIN**

Brand Names: **(Anti-Tuss, Baytussin, Breonesin, Glycotuss, Guiamid, Guiatuss, Halotussin, Hytuss, Malotuss, Nortussin, Robafen Syrup, Robitussin)**

FDA Pregnancy Category:—

ESTIMATED RISK SUMMARY:
   Time of Exposure throughout pregnancy
   Risk Risk assessment is not possible
   Pregnancy Outcome uncertain
   Documentation insufficient

← pre-conception	All or None	Organ Development – (in weeks)						Maturation – (in weeks)				
	1	2	3	4	5	6	7	8	9	10	12	20-36	38

conception   ←—— Time of Greatest Risk ——→   birth

Guaifenesin is an expectorant used to help relieve dry, nonproductive coughs. Expectorants work by loosening thick secretions so they can be removed naturally when you cough. However, most people with colds don't have thick secretions, so these products are of dubious value in most cases.

A number of medicines containing guaifenesin also contain alcohol. As you might already know, alcohol is a known teratogen, so it's a good idea to avoid products containing it (read the list of ingredients) (see alcohol, page 63). There has been one case of a child born with features of the fetal alcohol syndrome whose mother throughout her pregnancy consumed large amounts of a cough syrup containing both guaifenesin and alcohol.

Very little information about the effects of guaifenesin on a developing baby has been located. The Collaborative Perinatal Project, which evaluated pregnancy outcome in more than 50,000 mother-child pairs exposed to a wide variety of drugs, found an increase in the frequency of hernias in the groin area (inguinal hernias) among 197 children whose mothers were exposed during the first trimester.[1] When all exposures to guaifenesin were considered, no increase in the frequency of malformations was found among 1,336 mothers who used it at various times during pregnancy. The value of the information from this large prospective study for use in teratogen risk counseling has been questioned for several reasons: There were few controls for other possible causes. The critical issue of medication timing was not specified. Because of frequent multiproduct use, particularly of cold and allergy preparations, it is hard to determine which drugs, if any, could cause birth defects. When several substances are examined together, as they were in this study, an association between any of the drugs and birth defects may simply be a chance occurrence. Last, even if there is an association, it does not prove that the substance actually caused the defect.

Unlike the Collaborative Perinatal Project, a large retrospective investigation found no increase in the frequency of birth defects among the children of 241 women who took guaifenesin during their first trimester.[2] While the findings in this study are reassuring, the manner in which the research was conducted also has several faults. One limitation of the study is that all the information was gathered through pharmacy records of filled prescriptions. Therefore, the study only assumed that guaifenesin was used during pregnancy, but did not prove it. More research is needed before it can be stated conclusively that guaifenesin does not cause birth defects.

Long-term follow-up studies of children exposed before birth have not been located.

The rather-safe-than-sorry approach would be to avoid cold medications in early pregnancy. After the first trimester, you should take them only as indicated and when absolutely necessary. Most important, because guaifenesin is available without a prescription, please remember to check with your physician before self-prescribing any drug during pregnancy.

If you choose to take an expectorant, select one with the *lowest dose* (perhaps a children's preparation). And as with all over-the-counter medications, look for the product with the *fewest* ingredients!

References:

[1]O. P. Heinonen, D. Slone, and S. Shapiro, *Birth Defects and Drugs in Pregnancy* (Littleton, Mass.: Publishing Sciences Group, 1977).

[2]P. Aselton, H. Jick, A. Milunsky, J. R. Hunter, and A. Stergachis, First-trimester drug use and congenital disorders, *Obstetrics and Gynecology* 65 (1985): 451–55.

GENERIC NAME: **HALOPERIDOL**

Brand Name: **(Haldol)**

FDA Pregnancy Category:—

ESTIMATED RISK SUMMARY:

Time of Exposure throughout pregnancy

Risk No known risk*

Pregnancy Outcome appears favorable

Documentation inconclusive, based on very minimal data

← pre-conception	All or None		Organ Development – (in weeks)						Maturation – (in weeks)				
	1	2	3	4	5	6	7	8	9	10	12	20-36	38

conception　　←—Time of Greatest Risk—→　　birth

Haloperidol belongs to a therapeutic class of drugs known as antipsychotics. The primary use of these drugs is to treat psychiatric illness (psychosis). Haloperidol also has antiemetic (antinausea) properties, and has been used to treat nausea during pregnancy.

Two case reports describing arm and leg defects in infants whose mothers took haloperidol early in pregnancy prompted retrospective investigations of the drug as a possible cause. One study interviewed thirty-one mothers of children with severe limb defects regarding their drug use during pregnancy. It also reviewed the hospital records of a further seven mothers of similarly affected children.[1] In none of these pregnancies was haloperidol taken. A second study involved ninety-eight women taking haloperidol during the first (ninety women) or second (eight women) trimester for excessive vomiting during pregnancy (hyperemesis gravidarum). This study failed to find any adverse effects of drug treatment.[2] The rate and frequency of stillbirths, premature deliveries, early infant deaths, and birth defects were not significantly different from those in a group of women not taking haloperidol.

Adverse effects have not been observed in newborns when this drug was administered during labor.

Long-term follow-up studies of children exposed before birth have not been located.

References:

[1]J. W. Hansen and G. P. Oakley, Haloperidol and limb deformity, *Journal of the American Medical Association* 231 (1975): 26.

[2]A. Van Waes and E. Van de Velde, Safety evaluation of haloperidol in the treatment of hyperemesis gravidarum, *Journal of Clinical Pharmacology,* 9 (1969): 224–27.

*above the 4% background risk

GENERIC NAME: **HEPARIN**

Brand Names: **(Lipo-Heparin, Liquaemin)**

FDA Pregnancy Category: C

ESTIMATED RISK SUMMARY:

Time of Exposure*
Risk No measurable risk,** for birth defects
Pregnancy Outcome favorable
Documentation conclusive, based on current knowledge

Time of Exposure*
Risk Known risk,** for prematurity, stillbirths, and maternal complications
Pregnancy Outcome adverse
Documentation conclusive, based on current knowledge

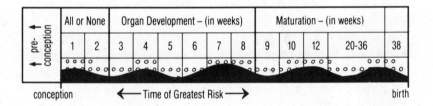

		All or None	Organ Development – (in weeks)						Maturation – (in weeks)				
← pre-conception ←		1	2	3	4	5	6	7	8	9	10	12	20-36	38

conception   ◄——— Time of Greatest Risk ———►   birth

Heparin is an anticoagulant—a drug that thins the blood by interfering with clotting (coagulation). Anticoagulants are used to treat and prevent blood clots (thrombophlebitis, pulmonary emboli), certian types of heart conditions, and stroke.

Unlike most substances, heparin cannot cross the placenta and enter the baby's bloodstream. Despite this fact, some adverse effects from its use during pregnancy have been reported. It is not clear, however, that heparin alone is responsible. Mothers who require an anticoagulant can be very ill and their poor health could certainly affect pregnancy outcome.

There is no record of increased incidence of birth defects, mental retardation, or growth retardation in children whose mothers required heparin during pregnancy. The greatest risks associated with its use are miscarriage and premature birth. One review of heparin-exposed pregnancies showed problems in one-third of them.[1] Twelve percent

---

*Insufficient data makes it impossible to calculate specific safe and at-risk exposure times during pregnancy.
**above the 4% background risk

of the babies were stillborn. Twenty percent were born prematurely, two-thirds of whom lived. However, some of the women studied received heparin experimentally for treating high blood pressure, a condition that may increase the risk for both stillbirths and premature births. Additional medications taken by these women might have also contributed to their pregnancy outcome. Without these causes, the rate of both stillbirths and premature deaths is cut by 50 percent.[2] Furthermore, some of these premature births date from as along ago as 1948. So they may reflect the limited medical knowledge of the past.

Two studies following women throughout their pregnancies have examined this issue further. One found twenty-five uncomplicated pregnancies and seven cases of premature labor.[3] The other study evaluated twenty treated women and twenty untreated controls.[4] It found more complications in the heparin-treated group but no increased incidence of stillbirth or death in prematurely born infants. Other similar studies are still in progress and will provide better information on the probabilities of such effects.

Heparin can also cause maternal bleeding, a decrease in blood platelets that are essential for coagulation (thrombocytopenia) and osteoporosis. To prevent these conditions, physicians reduce the dose of heparin as much as possible.

Long-term follow-up studies of children exposed before birth have not been located.

References:

[1]J. G. Hall, R. M. Pauli, and K. M. Wilson, Maternal and fetal sequelae of anticoagulation during pregnancy, *American Journal of Medicine* 68 (1980): 122–40; review.

[2]M. P. Nageotte, R. K. Freeman, T. J. Gartie, and R. A. Block, Anticoagulation in pregnancy, *American Journal of Obstetrics and Gynecology* 141 (1980): 472.

[3]M. Hellgren and E. B. Mygårds, Long-term therapy with subcutaneous heparin during pregnancy, *Gynecologic and Obstetric Investigation* 13 (1982): 76–89.

[4]R. Howell, J. Fidler, and E. Letsky. The risks of antinatal subcutaneous heparin prophylaxis: A controlled trial, *British Journal of Obstetrics and Gynecology* 90 (1983): 1124–28.

COMMON NAME: **HEPATITIS**

Brand Name/Chemical Name: **not applicable**

FDA Pregnancy Category: not applicable

ESTIMATED RISK SUMMARY:

All Forms of Hepatitis:

Time of Exposure throughout pregnancy

Risk No known risk* for birth defects
Pregnancy Outcome appears favorable
Documentation inconclusive, based on minimal data

Hepatitis A Virus:

Time of Exposure within 2 weeks of delivery
Risk Theoretical but unproven risk* for infection

Hepatitis B Virus:

Time of Exposure possibly throughout pregnancy
Risk Possible risk* for miscarriage, low birth weight, and prematurity (from acute
   infection)
Pregnancy Outcome uncertain: favorable and adverse outcomes observed
Documentation inconclusive

Time of Exposure throughout pregnancy, particularly during delivery
Risk Known risk* for infection
Pregnancy Outcome adverse
Documentation conclusive, based on current knowledge

Non-A, Non-B Hepatitis:

Time of Exposure during the last 3 months or during delivery
Risk Possible risk*
Pregnancy Outcome uncertain
Documentation inconclusive

pre-conception	All or None		Organ Development – (in weeks)						Maturation – (in weeks)				
	1	2	3	4	5	6	7	8	9	10	12	20-36	38

conception   ← Time of Greatest Risk →   birth

Hepatitis[1,2] is an inflammation of the liver. There are several types of this
infectious disease; three are discussed here:
• hepatitis A, formally called infectious hepatitis,

*above the 4% background risk

- hepatitis B, formally called serum hepatitis, and
- non-A, non-B hepatitis.

Hepatitis A virus is usually transmitted from contact with infected persons. Factors associated with transmission include poor sanitation, poor personal hygiene, and close personal (household and sexual) contact. Infection from contaminated food and water also occur.

Several studies have examined the effects of hepatitis A on a developing baby. None have found an increased incidence of birth defects or fetal infection associated with acute hepatitis A during pregnancy.[2] Nevertheless, if the mother contracts hepatitis within two weeks of delivery, the newborn faces a theoretical risk for infection. In such a situation clinical illness might be prevented by inoculating the baby, shortly after birth, with immune globulin (a product that contains antibodies against the hepatitis A virus).[3]

Hepatitis B virus (HBV) infection can be transmitted by contaminated needles, by transfusion with contaminated blood, through sexual contact or in settings of continuous close personal contact. Persons at risk for acquiring this form of hepatitis are described in Table 5–3 (page 180).

The most efficient mode of transmission of HBV is from the mother to her baby during pregnancy or delivery. Women who test positive for the hepatitis B surface antigen (HBsAg) can pass HBV on to their infants. HBsAg is found on the surface of the virus and is present in the blood of those with acute hepatitis and those who are chronic carriers of the infection. Transmission of HBV from mother to infant is highest when acute hepatitis occurs during the third trimester, particularly close to birth. The frequency of transmission is next highest when mothers are chronic HBsAg carriers at the time of birth and mother-to-infant transmission is rare when the mother has acute hepatitis early in pregnancy (first six months). There is no evidence that cesarean section will prevent HBV transmission to the infant.

Without treatment, up to 90 percent of the infected infants will become chronic HBsAG carriers. This is a serious concern because chronic carriers of the hepatitis B virus, especially those who acquire the infection at birth or early in life, are at an increased risk for developing cirrhosis (a liver disease) and liver cancer. Fortunately, though, two products are available that offer protection against HBV in the newborn: hepatitis B immune globulin (which contains antibodies against the hepatitis B virus) and hepatitis B vaccine (see hepatitis B vaccine, page 181). Preferably, both products should be administered to the baby within twelve hours of birth.

Infection appears to be the primary risk associated with HBV during pregnancy. Other problems associated with acute hepatitis include a possible increased frequency of miscarriages, low-birth-weight infants, and premature deliveries. An increased incidence of birth defects has not been observed.

At least two different agents cause *non-A, non-B hepatitis*. There are no diagnostic tests for this form of hepatitis; its diagnosis is made by exclusion. In the United States, non-A, non-B hepatitis is most commonly transmitted after intravenous drug abuse or blood transfusions. In Southeast Asia and North Africa, this form of hepatitis has occurred in epidemic proportions, reportedly spread through close personal contact or by water. In these epidemics an unusually high rate of death has been observed among infected pregnant women.[1]

Little is known about the risk of non-A, non-B hepatitis infection during pregnancy. Like hepatitis B virus, infection with non-A, non-B hepatitis can lead to a chronic carrier state. Some *indirect* evidence supports administering immune globulin to newborns of mothers with acute infection during the last trimester or during delivery.[2]

References:

[1]Centers for Disease Control, Recommendations for protection against viral hepatitis, *Morbidity and Mortality Weekly Report* 34 (1985): 313–35.

[2]J. S. Remington and J. O. Klein, (eds.), *Infectious Diseases of the Fetus and Newborn Infant*, 2d ed. (Philadelphia: W. B. Saunders, 1983), pp. 591–618.

[3]C. E. Stevens, S. Krugman, W. Szmuness, and R. P. Beasley, Viral hepatitis in pregnancy: Problems for the clinician dealing with the infant, *Pediatric Review* 2 (1980): 212–25.

Table 5–3

Persons at Risk of Acquiring Hepatitis B Virus Infection:

- newborns whose mothers are HBsAg positive
- health care workers (who are exposed to blood products and/or needles)
- clients and staff of institutions for the mentally retarded
- users of illicit injectable drugs
- homosexually active men
- household and sexual contacts of HBV carriers
- specific high-risk populations (Alaskan Eskimos, native Pacific islanders, immigrants and refugees from eastern Asia and sub-Saharan Africa)
- hemodialysis patients
- male prisoners
- international travelers (only to certain countries)

GENERIC NAME: **HEPATITIS B VACCINE**

Brand Name: **(Heptavax-B, Recombivax-HB)**

FDA Pregnancy Category: C

ESTIMATED RISK SUMMARY:

Time of Exposure throughout pregnancy
Risk assessment is not possible
Pregnancy Outcome uncertain
Documentation available information is insufficient

← pre-conception ←	All or None		Organ Development – (in weeks)						Maturation – (in weeks)				
	1	2	3	4	5	6	7	8	9	10	12	20-36	38

conception   ←——Time of Greatest Risk——→   birth

Hepatits B vaccine[1] provides protection against infection from the hepatitis B virus (formally called serum hepatitis). This infection is a major cause of acute and chronic hepatitis (inflammation of the liver), cirrhosis (a liver disease), and liver cancer (see hepatitis, page 177).

Hepatitis B vaccine is a noninfective product. Theoretically, then, vaccination during pregnancy should not present an increased risk to the unborn baby. The Centers for Disease Control supports this by stating, "Pregnancy should not be considered a contraindication of the use of this vaccine for persons who are otherwise eligible."[1] Unfortunately, this recommendation is not based on well-controlled scientific studies.

The only published information I could locate on hepatitis B vaccine during pregnancy was from a study designed to evaluate its efficacy.[2] In this investigation, eight pregnancies occurred in a total of 442 medical staff members who received the vaccine Heptavax-B. All eight babies were healthy at birth. The small number of women and infants in this investigation do not allow for definitive conclusions on the safety of hepatitis B vaccine during pregnancy.

Vaccination involves three doses of the vaccine. There is a one-month wait between the first and the second dose and six months between the first and the third. The vaccine recipient has optimal protection after the third dose is received. Still, the manufacturer (Merck Sharp & Dohme) suggests women becoming pregnant after the first two doses should consider delaying the third shot until after pregnancy.[3] (This recommendation is based not on documented adverse effects, but rather on the rather-safe-than-sorry approach.) If the delay is over a long period of time—a year, for example—a test to determine immunity to the virus should be performed.

Hepatitis B vaccine is also used to prevent hepatitis B in babies born to women who have acute hepatitis in the last trimester of pregnancy, particularly close to birth, or who are chronic carriers of the infection. Transmission of hepatitis B virus from mother to baby has been reported to occur up to 70 percent to 90 percent of the time. Without treatment, as many as 90 percent of these children will become chronic carriers of the hepatitis B virus. This is a serious concern because chronic carriers, especially those who acquire the infection at birth or early in life, are at an increased risk for developing cirrhosis and liver cancer. In addition to the vaccine, susceptible infants also receive hepatitis B immune globulin (which contains antibodies against the hepatitis B virus), and together these products offer the newborn the best protection available against the hepatitis B virus.

References:

[1]Centers for Disease Control, Recommendations for protection against viral hepatitis, *Morbidity and Mortality Weekly Report* 34 (1985): 313–35.

[2]W. Szmuness, C. E. Stevens, E. J. Harley, E. A. Zang, H. J. Alter, P. E. Taylor, A. DeVera, G. T. S. Chen, A. Kellner, and the Dialysis Vaccine Trial Study Group, Hepatitis B vaccine in medical staff of hemodialysis units, *New England Journal of Medicine* 302 (1982): 1481–86.

[3]Personal communication with Merck Sharp & Dohme, June 1987.

COMMON NAME: **HERBICIDES**

Chemical Names: **(dioxins (TCDD), 2,4,5-T and 2,4-D)**

FDA PREGNANCY CATEGORY: not applicable.

ESTIMATED RISK SUMMARY:

Time of Exposure before and during pregnancy

Risk No known risk* for birth defects

Pregnancy outcome appears favorable

Documentation inconclusive, based on minimal data

*above the expected 4% background risk

![pre-conception]	All or None	Organ Development – (in weeks)						Maturation – (in weeks)				
	1	2	3	4	5	6	7	8	9	10	12	20-36	38

conception   ⟵—Time of Greatest Risk—⟶   birth

The chemicals 2,4,5-T and 2,4-D are **herbicides**[1] used to control broadleaf plants and to clear away unwanted vegetation. These two products were also combined to formulate the well-known herbicide Agent Orange (see Agent Orange, page 55). During the manufacturing of 2,4,5-T, it is unfortunately contaminated by unwanted by-products called **dioxins.** The most toxic and the most studied of the dioxins is **TCDD** (2,3,7,8-TCDD). While dioxins are potent biological toxins, **2,4,5-T** and **2,4-D** have been shown to be relatively *nontoxic to humans* with the exception of chronic exposures.

Laboratory studies using rodents have shown all these substances to be potential teratogens. But dioxin is by far the most harmful. These findings have fueled the controversy surrounding the possible link between human exposure to herbicides and birth defects. However, the artificial circumstances under which the laboratory studies were conducted cannot be used to accurately predict human risks. Human studies must be relied upon for understanding this issue.

Human studies conducted in Europe, New Zealand, Australia, the United Kingdom, and the United States have failed to convincingly demonstrate a higher rate of abnormalities in children where one or both parents have been "exposed" to herbicides (dioxins [TCDD], 2,4,5-T, and 2,4-D). Collectively, these investigations included exposures in both males and females. They addressed populations exposed to herbicides during seasonal spraying or an industrial accident. And they looked at workers in herbicide manufacturing and in agriculture.

One of the most extensive experiences with human exposure to dioxin (TCDD) occurred in 1976 from an accident at a chemical plant in Sevesco, Italy. In the twelve months following the incident, 2,774 children were born in the area. A total of 38 (1.4%) malformations were recorded in these children. No specific pattern of abnormality was revealed, which is expected if there is a singular cause, and the percentage of abnormalities was within the expected 4 percent population incidence. While some feel an increased incidence of miscarriage occurred, documentation has proven difficult.

Other studies have also examined the question of increased miscarriage rates. A 1979 investigation conducted by the U.S. Environmental Protection Agency initially linked 2,4,5-T spraying on the forest regions of the state of Oregon with an increase in the frequency of miscarriages. The basis of these conclusions has, however, been severely criticized. Apparently the areas chosen in the original report did not truly reflect the ratio of land sprayed to land that was not sprayed. Also, the ways miscarriages were reported in the regions being studied differed greatly, which ultimately influenced the observed rates of pregnancy loss. Taking these factors into account, the conclusions reached by the EPA are not well founded. Additional attempts to evaluate miscarriage and stillbirth rates associated with herbicide exposures have had conflicting results, and to date this issue remains unresolved.

All of these investigations have been criticized as being flawed. The greatest criticism is that exposure to herbicides was often assumed and not proven. This would tend to camouflage the real risks by enlarging the study population to include both exposed and unexposed people. Researchers also find it very difficult, and sometimes impossible, to calculate how much herbicide an individual or a population actually came in contact with. Finally, the time during pregnancy when the exposure occurred was often not known, so researchers are unable to determine if an observed problem could be explained by the time of exposure.

Long-term follow-up studies of children exposed before birth have not been located.

Care should always be taken when using either herbicides or pesticides. Direct contact with the chemical should be avoided, and when necessary protective gear and clothing should be selected, a disposable face mask and gloves are the basics.

Reference:

[1] J. H. Pearn, Herbicides and congenital malformations: A review for the paediatrician, *Australian Paediatric Journal* 21 (1985): 237–42.

GENERIC NAME: **HEROIN**

Brand Names/Chemical name: **not applicable**

FDA Pregnancy Category: not applicable

ESTIMATED RISK SUMMARY:

Time of Exposure throughout pregnancy
Risk No known risk for birth defects*

*above the 4% background risk

Pregnancy Outcome appears favorable
Documentation inconclusive

Time of Exposure consistent doses, primarily in the last trimester of
pregnancy and up to the time of delivery
Risk Known risk* for a variety of complications, including low birth weight and
withdrawal syndrome
Pregnancy Outcome adverse
Documentation conclusive, based on current knowledge

pre-conception	All or None		Organ Development – (in weeks)						Maturation – (in weeks)				
	1	2	3	4	5	6	7	8	9	10	12	20-36	38

conception ←——Time of Greatest Risk——→ birth

Heroin is a narcotic that can relieve severe pain, but the drug is used for its
ability to elevate mood, induce euphoria, provide sedation, and permit sleep. There is a
high degree of tolerance for this drug and prolonged use results in physical and
pyschological dependence.

Pregnancy in the heroin-addicted woman is most trouble-free when she is on
maintenance doses of methadone (see methadone, page 233). Dose reduction, if
necessary, is advised only during the first two trimesters. Detoxification during the third
trimester presents a significant risk to the unborn child.

An increase in birth defects has not been seen in infants born to heroin addicts. But
fetal distress, stillbirths, premature births, and illness and death in newborns are more
frequent. Death rates in heroin-dependent infants are largely due to premature birth.
More than 80 percent of these infants may exhibit very severe complications, among
them: bleeding within their head (intracranial hemorrhage), life-threatening breathing
problems (hyaline membrane disease), growth retardation evident before birth, low
blood sugar (hypoglycemia), and severe infections.[1]

Heroin may accelerate lung maturation in the unborn baby because the incidence
of severe breathing problems in premature infants born to heroin-addicted mothers is
much lower than expected.[2]

Approximately 50 percent of infants born to heroin addicts weigh under 2,500 gms

---

*above the 4% background risk

(5.5 pounds),[3,4] due in part to slowed growth during gestation and in part to premature birth.[3,4,5,6] Premature delivery has been associated with more acute infections at the time of delivery in the heroin-addicted mother.[6] The continued use of cigarettes, alcohol, and other drugs during pregnancy certainly contributes to the incidence of small babies these women deliver. After birth, some of these children have grown more quickly to compensate for their smaller birth weight, according to some longitudinal studies. But other studies have not found this.

The impact of prenatal heroin exposure on motor development, intelligence, and behavior has not been determined. School-age children have not been evaluated, and the many other possible causes of developmental problems in this population have not been sorted out. Most studies focus on behavior in the newborn. Behavioral scores are influenced by withdrawal symptoms; as symptoms decrease, developmental gains increase. Few investigations into later motor and intellectual development focus on heroin only, and maintaining contact with these mothers and their children is difficult.

Twenty children aged 3 to 6 years born to women who predominantly abused heroin were compared to three matched, but drug-free groups.[7] While the overall performance of the heroin-exposed children was within normal limits, they scored lower than the compared groups on behavioral, intellectual, perceptual, and physical measures. The differences were not enough to impair mental development. Similarly, low-average or mildly retarded intellectual performances were seen in a small group of preschool-age children exposed before birth to heroin or methadone. But these scores were more related to health factors, amount of prenatal care received, and home environment than they were to maternal narcotic use.[8]

Withdrawal symptoms (neonatal abstinence syndrome) are observed in 70–90 percent of infants born to narcotic addicts. Neonatal abstinence syndrome is characterized by disturbed nervous system function that includes irritability, trembling, increased muscle tone, high-pitched crying, weak sucking, and frantic hand-to-mouth movements. Symptoms appear within twenty-four hours in more than 50 percent of those prenatally exposed to heroin. Withdrawal symptoms, such as agitation, restlessness, tremors, and sleep disturbances, may persist in some infants for three to four months.

There are case reports of sudden infant death syndrome (SIDS) in a small number of infants exposed to methadone, but less frequently to heroin. The relationship between SIDS and infant narcotic addiction remains unclear.[9]

Drug use is just one of a constellation of factors that affects the growth, development, and intellectual performance of the children born to heroin-addicted women. During pregnancy other risk factors include poor maternal health and nutritional habits, lack of prenatal care, obstetric complications (particularly infections), and the concomitant use of other drugs. After birth, the quality of the care-taking environment will ultimately influence the development of these children.

References:

[1]L. P. Finnegan, The effects of narcotics and alcohol on pregnancy and the newborn, *Annals of the New York Academy of Sciences* 362 (1981): 136–57.

[2]L. Glass, B. Rajegowda, and H. Evans, Absence of respiratory distress in premature infants of heroin-addicted mothers, *Lancet* 2 (1971): 685.

[3]L. P. Finnegan, Management of pregnant drug-dependent women, *Annals of the New York Academy of Sciences* 311 (1978): 135–46.

[4]G. C. Vargus, R. S. Pildes, D. Vidyasagar and L. G. Keith, Effect of maternal heroin addiction on 67 liveborn neonates, *Clinical Pediatrics* 14 (1975): 751–57.

[5]B. Stimmel, J. Goldberg, A. Reisman, R. J. Murphy, and K. Teets, Fetal outcome in narcotic-dependent women: The importance of the type of maternal narcotic used, *American Journal of Drug and Alcohol Abuse* 9 (1982–3): 383–95.

[6]R. L. Naeye, W. Blanc, W. Leblanc, and M. A. Khatamee, Fetal complications of maternal heroin addiction: Abnormal growth, infections and episodes of stress, *Journal of Pediatrics* 83 (1973): 1055–61.

[7]G. S. Wilson, R. McCreary, J. Kean, and J. C. Baxter, The development of preschool children of heroin-addicted mothers: A controlled study, *Pediatrics* 63 (1979): 135–41.

[8]M. H. Lifshitz, G. S. Wilson, E. Obrian-Smith, and M. M. Desmond. Factors affecting head growth and intellectual function in children of drug addicts, *Pediatrics* 75 (1985): 269–74.

[9]B. K. Rajegowda, S. R. Kandall, and H. Falciglia, Sudden unexpected death in infants of narcotic-dependent mothers, *Early Human Development* 2/3 (1978): 219–25.

COMMON NAME: **HERPES SIMPLEX VIRUS**

Brand Name/Chemical Name: **not applicable**

FDA Pregnancy Category: not applicable

ESTIMATED RISK SUMMARY:

Recurrent Infection
Time of Exposure about the first 19 weeks
Risk No known risk*
Pregnancy Outcome appears favorable
Documentation inconclusive

Primary Infection
Time of Exposure first trimester

*above the 4% background risk

Risk Suspected risk* for miscarriage and theoretical, but unlikely, risk for birth
 defects

Pregnancy Outcome uncertain: favorable and adverse outcomes obseved

Documentation inconclusive, based on minimal data

Time of Exposure after about 20 weeks

Risk Known risk* for prematurity and miscarriage

Pregnancy Outcome adverse

Documentation conclusive, based on current knowledge

Active Herpes

Time of Exposure during vaginal delivery

Risk Known risk* for severe infection of the newborn

Pregnancy Outcome adverse

Documentation conclusive, based on current knowledge

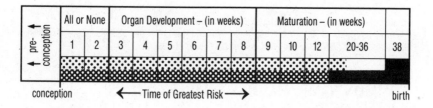

pre-conception	All or None		Organ Development – (in weeks)						Maturation – (in weeks)				
	1	2	3	4	5	6	7	8	9	10	12	20-36	38

conception   ← Time of Greatest Risk →   birth

Herpes simplex virus[1,2] (also called **HSV**) is a common viral infection. There
are two types of herpes: **HSV-I** and **HSV-II.** HSV-I, or oral herpes, usually appears
around the mouth as fever blisters and canker sores. HSV-II, or genital herpes, is
sexually transmitted, and oral-genital contact with the infection could also transmit
HSV-II to the mouth or lips. Herpes, once contracted, tends to persist within your body
for an indefinite period of time, resulting in recurrent episodes of infection. This is in
contrast to other viral infections, such as the German measles (rubella) or the mumps.

Research indicates that an unborn child does not have an increased risk of birth
defects or infection if the mother's old herpes infection recurs during the first nineteen
weeks of pregnancy (although, recently, a mother who had recurrent episodes of
herpes at various times during pregnancy gave birth to a baby with evidence of herpes
infection acquired in the womb).[3] A new infection (primary infection) during the first
trimester may increase the risk for miscarriage. A theoretical risk for birth defects also

*above the 4% background risk

exists for women with a primary infection during the first trimester; however, recorded instances are extremely rare.[3]

A new herpes infection after the twentieth week of pregnancy results in a 35 percent chance of premature labor and fetal loss. However, no increased risk of premature birth exists when a chronic herpes infection recurs.

The risk of a newborn baby acquiring a herpes infection during the birth process, as they pass through the cervix, vagina, or vulva, is 50 percent. Three-quarters of the infections result from HSV-II, and the rest are from HSV-I. The infections from the two strains are equally severe, and it does not matter whether it is the mother's first infection or a recurrence of an old one.

Almost all newborn babies with herpes infections contract it during birth. Between 60 percent and 90 percent of all babies with such infections die or become permanently disabled. Such infections cause the deaths of approximately one thousand infants yearly in the United States.

Any woman with an active HSV infection, whether recurrent or new, or whose sexual partner is infected, should undertake weekly laboratory tests from thirty-four to thirty-six weeks until the time of delivery. If laboratory tests are negative within one week of the baby's birth and signs of the infection are not detected upon examination, a vaginal delivery is considered safe. If laboratory tests are positive, or if the mother's water breaks four to six hours before delivery, a cesarean section could prevent infection in the newborn baby.

At the present time there is no way to completely prevent herpes from recurring. Although it has not been proven, some people claim that taking supplemental lysine (an amino acid) reduces the frequency of herpes episodes. Because the effects of supplemental lysine in pregnancy have not been studied, the rather-safe-than-sorry approach would be to avoid unnecessary doses of this compound. A drug called acyclovir has been shown to be helpful in reducing the duration of initial herpes infections, but it is not as effective for treating or preventing recurrent episodes (see acyclovir, page 54).

References:

[1]R. H. Kaufman and S. Faro, Herpes genitalis: Clinical features and treatment, *Clinical Obstetrics and Gynecology* 28 (1985): 152–62.

[2]S. Kibrick, Herpes simplex infection at term: What to do with mother, newborn and nursery personnel, *Journal of the American Medical Association* 243 (1980): 157–60.

[3]C. Hutto, A. Arvin, R. Jacobs, R. Steele, S. Stagno, R. Lyrene, et al., Intrauterine herpes simplex virus infections, *Journal of Pediatrics* 110 (1987): 97–101.

COMMON NAME: **HERPES ZOSTER (SHINGLES)**

Brand Name/Chemical Name: **not applicable**

FDA Pregnancy Category: not applicable

ESTIMATED RISK SUMMARY:
   Time of Exposure throughout pregnancy
   Risk Risk assessment is not possible
   Pregnancy Outcome uncertain
   Documentation insufficient

← pre-conception	All or None		Organ Development – (in weeks)						Maturation – (in weeks)				
	1	2	3	4	5	6	7	8	9	10	12	20-36	38

conception   ← Time of Greatest Risk →   birth

Herpes zoster (shingles),[1] caused by the same virus as is chicken pox, is the result of a "reactivated chicken pox infection" (see varicella, page 336). The virus responsible for these infections is called varicella-zoster and it is one of the five known herpesviruses. (Other herpesviruses include: cytomegalovirus [CMV], Epstein-Barr virus [mononucleosis], and herpes simplex virus I and II [oral and genital herpes].) Unlike other viral infections such as the German measles (rubella) or the mumps, the varicella-zoster virus tends to persist within your body for an indefinite time and can be reactivated later. Herpes zoster is not the same as the herpes simplex infection that has received so much attention in recent years (see herpes, page 187).

The incidence of herpes zoster increases with age, with most cases occurring in those over 50 years. Herpes zoster is an uncommonly reported disease in women of childbearing age.

No more than fifty cases of herpes zoster occurring in pregnancy have been located.[2,3,4] Several early instances are poorly documented, meaning that diagnosis was made clinically rather than confirmed by laboratory tests. Because of this, there is no way of knowing whether the infection was actually herpes zoster. Nevertheless, the majority of babies born to women with herpes zoster during early and later pregnancy have had normal development with no birth defects. The few cases of detected abnormalities have been attributed to other causes, including exposure to the viral teratogen rubella. There is one possible exception, a woman who had chicken pox as a little girl suffered from herpes zoster at twelve weeks gestation and gave birth to a child with a scarred and underdeveloped leg. According to one group of physicians, the birth defect seems to be linked to the mother's herpes zoster infection.[4]

Occasionally a patient with herpes zoster may exhibit chicken-pox-like eruptions. In such a case the unborn child faces a theoretical risk of infection.

References:

[1]J. S. Remington and J. O. Klein (eds.) *Infectious Diseases of the Fetus and Newborn Infant* 2nd ed. (Philadelphia: W. B. Saunders, 1983), pp. 376–402.

[2]S. G. Paryani and A. M. Arvin, Intrauterine infection with varicella-zoster virus after maternal varicella, *New England Journal of Medicine* 314 (1986): 1542–46.

[3]A. Eyal, M. Friedman, B. A. Peretz, and E. Paldi, Pregnancy complicated by herpes zoster: A report of two cases and literature review, *Journal Reproductive Medicine* 28 (1983): 600–603.

[4]K. Higa, K. Dan, and H. Manabe, Varicella-zoster virus infections during pregnancy: Hypothesis concerning the mechanisms of congenital malformations, *Obstetrics and Gynecology* 69 (1987): 214–22.

MEDICATION CLASSIFICATION: **HYDANTOINS**

GENERIC NAMES: **ETHOTOIN, MEPHENYTOIN, PHENYTOIN**

Brand Names: **(Dilantin, Mesantoin, Peganone)**

FDA Pregnancy Category: D

ESTIMATED RISK SUMMARY:

Time of Exposure potentially throughout pregnancy

Risk Known risk*

Pregnancy Outcome adverse

Documentation conclusive, based on current knowledge

pre-conception	All or None	Organ Development – (in weeks)						Maturation – (in weeks)				
	1	2	3	4	5	6	7	8	9	10	12	20-36	38

conception   ←— Time of Greatest Risk —→   birth

*above the 4% background risk

Hydantoins (ethotoin, mephenytoin, phenytoin) are anticonvulsant drugs used to control epileptic seizures.

Opinions differ about the specific risk of hydantoins. Many experts say there is two to three times the risk of major malformations in the children of epileptic women as in the general population. Some think the underlying disease is the cause. Others believe this statistic reflects a population of women who are exposed more often to hydantoins and other potentially teratogenic anticonvulsants. This difference of opinion arises, in part, from the variation in types of defect, and in their incidence. The best explanation of this variation is the way the genetics of the mother and fetus influence drug reaction.[1] (First Principle of Teratology).

The spectrum of defects caused by these drugs is usually called the "fetal hydantoin syndrome."[2] Its principal features are:

• *abnormalities of the head and face*: short nose, bowed upper lip, broad nose bridge, eyes spaced wider than normal (mild ocular hypertelorism), and cleft lip and/or cleft palate,
• *minor hand malformations*: slight underdevelopment of the fingertips, with small or absent nails,
• *growth deficiency both before and after birth*, including an abnormally small head size (microcephaly),
• *performance abnormalities*, including developmental delay and mild to moderate mental retardation, and,
• less frequently, *heart defects*
• Occasionally, hernias and hypospadias (the abnormal placement of the urethral opening on the penis) occur.

Some of these minor malformations may be apparent at birth only in severely affected children. Otherwise, they may go unnoticed.

The scientists who defined the fetal hydantoin syndrome believe that children of women who use hydantoins during pregnancy have an 11 percent risk for the full-blown syndrome.[2] The risk of a subtle or nonserious effect is 30 percent.

Most studies have focused on phenytoin, the most commonly used hydantoin. Mephenytoin and ethotoin are also teratogens, causing the same pattern of malformation as phenytoin.[2,3] The American Academy of Pediatrics states that women taking phenytoin have a 90 percent chance of having a normal child, and that the risk of mental retardation among their children is two to three times greater than average.[4]

There are reports of tumors in ten children exposed before birth to phenytoin and a barbiturate (plus alcohol in two cases).[5] From this evidence, some suspect that prenatal exposure to these drugs may cause cancer. But because of the small number of cases, it is impossible to know this for sure.

Phenytoin is associated with a blood coagulation defect in newborns, which can cause severe bleeding (usually within the first twenty-four hours). To help prevent this, your physician will usually administer vitamin K_1 to you some weeks before delivery, and during labor. (Vitamin K_1 is required for normal blood-clotting.) At birth, your baby will also receive vitamin K_1.

Using hydantoins might reduce your level of one of the B-complex vitamins, folic acid or folate. The need for folate increases greatly during pregnancy, as it is required for fetal growth and development. Some experts suggest that taking folic acid supplements during pregnancy might reduce the risk for abnormalities.[6]

Investigations of hydantoins have focused on women who take phenytoin *throughout* pregnancy. As yet, no studies have been conducted on limited or first trimester exposures. This is important because abnormalities can occur at various times within the embryonic and fetal periods: Hydantoins can harm organs that develop in the first trimester. They also affect growth early or late in pregnancy. And they can potentially damage the baby's brain anytime during pregnancy.

Theoretically, exposures limited to early pregnancy would affect only those organs which are developing at the time. This would reduce the risk for growth retardation and mental deficiency.

Expert opinion is divided about switching from hydantoins to other anticonvulsant drugs during pregnancy. The American Academy of Pediatrics,[4] and other experts, advise against switching. But some believe that even after the first trimester, changing to another effective drug will reduce the risk to the child. Unfortunately, the safety of most alternative drugs has not been determined.

Most women continue taking anticonvulsant medication during pregnancy, unless they have been seizure free for many years. *Under no circumstances should you ever discontinue your anticonvulsant medication, unless under the direction and supervision of the prescribing physician.* Sudden withdrawal could cause a seizure. And while seizures are not known to cause malformations, they do present a possible risk to both you and your unborn baby.

Many women question how epilepsy or anticonvulsant medication in the father might affect their baby. Although not all scientists agree, most experts think this presents no increased risk. They believe that children fathered by men taking these drugs have the same chance of being normal and healthy as anyone else's, and well-conducted animal research confirms this belief.[7] (For more information on this see Risks from Exposures in the Baby's Father, page 14.)

Finally, remember: If you have to take this drug during pregnancy, your odds are in favor of giving birth to a normal, healthy baby.

References:

[1]R. H. Finnell and G. F. Chernoff, Genetic background: The elusive component of the Fetal Hydantoin Syndrome, *American Journal of Medical Genetics* 19 (1984): 459–62.

[2]J. W. Hanson, N. C. Myrianthropoulos, M. A. Sedgewick-Harvey, and D. W. Smith, Risks to offspring of women treated with hydantoin anticonvulsants, with emphasis on the fetal hydantoin syndrome, *Journal of Pediatrics* 89 (1976): 62–68.

[3]M. Zablen, and N. Brand, Cleft lip and palate with the anticonvulsant ethotoin, *New England Journal of Medicine* 298 (1970): 285.

[4]American Academy of Pediatrics, Committee on Drugs, Anticonvulsants and pregnancy, *Pediatrics* 63 (1979): 331–33.

[5]A. Lipson and P. Bale, Ependymoblastoma associated with prenatal exposure to Diphenylhydantoin and methylphenobarbitone, *Cancer* 55 (1985): 1859–62.

[6]Y. Biale and H. Lewenthal, Effect of folic acid supplementation on congenital malformations due to anticonvulsive drugs, *European Journal of Obstetrics, Gynecology and Reproductive Biology* 18 (1984): 211–16.

[7]R. H. Finnell and J. F. Baer, Congenital defects among the offspring of epileptic fathers: Role of the genotype and phenytoin therapy in a mouse model, *Epilepsia* 25 (1986): 697–705.

GENERIC NAME: **HYDRALAZINE**

Brand Names: **(Alazine, Apresoline)**

FDA Pregnancy Category:—

ESTIMATED RISK SUMMARY:

Time of Exposure throughout pregnancy

Risk No known risk* for birth defects

Pregnancy Outcome appears favorable

Documentation inconclusive, based on minimal data

		All or None	Organ Development – (in weeks)						Maturation – (in weeks)				
← pre-conception ←		1	2	3	4	5	6	7	8	9	10	12	20-36	38

conception   ←——Time of Greatest Risk——→   birth

*above the 4% b ckground risk

Hydralazine[1] is used to treat low blood pressure (hypotension). Currently there is no information implicating this drug as a teratogen. The majority of studies report normal pregnancy outcomes following hydralazine use by pregnant women, and only occasionally have fetal complications been observed. These include hypothermia (low body temperature) and thrombocytopenia (a decrease in blood platelets, which are essential for blood coagulation) in some newborns. Also, changes in fetal heart rate were seen after an acute dose. It is important to be aware that the mother's illness and the other medications she might also be taking could contribute to some of these problems.

In addition, it is not certain whether hydralazine reduces blood flow between the uterus and the placenta. If this is so, it becomes a problem, because this blood flow determines how much oxygen the unborn child receives.

Long-term follow-up studies of children exposed before birth have not been located.

Reference:

[1]A. L. Wilson and G. R. Matzke, The treatment of hypertention in pregnancy, *Drug Intelligence and Clinical Pharmacy* 15 (1981): 21–26.

GENERIC NAME: **HYDROCODONE**

Brand Names: **(Hycodan, ◇ Lortab Liquid, ◇ Norcet, ◇ Vicodin)**

FDA Pregnancy Category: C

ESTIMATED RISK SUMMARY:
   Time of Exposure throughout pregnancy
   Risk Risk assessment is not possible
   Pregnancy Outcome uncertain
   Documentation unavailable

← pre- conception →	All or None		Organ Development – (in weeks)						Maturation – (in weeks)				
	1	2	3	4	5	6	7	8	9	10	12	20-36	38

conception   ←—Time of Greatest Risk—→   birth

◇ = also contains acetaminophen

Hydrocodone is a semisynthetic narcotic. This drug is used to relieve coughs and to treat moderate and moderately severe pain. As with other narcotics, prolonged use of hydrocodone can result in physical and psychological dependence.

Hydrocodone has not been evaluated for any possible effects it might have on the unborn baby. Theoretically, the consistent use of any narcotic agent near birth could cause addiction and withdrawal symptoms in the newborn.

Long-term follow-up studies of children exposed before birth have not been located.

GENERIC NAME: **HYDROXYZINE**

Brand Names: **(Anxanil, Atarax, Atozine, Durax)**

FDA Pregnancy Category:—

ESTIMATED RISK SUMMARY:
   Time of Exposure throughout pregnancy
   Risk Risk assessment is not possible
   Pregnancy Outcome uncertain
   Documentation insufficient

← pre-conception ←	All or None		Organ Development – (in weeks)						Maturation – (in weeks)				
	1	2	3	4	5	6	7	8	9	10	12	20-36	38

conception   ←—Time of Greatest Risk—→   birth

Hydroxyzine is used to relieve anxiety and tension and it is used as a sedative. Hydroxyzine has also been used as an antinauseant. This drug is related to buclizine (see page 92), cyclizine (see page 130), and meclizine (see page 226).

Only limited information is available on the effects of hydroxyzine on the unborn baby. For this reason, the drug manufacturer has recommended against its use in early pregnancy. The Collaborative Perinatal Project, which evaluated pregnancy outcome in more than 50,000 mother-child pairs exposed to a wide variety of drugs, found an increase in the frequency of birth defects among fifty children whose mothers used hydroxyzine during the first trimester.[1] The very small number of exposures makes the significance of the observation difficult to determine. In addition, the value of the information from this large prospective study for use in teratogen risk counseling has been questioned for several reasons: There were few controls for other possible causes. The critical issue of medication timing was not specified. When several substances are examined together, as they were in this study, an association between any of the drugs and birth defects may simply be a chance occurrence. Last, even if there is an association, it does not prove that the substance actually caused the defect.

Another study investigated the use of this drug in one hundred women who were treated with hydroxyzine for nausea and vomiting during their first three months of pregnancy.[2] When they were compared to women who received no treatment, there were no significant differences in the frequency of miscarriages or birth defects.

Additional studies are needed before the effects of hydroxyzine during pregnancy can be fully understood.

Long-term follow-up studies of children exposed before birth have not been located.

References:

[1]O. P. Heinonen, D. Slone, and S. Shapiro, *Birth Defects and Drugs in Pregnancy* (Littleton, Mass.: Publishing Sciences Group, 1977).

[2]S. Erez, B. S. Schifrin, and O. Dirim, Double-blind evaluation of hydroxyzine as an antiemetic in pregnancy, *Journal of Reproductive Medicine* 7 (1971). 57–59.

COMMON NAME: **HYPERTHERMIA**

Brand Name/Chemical Name: **not applicable**

FDA Pregnancy Category: not applicable

ESTIMATED RISK SUMMARY:

Time of Exposure primarily 2–12 weeks after conception

Risk Possible risk*

Pregnancy Outcome very uncertain: favorable and adverse outcomes observed

Documentation inconclusive, based on minimal data

*above the 4% background risk

← pre-conception ←		All or None		Organ Development – (in weeks)						Maturation – (in weeks)				
		1	2	3	4	5	6	7	8	9	10	12	20-36	38

conception   ← Time of Greatest Risk →   birth

Hyperthermia[1,2] is defined as an abnormally high body temperature. Causes of hyperthermia include fever, hot tubs (Jacuzzis), sauna bathing, and extremely strenuous exercise.

In the first studies of hyperthermia-related birth defects, laboratory animals were subjected to high temperatures during the first one-third to one-half of their pregnancies. They showed higher rates of miscarriage, and their offspring had various abnormalities, particularly central nervous system (CNS) defects.

These observations prompted a closer look at the relationship between hyperthermia during human pregnancy and birth defects. Only a limited number of such investigations have been conducted. Most are retrospective studies, which tend to overrepresent the frequency of abnormalities (see retrospective studies, page 43). In some cases researchers had to depend on the mother's memory to record whether or not she had a fever and specifically when during pregnancy it occurred. It is a well-known fact that people seldom remember even recent historical events accurately. Mothers of babies with birth defects recall the events during their pregnancies much differently than do mothers of normal children. Therefore, relying on mothers' memories can affect the reliability of the conclusions drawn from the study.

With such cautions in mind, these studies showed a variety of defects similar to those in laboratory animals. And the types of malformations in the children seemed to correspond to the time during pregnancy when the hyperthermia occurred. To date, only a limited number of prospective studies, conducted before the birth outcome is known, have been attempted. These have failed to associate elevated body temperature during pregnancy with birth defects.

In animals, the effects of temperature are related to how hot it is, the length of the exposure, and when during pregnancy it occurs.

In humans, hyperthermia is defined as a body temperature of at least 102°F (38.9°C). Our normal body temperature is 98.6°F (37°C), so this is an increase that would not go unnoticed. Experts believe that the temperature must also be prolonged, but an exact definition of this does not exist. Based on reported cases, exposures that occur between fourteen to twenty-eight days (primarily twenty-one to twenty-eight days) after conception might pose an increased risk for neural tube defects (spina bifida and anencephaly). Luckily, these birth defects can be screened for during pregnancy with a simple test performed on blood drawn from the mother's arm (see maternal serum alpha-fetoprotein, page 25). Maternal hyperthermia between four and fourteen weeks of gestation* might increase the risk of mental deficiency, altered muscle tone, and facial defects (cleft lip and/or cleft palate, external ear abnormalities, abnormally small eyes and chin, and slight underdevelopment of the mid-facial area).[3] In addition to birth defects, miscarriages coinciding with an episode of fever have also been documented.

In most cases where a birth defect has been reported, the source of the hyperthermia was fever, usually over several days but always lasting at least one day. According to one researcher, brief episodes of high fever are not sufficient to produce permanent damage.[4]

If fever were a major cause of malformations, we could expect short-term epidemics of hyperthermia-related birth defects associated with the flu and its fevers. But there is no evidence of this. Some experts have rejected fever as an independent cause of birth defects. This is because it is so difficult to separate the fever from the illness that causes it, especially since some illnesses (rubella infection, for example) are themselves teratogenic.

In a few instances the source of maternal hyperthermia has been prolonged use of a hot tub (Jacuzzi) or sauna. An investigation was undertaken in Finland to examine further the customary habit of sauna bathing. It found that sauna bathing during pregnancy did not influence the rate of facial clefts or CNS defects. In fact, in Finland, CNS defects are among the lowest reported in the world. I suppose it is possible that this population is genetically less susceptible to hyperthermia-induced birth defects (see the First Principle of Teratology, page 33), but this concept has not been explored.

Even the most theoretical risk warrants a better-safe-than-sorry approach. An attempt to establish "safe" limits to hot tub and sauna bathing discovered that it took fifteen minutes to raise body temperature to 102° in a hot tub of 102° and ten minutes in a hot tub of 106°.[5] This experiment required all subjects (none of them pregnant) to keep all of the body except the head immersed for the entire time. Normally in a hot tub people expose a portion of their bodies, which slows heating. This same study

---

*The term *gestation* often is used to describe the time from the first day of the last menstrual period to birth, rather than the period from conception to birth.

found that it was too uncomfortable for women to remain in a sauna of 178° long enough to raise their body temperature to 102°. Conservatively, then, use of a hot tub or sauna should be limited to ten minutes, preferably with the temperature considerably below 102°.

Women who train to run marathons competitively need to know that this activity can raise body temperature into the "high fever" range. Since a marathon is twenty-six miles, its effect on the body is very different from that of recreational running or jogging. The actual effects of exercise-induced hyperthermia during pregnancy have not been studied (see exercise, page 159).

In summary, hyperthermia is a proven cause of malformation in laboratory animals. But these results cannot be directly applied to human situations because pregnant women are not subjected to the conditions used in animal studies. In humans, there is no consensus among experts on the teratogenicity of hyperthermia. Despite several reports of hyperthermia in mothers with malformed children, there is no actual proof of cause-and-effect. So until more evidence becomes available, pregnant women should avoid situations that could cause hyperthermia. Although a fever cannot be avoided, it should be treated, preferably under a physician's care. There is no evidence that very hot baths and showers are risky. But avoiding this practice, particularly during the early weeks of pregnancy, might be the safest approach.

References

[1] D. W. Smith, *Recognizable Patterns of Human Malformation* (Philadelphia: W. B. Saunders, 1982), p. 418.

[2] J. Warkany, Teratogen update: Hyperthermia, *Teratology* 33 (1986): 365–71.

[3] H. Pleet, J. M. Graham, and D. W. Smith, Central nervous system and facial defects associated with maternal hyperthermia at 4 to 14 weeks gestation, *Pediatrics* 61 (1981): 785–89.

[4] S. K. Clarren, D. W. Smith, M. A. S. Harvey, and R. H. Ward, Hyperthermia—A prospective evaluation of a possible teratogenic agent in man, *Journal of Pediatrics* 95 (1979): 81–82.

[5] M. A. S. Harvey, M. M. McRosie, and D. W. Smith, Suggested limits to the use of hot tub and sauna by pregnant women, *CMA Journal* 125 (1981): 50–53.

COMMON NAME: **INFLUENZA (the "FLU")**

Brand Name/Chemical Name: **not applicable**

FDA Pregnancy Category: not applicable

ESTIMATED RISK SUMMARY:
   Time of Exposure throughout pregnancy

Risk No known risk*
Pregnancy Outcome appears favorable
Documentation inconclusive

← pre-conception	All or None		Organ Development – (in weeks)						Maturation – (in weeks)				
	1	2	3	4	5	6	7	8	9	10	12	20-36	38

conception   ←—Time of Greatest Risk—→   birth

Influenza[1] infection, commonly referred to as the "flu," is an illness caused by a number of different viruses.

Some researchers have considered influenza as a possible cause of birth defects, but the evidence is confusing and inconclusive. One problem is the difficulty of using mothers' recollections to verify that the illness did actually occur. In fact, one study showed that 60 percent of women stating they did not have the flu had been recently infected, and 35 percent of those lacking evidence of infection stated that they did have the flu.[2] In addition, mothers of children with abnormalities recall events more readily than do mothers of normal children. The result is an increased likelihood of associating birth defects with an event during pregnancy, in this case—the flu.

Some investigations have raised the question of influenza-related neural tube defects (anencephaly and spina bifida). Studies specifically focusing on this issue have produced conflicting results, the majority failing to demonstrate a causal relationship. Nevertheless, one possible explanation for the reported defects should be considered—fever.

Fever (hyperthermia) frequently accompanies the flu. Studies, primarily with laboratory animals, have shown that elevated body temperature during the time of neural tube formation causes defective development (see hyperthermia, page 197).

In summary:

The abnormalities described and the frequency with which they have been reported are not sufficient to link influenza infection during pregnancy with an increase in abnormal births.

High fever as a cause of birth defects in human pregnancy is suspected but not proven.

*above the 4% background risk

To reduce the likelihood of contracting the flu, pregnant women may wish to avoid crowded areas during an influenza outbreak (see also influenza vaccine, page 202).

References:

[1]J. S. Remington and J. O. Klein (eds.), *Infectious Diseases of the Fetus and Newborn Infant* (2d ed.) (Philadelphia: W. B. Saunders, 1983), pp. 547–49.

[2]M. G. Wilson and A. M. Stein, Teratogenic effects of Asian influenza, *Journal of the American Medical Association* 210(1969): 336.

GENERIC NAME: **INFLUENZA VACCINE**

Brand Names: **(Influenza Virus Vaccine, Trivalent, Types A & B, Fluogen, Fluzone)**

FDA Pregnancy Category: C

ESTIMATED RISK SUMMARY

Time of Exposure throughout pregnancy

Risk No known risk*

Pregnancy Outcome appears favorable

Documentation inconclusive

pre-conception	All or None		Organ Development – (in weeks)						Maturation – (in weeks)				
	1	2	3	4	5	6	7	8	9	10	12	20-36	38

conception   ←— Time of Greatest Risk —→   birth

Influenza vaccine[1] provides protection against contracting influenza infection, commonly referred to as the "flu" (see influenza, page 200). Under ordinary circumstances pregnancy is not a routine indication for vaccination against the flu, though influenza vaccine is generally considered to be safe for pregnant women. Despite this, if you are going to be vaccinated while pregnant, postponing vaccination until after the first trimester is recommended.

Reference:

[1]Centers for Disease Control, Prevention and control of influenza. Recommendation of the immunization practices advisory committee. *Annals of Internal Medicine* 103 (1985): 560–65.

*above the 4% background risk

MEDICATION CLASSIFICATION: **IODINE (or IODIDE)**

GENERIC NAMES: **HYDRIODIC ACID, IODINE, IODINATED GLYCEROL, POTASSIUM IODIDE, POVIDONE-IODINE, SODIUM IODIDE**

Brand Names: **(ACU-dyne, Betadine, Biodine Topical, Efodine, Hydriodic Acid, Iodex Regular, Iodine Tincture, Iodo-Niacin, Iodopen, Isodine, Pharmadine, Pima, Polydine, Povadyne, Operand, Organidin, Sepp Antiseptic, SSKI)**

FDA Pregnancy Category: C and D (Iodinated Glycerol: X)

ESTIMATED RISK SUMMARY:
Excess Iodine
Time of Exposure potentially from 10 weeks on
Risk Known, related to duration and dose*
Pregnancy Outcome adverse
Documentation conclusive, based on current knowledge

Severe Iodine Deficiency
Time of Exposure during the first third to half of pregnancy
Risk Known risk*
Pregnancy Outcome adverse
Documentation conclusive, based on current knowledge

pre-conception	All or None		Organ Development – (in weeks)						Maturation – (in weeks)				
	1	2	3	4	5	6	7	8	9	10	12	20-36	38

conception   ←—Time of Greatest Risk—→   birth

Iodine or *iodide*,[1] as it is also called, is a mineral that concentrates in the thyroid gland. Either too much of it or too little can impair normal thyroid functioning. Without sufficient thyroid hormone, the fetus cannot develop normally, suffering mental and physical retardations.

Iodine does cross the placenta.

*above the 4% background risk

Severe iodine deficiency during pregnancy is teratogenic. In affected children, it retards physical and mental development (cretinism), enlarges the thyroid (goiter), and decreases the functioning of the thyroid gland (hypothyroidism).[2] Today in the United States there is little concern for iodine deficiency. Our food, such as iodized salt, supplies an adequate amount. But in isolated parts of the world (areas of New Guinea, the Himalayas, and the Andes), severe iodine intake deficiency still exists. Various sources of iodine can be administered prior to pregnancy, thus completely preventing the disabling effects of fetal iodine deficiency.

Excess iodine intake during pregnancy, for prolonged periods of time or near the time of delivery, can contribute to the formation of goiter and hypothyroidism in the newborn. How much iodine is needed to produce these complications in babies is not known. Fortunately, hypothyroidism, which can interfere with development of the brain, can easily be detected in the newborn, through a simple blood test. Once detected, the condition can be treated. Routine screening of newborns for hypothyroidism is now required by many states.

Excess iodine intake is not known to interfere with development of the unborn baby's thyroid gland until it begins to function, at about ten weeks. After this time the gland takes up increasing amounts of iodine.

There are many sources of iodine. Dairy products, meat, poultry, fish, and grains contribute significantly to our dietary intake of iodine, as does iodized salt. Many prescription and nonprescription drugs are also sources of iodine. Various **vitamin** and **mineral pills** contain the recommended dietary allowance (RDA) of iodine. **Topical antiseptics** often contain betadine (providone-iodine). **Iodine crystals** and **tablets** (tetraglycine hydroperiodide) containing high doses of the mineral are used by campers for water purification. Just to be on the safe side, you should probably avoid using these iodine-containing products during pregnancy (excluding the dietary sources), particularly after your tenth week. However, if you have used any of these products, not realizing you were pregnant, very minimal exposures would not be expected to increase your risk. Please remember that in order to assess fully any potential risks, you must consult your health care provider and possibly someone who specializes in this area.

Many **vaginal douche products** contain iodine, and this mineral is rapidly absorbed into your bloodstream through the vagina. Chronic use can result in persistent and often high blood levels of iodine. For this reason, such products should be avoided during pregnancy. Certain **expectorants** and **bronchodilators** used to control asthma also contain iodine. If you use these, it's a good idea to check with your doctor about their safety during pregnancy.

The recommended dietary allowance during pregnancy for iodine is 175 micrograms.

But most people's diets contain four to six times that amount. The upper safe limit is not precisely known, especially over the long term. However, 2,000 micrograms per day is considered safe for nonpregnant adults with no health problems.[1]

References:

[1]P. S. Mehta, S. J. Mehta, and H. Vorherr, Congenital Iodide goiter and hypothyroidism: A review, *Obstetrical and Gynecological Survey* 38 (1983): 237–47.

[2]J. Warkany, Teratogen update: Iodine deficiency, *Teratology* 31 (1985): 309–11.

GENERIC NAME: **ISONIAZID**

Brand Names: **(Laniazid, Teebaconin, Nydrazid)**

FDA Pregnancy Category:—

ESTIMATED RISK SUMMARY:
   Time of Exposure throughout pregnancy
   Risk No known risk*
   Pregnancy Outcome appears favorable
   Documentation inconclusive

← pre- conception →		All or None		Organ Development – (in weeks)						Maturation – (in weeks)				
		1	2	3	4	5	6	7	8	9	10	12	20–36	38

conception ◄——Time of Greatest Risk——► birth

Isoniazid is the most widely used agent for the treatment of tuberculosis during pregnancy.

An extensive review of the medical literature on pregnant women treated with various antitubercular medications was conducted in an effort to discover the effect of these drugs on the developing baby.[1] The investigators located information on the pregnancies of 2,787 women and found that 94 percent of them had full-term infants who appeared normal at birth. Approximately 3 percent of the pregnancies resulted in miscarriages, stillbirths, or premature births, while 2.89% resulted in birth defects. The reported frequency of problems is within the expected range. As abnormalities are likely

*above the expected 4% background risk

to be overrepresented in the literature, the small incidence of adverse pregnancy outcomes is particularly reassuring.

In this literature review, isoniazid was *not* identified as a teratogen. Of 1,480 reported isoniazid exposures before birth, there were 1,417 normal term infants (95.7%), 5 miscarriages (0.3%), 9 stillbirths (0.6%), 27 premature births (1.8%), and 16 birth defects (1%) varying from very minor to major in a couple of cases. While the percentage of malformations was well within the expected incidence, several of the reported defects did involve the central nervous system.

In some adults, high doses of isoniazid have been associated with a deficiency in vitamin B_6 (pyridoxine). In order to avoid this possibility, one expert has recommended that pregnant women using isoniazid also take vitamin B_6.[2]

Investigations into the long-term effects of this agent have not commented on an increase in developmental problems. However, one case of cancer (malignant mesothelioma) has been reported—that of a 9-year-old whose mother took isoniazid during pregnancy.[3] This appears to be an isolated instance, as cancer was not observed in a study on isoniazid therapy that followed 660 children to age 16.[4]

References:

[1]D. E. Snider, P. M. Layde, M. W. Johnson, and M. A. Lyle, Treatment of tuberculosis during pregnancy, *American Review of Respiratory Diseases* 122 (1980): 65–79.

[2]P. Monnet, J. C. L. Kalb, and M. Pujol, Doit-on craindre une influence teratogene eventuelle de l'isoniazide? *Revue de la Tuberculose* 31 (1967): 845–48.

[3]K. J. Tuman, R. R. Chilcote, R. I. Gerkow, and J. W. Moohr, Mesothelioma in a child with prenatal exposure to isoniazid, *Lancet* 2 (1980): 362.

[4]D. C. Hammond, I. J. Silidoff, and E. H. Robitzek, Isoniazid therapy in relation to later occurrence of cancer in adults and in infants, *British Medical Journal* 2 (1967): 792–95.

GENERIC NAME: **ISOTRETINOIN**

Brand name: **(Accutane)**

FDA Pregnancy Category: X

ESTIMATED RISK SUMMARY:

> *Time of Exposure* not known for certain, most exposures are confined to the first 10 weeks, critical period appears to be 2–5 weeks after conception
>
> *Risk* Known risk*
>
> *Pregnancy Outcome* adverse
>
> *Documentation* conclusive, based on current knowledge

*above the 4% background risk

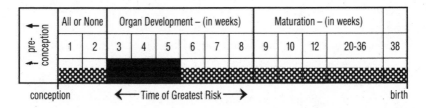

pre-conception	All or None		Organ Development – (in weeks)						Maturation – (in weeks)				
	1	2	3	4	5	6	7	8	9	10	12	20-36	38

conception   ←— Time of Greatest Risk —→   birth

Isotretinoin[1] is a vitamin A derivative used to treat a very severe form of acne (see vitamin A, page 341). In high doses, vitamin A derivatives, including vitamin A itself, have long been known to be teratogens in animals. The premarketing studies conducted on isotretinoin with pregnant rodents confirmed that isotretinoin, too, caused birth defects in animals. These findings led the drug company to release isotretinoin with a warning, contraindicating its use during pregnancy. Despite these warnings, accidental exposures to isotretinoin occurred. In August 1983, less than one year after the drug's release, the FDA reported its suspected teratogenicity in humans.[2]

Isotretinoin, like vitamin A, is fat soluble. This means that such products are not readily excreted from your system and instead are stored in your body fat. Isotretinoin remains in the body for about five days, but the effects of this drug are thought to persist beyond the time it takes to clear them from the system. This is why it's best to wait at least one month after you discontinue the drug before becoming pregnant.

Isotretinoin appears to be most harmful to the unborn during early pregnancy. Initial evidence revealed that all the exposures occurred during the first ten weeks of pregnancy.[3] Further information from a small "semi-prospective" study indicates that the critical period for malformation could be between two to five weeks after conception[1] although it is important to understand that this is not exact. Also of interest are three isotretinoin-related birth defects linked to exposures which occurred during the first two weeks of pregnancy. This might mean that the usual "all or none" time of lethal damage or no effect might not apply to isotretinoin exposures. (See Chapter 3: How Substances Cause Birth Defects, page 34.) For this reason, women who discontinue using isotretinoin during the first two-weeks post conception might still be at risk.

Major malformations associated with isotretinoin are generally confined to the brain, the ears, the heart, and the thymus. In addition to defects involving these organs, blindness and facial peculiarities have also been reported. How often all of these problems occur in relation to a prenatal isotretinoin exposure can only be guessed. One report estimated the relative risk for birth defects from this drug to be 25.6%.[3]

There has been an isolated report of a child with reduction abnormalities of both arms and both legs.[4] Because other problems of this nature have not been observed, it is not at all clear that the limb defects were caused by isotretinoin. Also, another medical explanation for this child's birth defects has been offered.[5]

In addition to causing birth defects, isotretinoin has been held responsible for a number of miscarriages. The risk of such occurrences has not been established, but it is expected to be high. The frequency of miscarriages attributable to isotretinoin, or any drug for that matter, is difficult to determine accurately. This is because miscarriages are fairly common and some of them are early enough to be confused with a late period.

Further research is required before more specific information is known. But it is hoped that pregnant women will heed the warnings issued with this drug and avoid it during pregnancy. If all pregnant women did so, such research might not be necessary.

Follow-up of all isotretinoin-exposed infants, particularly those appearing normal, is very important, since in several cases abnormalities have been found later. Among these infants were three who became blind and one who died unexplainably at 7 weeks of age.

Three unusual defect outcomes with only the father exposed have been reported.[1] Because they were so different, chance probably explains them. It is also reassuring to know that no abnormalities in sperm count, sperm mobility and in the form and structure of the sperm have been reported.[6] At this time, there is no reason to suspect that the use of this drug by men and non-pregnant women will interfere with future reproduction.

In summary: Isotretinoin is a very potent teratogen and its use must be completely avoided during pregnancy. A pregnancy test should be performed within two weeks prior to isotretinoin therapy and a very effective form of contraception should be used while taking it, and for at least one month before and after the course of therapy.

If you accidentally become pregnant while using this drug, you should immediately notify your doctor. While prenatal diagnosis can detect some of the birth defects caused by isotretinoin, the malformations are very severe. For this reason it is best to discuss continuing the pregnancy with your doctor.

Mariessa's Story:

Even though I wasn't planning to become pregnant, I had to have a pregnancy test before my doctor prescribed Accutane to me. My dermatologist explained that the drug that would help heal my acne had caused severe birth defects in children born to mothers who had accidentally continued the drug while pregnant. It made me a little nervous to hear this, not because I was worried about getting pregnant—I was on the Pill and planned to continue while taking Accutane. What I wondered about was the future. After I stopped taking the drug, would my chances of having a normal baby be any different? Could Accutane taken years earlier malform a developing baby?

I posed this question to several experts. They told me that specific research on this issue had not been conducted, but they reassured me that there was no evidence suggesting a risk for future pregnancies.

References:

[1]F. W. Rosa, A. L. Wilk, and F. O. Kelsey, Teratogen update: Vitamin A congeners, *Teratology* 33 (1986): 355–64.

[2]F. W. Rosa, Teratogenicity of isotretinoin, *Lancet* 2 (1983) 513.

[3]E. J. Lammer, D. T. Chen, R. M. Hoar, N. D. Agnish, P. J. Benke, J. T. Braun, C. J. Curry, P. M. Fernhoff, A. W. Grix, I. T. Lott, J. M. Richard, and S. C. Sun, Retinoic acid embryopathy, *New England Journal of Medicine* 313 (1985): 837–41.

[4]W. G. McBride, Limb reduction deformities in child exposed to isotretinoin in utero on gestation days 26–40 only, *Lancet* 1: (1985) 276.

[5]E. J. Lammer, D. B. Flannery, and M. Barr, Does isotretinoin cause limb reduction defects? *Lancet* 2 (1985): 328.

[6]S. B. Millan, F. P. Flowers, and E. F. Sherertz, Isotretinoin, *Southern Medical Journal* 80 (1987): 494–99.

GENERIC NAME: **ISOXSUPRINE**

Brand Names: **(Vasodilan, Voxsuprine)**

FDA Pregnancy Category:—

ESTIMATED RISK SUMMARY:

Time of Exposure throughout pregnancy
Risk Risk assessment for birth defects is not possible
Pregnancy Outcome uncertain
Documentation insufficient

Time of Exposure during labor
Risk Suspected risk* for complications from high doses
Pregnancy Outcome uncertain: favorable and adverse outcomes observed
Documentation inconclusive, based on minimal data

*above the 4% background risk

← pre- conception ←	All or None		Organ Development – (in weeks)						Maturation – (in weeks)				
	1	2	3	4	5	6	7	8	9	10	12	20-36	38

conception   ←— Time of Greatest Risk —→   birth

Isoxsuprine belongs to a group of drugs called vasodilators, which increase blood flow by expanding (dilating) the blood vessels. In addition to this purpose, isoxsuprine has also been used to inhibit premature labor.

Most of the data on isoxsuprine use by pregnant women relates to the prevention of premature labor in the latter part of pregnancy. So, while birth defects have not been reported, there is little experience with use of this drug during organ development (organogenesis). Investigations into the use of isoxsuprine during early pregnancy are required before its teratogenic potential can be determined.

When *high* doses of isoxsuprine are used to delay labor, there can be complications in the newborn child.[1] These include low blood sugar (hypoglycemia), low blood calcium (hypocalcemia), intestinal blockage (ileus), rapid heart rate (tachycardia), low blood pressure (hypotension), and death. Some of these findings were dose related, occurring more often in infants with higher blood concentrations of isoxsuprine. However, some of these children were born prematurely, a fact that itself predisposes an infant to many problems and in some cases, it can lead to death.

Long-term follow-up studies of children exposed before birth have not been located.

Reference:

[1]J. E. Brazy, V. Little, and J. Grimm, Isoxsuprine in the perinatal period. II. Relationships between neonatal symptoms, drug exposure, and drug concentration at the time of birth, *Journal of Pediatrics* 98 (1981) 146–51.

GENERIC NAME: **LABETALOL**

Brand Names: **(Normodyne, Trandate)**

FDA Pregnancy Category: C

ESTIMATED RISK SUMMARY:
   Time of Exposure first 3 months
   Risk Risk assessment is not possible

Pregnancy Outcome uncertain
Documentation insufficient

Time of Exposure last 6 months of pregnancy
Risk No known risk*
Pregnancy Outcome appears favorable
Documentation inconclusive

← pre-conception ←	All or None		Organ Development – (in weeks)						Maturation – (in weeks)				
	1	2	3	4	5	6	7	8	9	10	12	20-36	38

conception   ← Time of Greatest Risk →   birth

Labetalol[1] is classified an alpha/beta-adrenergic blocking agent and is given both by mouth and intravenously (IV) to control high blood pressure (hypertension). This drug has been successfully used during pregnancy with no reported ill effects. However, information relative to the effects of its use during the first three months of pregnancy is lacking

As with other antihypertensive drugs, there have been case reports of slower than normal heartbeat (bradycardia) in infants whose mothers received IV labetalol during pregnancy (see acebutolol, page 50 and atenolol, page 89). However, most newborns prenatally exposed to labetalol show no such effects.

A small number of infants exposed before birth to labetalol were evaluated at 6 months of age. All ten infants appeared normal in terms of both their growth and their development. Unfortunately, long-term follow-up studies of prenatally exposed children have not been located.

Reference:

[1]R. P. Naden and C. W. Redman, Antihypertensive drugs in pregnancy, *Clinics in Perinatology* 12 (1985): 521–38.

MEDICATION CLASSIFICATION: **LAXATIVES**
GENERIC NAMES: **BISACODYL, CASCARA SAGRADA,**

*above the 4% background risk

DANTHRON, DOCUSATE SODIUM, MAGNESIUM HYDROXIDE, MINERAL OIL, PHENOLPHTHALEIN, PSYLLIUM, SENNA

Brand Names: (Akshun, Bu-Lax, Cascara Sagrada, Citroma, Citrate of Magnesia, Colace, Correctol, Danthron, Docusate, Dorbane, Effersyllium Instant Mix, Ex-Lax, Feen-a-Mint, Fiberall, Magnesium Sulfate, Milk of Magnesia, Metamucil, Modane, Neoloid, Perdiem, Purge, Senexon, Senokot, Senolax, Serutan)

FDA Pregnancy Category:—

ESTIMATED RISK SUMMARY:

Time of Exposure short-term use during pregnancy

Risk No known risk* for birth defects

Pregnancy outcome appears favorable

Documentation inconclusive, based on minimal data and clinical experience

Time of Exposure near term

Risk Suspected risk* for castor oil

Pregnancy Outcome uncertain: favorable and adverse outcomes observed

Documentation inconclusive, based on minimal data

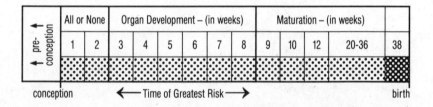

pre-conception	All or None		Organ Development – (in weeks)						Maturation – (in weeks)				
	1	2	3	4	5	6	7	8	9	10	12	20-36	38

conception   ←——Time of Greatest Risk——→   birth

Constipation is not an unusual complaint of pregnancy. This may first arise early in your pregnancy due to increasing levels of the female hormone, progesterone. Iron, an ingredient in prenatal vitamins, can also contribute to this condition. The best way to remedy constipation is to change your diet. For some pregnant women this natural approach might not provide sufficient relief, so the issue of the safety of laxatives[1] becomes a question.

---

*above the 4% background risk

Laxatives are commonly taken by pregnant women, so it is surprising that well-controlled studies of the safety of their use during pregnancy have not been conducted. To my knowledge, none of these products is suspected of increasing the risk for birth defects, but based on how they work, some are better than others for use in pregnancy. (These products are intended for *short-term* use; chronic use can lead to laxative dependency.)

Saline laxatives (Magnesium Sulfate, Milk of Magnesia, Citroma, and Citrate of Magnesia), if not used properly, can lead to sodium retention.

Caster oil should be avoided because it has been suspected of initiating premature labor.

Continued use of lubricants, like **mineral oil**, can interfere with your body's ability to absorb fat-soluble vitamins A, D, E, and K.

Not much is known about the **stimulant laxatives** (Cascara Sagrada, Danthron, Modane, Senexon, Senokot, Ex-Lax, and Correctol), although Cascara Sagrada was taken during the first trimester by fifty-three mothers without apparent adverse effects.[2] This information is reassuring but by no means conclusive. Both Cascara Sagrada and Danthron are also excreted into breast milk and may cause diarrhea in the nursing infant.

Docusate sodium (Bu-Lax, Colace, Docusate) is a stool softener. A large prospective study reported no birth defects in the children of 116 mothers who took this laxative during pregnancy.[2] There are some shortcomings of this investigation, but again, the information is reassuring.

Most sources recommend that **bulk-forming laxatives** (Metamucil, Effer-syllium, Perdeim, Fiberall) are the best products for pregnant women.

Long-term follow-up studies of children exposed before birth have not been located.

Natural Remedies*

Because of changes in your intestinal functioning, you may become constipated during pregnancy. Here are some nonmedicinal methods[3] you may find effective in coping with this problem:

- Drink 6–8 glasses of fluid each day.
- Walk or perform other appropriate exercise every day.
- Eat raw vegetables and cooked fruit.
- Chew your food thoroughly.

---

*None of these commonsense remedies have been medically proven. They are listed here because I have found them useful.

• Don't try to force a bowel movement, but go when you feel the need.
• Relax and avoid straining; putting your feet on a box or footstool may help.
• Very hot or very cold liquids on an empty stomach may encourage bowel movements.

References:

[1]J. H. Lewis and A. B. Weingold, The uses of gastrointestinal drugs during pregnancy and lactation, *American Journal of Gastroenterology* 80 (1985): 912–23.

[2]O. P. Heinonen, D. Slone, and S. Shapiro, *Birth Defects and Drugs in Pregnancy*. (Littleton, Mass.: Publishing Sciences Group, 1977).

[3]The Over-the-Counter-Drug Committee of the Coalition for the Medical Rights of Women, *Safe and Natural Remedies for Discomforts of Pregnancy* (San Francisco, Calif.: January 1981, rev. 1982).

COMMON NAME: **LEAD**

Brand Name/Chemical Name: **not applicable**

FDA Pregnancy Category: not applicable

ESTIMATED RISK SUMMARY:

Time of Exposure throughout pregnancy
Risk Risk assessment is not possible for low-level exposures
Pregnancy Outcome uncertain
Documentation insufficient

Time of Exposure possibly before and throughout pregnancy
Risk Known risk* from very high-level exposures
Pregnancy Outcome adverse
Documentation conclusive, based on current knowledge

← pre-conception	All or None		Organ Development – (in weeks)						Maturation – (in weeks)				
	1	2	3	4	5	6	7	8	9	10	12	20-36	38

conception   ←—Time of Greatest Risk—→   birth

Lead[1] is a heavy, toxic metal. It is present in the environment from many sources, including old house paint, polluted soil and drinking water, and automobile

*above the 4% background risk

emissions. Because lead is involved in manufacturing a variety of products, some people also encounter it in the workplace (see paint, page 254).

Late in the nineteenth century, sterility was often seen in women working in the lead industry, along with menstrual problems and miscarriages. Lead was used as an agent in criminal abortions early in the twentieth century, presenting an added risk to the woman. More recently, high-level lead exposures through accidental intoxication or through contaminated drinking water has been associated with both growth retardation and mental retardation in infants of exposed mothers.

Today, the lead levels in industry are regulated and cases of actual lead intoxication are rare. More commonly, people are exposed to lead through inhalation of "polluted" air. Evidence as to whether these types of low-level lead exposures are teratogenic are less clear.

Studies have attempted to link the lead levels in the blood of newborn babies to an increase in minor birth defects[2] and delayed early development.[3] Whether these problems were due to lead exposure before birth or to other risk factors is difficult to sort out. Another unresolved issue is whether the toxic effects of lead are more dangerous in the early part of pregnancy, or later on.

Long-term follow-up studies of children exposed before birth have not been located.

Because we are all exposed to lead to some extent, the effects of low-level lead exposures are widespread. Further study into their effects on the entire population, including unborn children, is needed.

If you think that your working environment might have unsafe levels of lead in the air, you should ask for proof that health-monitoring codes are being observed. The Occupational Safety and Health Administration (OSHA) may be consulted regarding the recommended safety precautions for working with this metal, though not specifically during pregnancy.

References:

[1]G. B. Gerber, A. Léonard, and P. Jacquet. Toxicity, mutagenicity and teratogenicity of lead, *Mutation Research* 76 (1980): 115–41.

[2]H. L. Needleman, M. Rabinowitz, A. Leviton, S. Linn, and S. Schoenbaum, The relationship between prenatal exposure to lead and congenital anomalies, *Journal of the American Medical Association* 252 (1984): 2956–59.

[3]D. Bellinger, A. Leviton, H. L. Needleman, C. Waternaux, and M. Rabinowitz, Low-level lead exposure and infant development in the first year, *Neurobehavioral Toxicology and Teratology* 8(1986): 151–61.

GENERIC NAME: **LIDOCAINE**

Brand Names: **(BayCaine, Dalcaine, Dilocaine, L-Caine, Lido-ject, Nervocaine, Nulicaine, Octocaine, Ultracaine, Xylocaine)**

FDA Pregnancy Category: B

ESTIMATED RISK SUMMARY:

Time of Exposure throughout pregnancy
Risk Risk assessment for birth defects is not possible
Pregnancy outcome uncertain
Documentation unavailable

Time of Exposure during labor and delivery
Risk No known risk*
Pregnancy Outcome appears favorable
Documentation inconclusive, based on minimal data

← pre-conception	All or None		Organ Development – (in weeks)						Maturation – (in weeks)				
	1	2	3	4	5	6	7	8	9	10	12	20-36	38

conception   ← Time of Greatest Risk →   birth

Lidocaine[1] is used as a local anesthetic and in the treatment of abnormal heartbeat rhythms (arrhythmias). Lidocaine has replaced Novocaine (procaine) as the local anesthetic most often used in dental procedures today. Most of the data on lidocaine use during pregnancy relates to its use as a local anesthetic to relieve pain during labor and delivery. Other drugs used for this purpose can cause the baby's heart rate to slow down (bradycardia). This undesirable side effect can be a particular problem if the delivery is premature or if there have already been signs of fetal distress. However, research has found that only low amounts of lidocaine appear in the blood of the fetus and newborn, which reduces the possibility that it will harm the baby.

There is little documentation of the effects of lidocaine when used during organ development. Investigations into its use during early pregnancy are required before its teratogenic potential can be determined. It is reassuring that despite the drug's widespread use, no anecdotal reports of birth defects resulting from exposure during this vulnerable time have been published.

Long-term follow up studies of children exposed before birth have not been located.

---

*above the 4% background risk

Reference:

[1]H. H. Rotmensch, U. Elkayam, and W. Frishman, Antiarrhythmic drug therapy during pregnancy, *Annals of Internal Medicine* 98 (1983): 487–97.

GENERIC NAME: **LINCOMYCIN**

Brand Name: **(Lincocin)**

FDA Pregnancy Category:—

ESTIMATED RISK SUMMARY:

Time of Exposure throughout pregnancy

Risk Risk assessment is not possible

Pregnancy Outcome uncertain

Documentation insufficient; more studies needed

pre-conception		All or None		Organ Development – (in weeks)						Maturation – (in weeks)				
		1	2	3	4	5	6	7	8	9	10	12	20-36	38

conception　　←—Time of Greatest Risk—→　　birth

Lincomycin is an antibiotic usually reserved for serious infections. To date there is no evidence that birth defects are a risk from its use during pregnancy.[1]

One study evaluated ninety-two children whose mothers received lincomycin during various stages of pregnancy. The children were examined a number of times up to the age of 7½ years and showed no physical or developmental defects.[2]

References:

[1]A. W. Chow and P. J. Jewesson, Pharmacokinetics and safety of antimicrobial agents during pregnancy, *Reviews of Infectious Diseases* 7 (1985): 287–313.

[2]A. Mickal and J. D. Panzer, The safety of lincomycin in pregnancy, *American Journal of Obstetrics and Gynecology* 121 (1975): 1071–74.

GENERIC NAME: **LINDANE**

Brand Names: **(G-well, Kwell, Kwildane, Scabene)**

FDA Pregnancy Category: B

ESTIMATED RISK SUMMARY:

Time of Exposure throughout pregnancy
Risk Risk assessment is not possible
Pregnancy Outcome uncertain
Documentation insufficient

pre-conception	All or None		Organ Development – (in weeks)						Maturation – (in weeks)				
	1	2	3	4	5	6	7	8	9	10	12	20-36	38

conception   ←—Time of Greatest Risk—→   birth

Lindane[1] is used to treat head lice, crab lice, and scabies. Controlled studies evaluating the safe use of lindane during human pregnancy have not been conducted. Pregnant rodents treated with this product have not produced abnormal offspring.

Investigations have found traces of lindane in human placental and fetal tissue, but this does not necessarily mean that it interferes with prenatal development. A comparison of problem pregnancies with normal pregnancies did, however, find higher traces of lindane in the maternal blood and the fetal tissue of spontaneous abortions (miscarriages) and premature deliveries. Whether or not these observations were actually caused by lindane is not known, and further investigation is required.

The manufacturer recommends no more than two treatments during pregnancy, using as little of the product as is necessary. In addition, avoid applying creams, ointments, or oils to treated areas, as they may increase the absorption of lindane. Normally only small amounts of lindane are absorbed through the skin.

Accidental oral ingestion and overexposure from *misusing* lindane have been associated with toxic symptoms, including convulsions. Such observations are the basis for recommending judicious use of this product by pregnant women, infants, and children. Adverse reactions are not expected to occur when lindane is used as directed.

Long-term follow-up studies of children exposed before birth have not been located.

Reference:

[1]Reproductive Toxicology, a medical letter on Environmental Hazards to Reproduction, Lindane, Reproductive Toxicology Center, Washington, D.C. 2(3) (1983): 11–12.

GENERIC NAME: **LITHIUM**

Brand Names: **(Cibalith-S, Eskalith, Lithane, Lithobid, Lithonate, Lithotabs)**

FDA Pregnancy Category: D

ESTIMATED RISK SUMMARY:

Time of Exposure first trimester (primarily 3–8 weeks)
Risk Highly suspected risk* for heart defects
Pregnancy Outcome uncertain: favorable and adverse outcomes observed
Documentation inconclusive

Time of Exposure near the time of delivery
Risk Known risk* for toxicity
Pregnancy Outcome adverse
Documentation conclusive, based on current knowledge

pre-conception	All or None		Organ Development – (in weeks)						Maturation – (in weeks)				
	1	2	3	4	5	6	7	8	9	10	12	20-36	38

conception   ← Time of Greatest Risk →   birth

Lithium is an antipsychotic drug. It is used to treat a specific psychiatric illness called manic-depression, in which the patient alternates episodes of mania (a state of extreme excitement) and depression. Lithium helps prevent the manic phase.

The Register of Lithium Babies (or Lithium Register) has collected retrospective information on 225 infants who were exposed to lithium at least during the first trimester.[1] Among the outcomes were seven reported stillbirths and twenty-five (11.1%) malformed infants. Eight percent of these 225 infants (a total of eighteen children) had heart defects, where the rate expected in the general population is 0.04 percent. Six of the eighteen children with cardiac defects (2.8% of the total) had a very rare heart valve malformation called Ebstein's Anomaly, for which the expected risk is 0.005 percent.

In addition to those recorded by the Lithium Register, other cases of cardiac

---

*above the 4% background risk

defects in lithium-exposed infants (including Ebstein's Anomaly) have also been reported.[2,3,4]

The reliability of the data from the Lithium Register is overshadowed by three factors: the lack of a control population, the likely over-reporting of abnormal children, and, in many cases, the use of other drugs during pregnancy. While definitive conclusions will require more research, the repeated observation of heart defects, particularly the rare Ebstein's Anomaly, appears to be more than coincidental.

The heart develops early in pregnancy, primarily during the third through the eighth week. Therefore, this is the time of greatest risk for injury to the developing heart. Lithium taken in later pregnancy poses no known increased risk for cardiac defects.

Some physicians recommend prenatal examination for Ebstein's Anomaly by means of echocardiography (see fetal echocardiography, page 26). This procedure has been performed as late as the twenty-third week, and has been found effective before twenty weeks gestation.[5] Fetal echocardiography is by no means routinely performed on all women taking lithium during pregnancy. The woman and her physician must carefully consider the value of having this information as late as the second trimester.

Lithium toxicity (poisoning) in the newborn has occurred when the drug is used near term. The symptoms do disappear as lithium is excreted from the infant's system. Lithium toxicity has been characterized by lethargy, decreased muscle tone (hypotonia), poor reflexes, and abnormal heartbeat rhythms (arrhythmias). Thyroid dysfunction has also been observed. While discontinuing the drug before delivery would reduce the likelihood of such adverse effects, the mother's psychiatric condition may worsen. Therefore, the decision to continue or to discontinue lithium before delivery or when labor begins must be made by the physician on an individual basis.

One study followed sixty lithium-exposed children born with no apparent defects. At age 5 or older, the children showed no more physical or mental deficits than did their brothers or sisters who were not exposed.[6] The drawbacks of this study are its small sample size, short follow-up period, and method of data collection (questionnaires completed by the mothers). These make it hard to interpret the study's significance (see retrospective studies, page 43).

A child exposed to lithium throughout the pregnancy was born apparently normal. However, at 1 year of age she showed delayed development. At birth the child exhibited short-lived functional impairment of the heart, kidneys, and muscles.[7]

The American Academy of Pediatrics Committee on Drugs advises, for women trying to become pregnant, that when possible, lithium medication be switched to a less hazardous alternative.[8] It is up to your doctor to determine whether it is appropriate to change your medication and if so, what drug would be best. Because of the suspected risks with lithium use during pregnancy, it is very important to let your doctor know when you become pregnant. Ideally, you should inform your doctor when planning to have a baby.

References:

[1]M. R. Weinstein, Lithium treatment of women during pregnancy and in the post-delivery period, in F. N. Johnson, (ed.), *Handbook of Lithium Therapy* (XXXXX: University Park Press, 1980), pp. 421–32.

[2]J. M. Park, S. Sridaromont, E. O. Ledbetter, and W. M. Terry, Ebstein's Anomaly of the tricuspid valve associated with prenatal exposure to lithium carbonate, *American Journal of Diseases of Children* 134 (1980): 703.

[3]R. G. Arnon, J. Marin-Garcia, and J. N. Peeden, Tricuspid valve regurgitation and lithium carbonate toxicity in a newborn infant, *American Journal of Diseases of Children* 135 (1981): 941–43.

[4]A. Rane, G. Tomson, and B. Bjarke. Effects of maternal lithium therapy in a newborn infant, *Journal of Pediatrics* 93 (1978): 296–97.

[5]L. D. Allan, G. Desai, and M. J. Tynan, Prenatal echocardiographic screening for Ebstein's Anomaly for mothers on lithium therapy, *Lancet* 2 (1982): 875–76.

[6]M. Shou, What happened later to the lithium babies? A follow-up study of the children born without malformations, *Acta Psychiatrica Scandinavica* 54 (1976b): 193–97.

[7]P. Morrell, G. R. Sutherland, P,. K. Buamah, M. Oo, and H. H. Bain, Lithium toxicity in a neonate. Archives of Disease in Childhood 58 (1983): 539–41.

[8]American Academy of Pediatrics, Committee on Drugs, Psychotropic drugs in pregnancy and lactation, *Pediatrics* 69 (1982): 241–44.

COMMON NAME: **MARIJUANA**

Brand name/Chemical Name: **not applicable**

FDA Pregnancy Category: not applicable

ESTIMATED RISK SUMMARY:

Time of Exposure throughout pregnancy

Risk No known risk* for birth defects

Pregnancy Outcome appears favorable

Documentation inconclusive, based on minimal data

Time of Exposure cannot specify (theoretically in the last few months)

Risk Possible risk* for problems in labor, low birth weight, effect on early behavior

Pregnancy Outcome uncertain: favorable and adverse outcomes observed

Documentation inconclusive, based on minimal data

*above the 4% background

← pre-conception		All or None		Organ Development – (in weeks)						Maturation – (in weeks)				
		1	2	3	4	5	6	7	8	9	10	12	20-36	38

conception   ← Time of Greatest Risk →   birth

Marijuana originates from the Indian hemp plant cannabis sativa. "Hash" or hashish is a resin processed from the flowers and top leaves of the plant. The major psychoactive component of marijuana is tetrahydrocannabinol (THC).

According to recent estimates, 10–13 percent of pregnant women use marijuana to some degree. Despite a large number of investigations in recent years into birth defects among the children of marijuana users, the drug's effects on the unborn baby are still uncertain. Factors such as small sample size, socioeconomic status, maternal health factors, the reliability of self-reported drug use, and the use of marijuana in combination with cigarettes and alcohol influence the observed pregnancy outcomes.

One study found that the length of pregnancy was decreased by 0.8 week among women who smoked marijuana on the average of six or more times per week.[1]

Hazardous labor, either prolonged and difficult or unexpectedly quick, has been observed more frequently in women who smoked marijuana at least once a month (most smoked once per week).[2] An increase in meconium passage, which is when the baby has a bowel movement before birth, was observed in this same study. Meconium problems are associated with fetal distress; however, in this study, one less case of meconium would render the observation statistically insignificant. The thirty-five women in this small sample were of lower socioeconomic status and most of them used alcohol and cigarettes—all factors that influence the results. A second study, designed to reproduce these observations, failed to do so.[3] One possible explanation for this is that the women in the second study were of better health and had better living conditions.

In an ongoing prospective investigation, birth weight differences were not observed between infants born to marijuana users and those born to nonusers.[4,5,6] Retrospective studies that observed lower birth weight found that other possible causes, including alcohol consumption, low socioeconomic status, and maternal health factors effectively canceled the importance of the observation.[7] Another retrospective investigation did discover a decrease in birth weight and an increase in premature deliveries. But the differences were seen only among white women who used marijuana regularly during pregnancy (two to three times per month or more, of which about 20% reported daily use).[8] Nonwhite women who also smoked marijuana during pregnancy faced additional risk factors that might have made it difficult to isolate marijuana's effect.

A retrospective study designed to investigate the prenatal effects of *alcohol* found that children born to women who smoked marijuana were five times more likely than those born to nonusers to have features compatible with the fetal alcohol syndrome.[7] The researchers tried to account for various other causes, including drinking. But there is no way to know for certain how possible alcohol consumption by the mother contributed to their observations. Also there is the possibility that marijuana and alcohol interact together in a way that increases the risk to the developing baby. Of interest is one investigator who discovered that marijuana smoking was associated with features of the fetal alcohol syndrome in six infants born to women who denied using alcohol during pregnancy.[9] On the other hand, another study found no overall difference between the number of minor physical abnormalities or fetal alcohol syndrome–type features when the babies of marijuana users were compared to nonusers.[6,8] Case reports of children with birth defects born to women who use many drugs, could not single out marijuana as a cause of birth defects.[10,11]

Differences in neurological behavior, such as increased tremors and altered visual responses, were observed in 60-to-80-hour-old babies who were exposed to marijuana before birth. The differences were less distinguishable by 9 days of age and had disappeared by 30 days.[4,5] These effects were most marked in babies whose mothers were heavy marijuana users (smoked more than six times per week). The abnormal neurological behaviors could be evidence of an immature nervous system or they could be drug withdrawal symptoms.

Infant development tests (Bayley scale) conducted at 6, 12, 18, and 24 months revealed no differences between children born to marijuana users and those born to nonusers.[12] However, these observations must be interpreted cautiously. This is because the tests might not be sensitive enough to detect a subtle problem that might appear later on, perhaps when the children are school age. Long-term follow-up of these children is still needed before the effect of marijuana on the unborn is really known.

References:

[1]P. A. Fried, B. Watkinson and A. Willan, Marijuana use during pregnancy and decreased length of gestation, *American Journal of Obstetrics and Gynecology,* 150 (1984): 23–27.

[2]S. Greenland, K. J. Staisch, N. Brown, and S. J. Gross, The effects of marijuana use during pregnancy I. A preliminary epidemiology study, *American Journal of Obstetrics and Gynecology,* 143 (1982): 408–13.

[3]S. Greenland, K. J. Staisch, N. Brown, and S. J. Gross, Effects of marijuana on human pregnancy, labor, and delivery, *Neurobehavioral Toxocology and Teratology* 4 (1983): 447–50.

[4]P. A. Fried, Marijuana use by pregnant women: Neurobehavioral effects in neonates. *Drug and Alcohol Dependence* 6 (1980): 415–24.

[5]P. A. Fried, Marijuana use by pregnant women and effects on offspring: An update, *Neurobehavioral Toxicology and Teratology* 4 (1982): 451–54.

[6]C. M. O'Connell and P. A. Fried, An investigation of prenatal cannabis exposure and minor physical anomalies in a low risk population, *Neurobehavioral Toxicology and Teratology,* 6 (1984): 345–50.

[7]S. Linn, S. C. Schoenbaum, R. R. Monson, R. Rosner, P. C. Stubblefield, and K. J. Ryan, The association of marijuana use with outcome of pregnancy,*American Journal of Public Health* 73 (1983): 1161–64.

[8]E. E. Hatch and M. B. Bracken, Effect of marijuana use in pregnancy on fetal growth, *American Journal of Epidemiology,* 124 (1986): 986–93.

[9]Q. Qazi, E. Marlane, E. Beller, D. Milman, and W. Crumbleholme, Is marijuana smoking fetotoxic? *Pediatric Research* 16 (1982): 272a.

[10]F. Hecht, R. Beals, M. Lees, H. Jolly, and P. Roberts, Lysergic-acid-diethylamide and cannabis as possible teratogens in man, *Lancet* (2) 577 (1968): 1037.

[11]G. Carakushansky, R. New, and L. Gardner, Lysergide and cannabis as possible teratogens in man, *Lancet* (1) 586 (1969): 150–51.

[12]P. A. Fried, Postnatal consequences of maternal marijuana use, National Institute on Drug Abuse Research Monograph Series (1985), pp. 61–72.

COMMON NAME: **MEASLES (RUBEOLA)**

Brand Name/Chemical Name: not applicable

FDA Pregnancy Category: not applicable

ESTIMATED RISK SUMMARY:
Time of Exposure first trimester
Risk risk assessment for birth defects is not possible
Pregnancy Outcome uncertain
Documentation insufficient

Time of Exposure first trimester, early second trimester, and near term
Risk Suspected risk* premature births, low birth weight, and possibly miscarriages
Pregnancy Outcome uncertain: favorable and adverse outcomes observed
Documentation inconclusive, based on minimal data

Time of Exposure at the time of delivery
Risk Known risk* for infection of the newborn
Pregnancy Outcome adverse
Documentation conclusive, based on current knowledge

*above the 4% background risk

← pre-conception	All or None	Organ Development – (in weeks)						Maturation – (in weeks)				
← pre-conception	1	2	3	4	5	6	7	8	9	10	12	20-36	38

conception   ←—Time of Greatest Risk—→   birth

Measles (rubeola)[1] is a very contagious infection that is highly communicable among children. Today this infection is extremely rare in pregnancy, because most women of childbearing age have either been vaccinated or have had the disease itself.

For this reason, it is difficult to prove definitively whether or not measles is a teratogen. There is some evidence that measles during pregnancy is responsible for an increase in premature births, and low birth weight. There is less certainty that it may cause miscarriages. Occasional instances of abnormalities following measles in pregnancy reveal no specific pattern of birth defects. Such a pattern is usually present if there is a singular cause. In these cases, documentation that the mother had measles and not rubella (a known teratogen) or another illness is often lacking. Studies conducted on pregnant women during various outbreaks of the measles, have failed to demonstrate that having measles increases the risk of birth defects.

Having the measles near the time of delivery can cause infection in the newborn, which can vary from mild illness to fatal disease. It appears that measles in babies born prematurely is more often a life-threatening condition.

Measles can be prevented through the use of the vaccine (see measles vaccine, page 225).

Reference:

[1] J. S. Remington and J. O. Klein (eds.), *Infectious Diseases of the Fetus and Newborn Infant*, 2d ed. (Philadelphia: W. B. Saunders, 1983), pp. 402–15.

GENERIC NAME: **MEASLES VACCINE**

Brand Name: **(Attenuvax)**

FDA Pregnancy Category:—

ESTIMATED RISK SUMMARY:
    Time of Exposure throughout pregnancy
    Risk Risk assessment is not possible

Pregnancy Outcome uncertain
Documentation insufficient

pre-conception	All or None		Organ Development – (in weeks)						Maturation – (in weeks)				
	1	2	3	4	5	6	7	8	9	10	12	20-36	38

conception   ← Time of Greatest Risk →   birth

Measles (rubeola) can be prevented through the use of the vaccine (see measles, page 224). Vaccine control programs directed at preschool and elementary school children have dramatically reduced the prevalence of this disease. *Measles vaccine*[1] contains the live virus, which has been made noninfectious—what is called a live attenuated vaccine. Measles vaccine cannot cause measles. But since it contains a form of the live virus, it should not be used for pregnant women. The only experience with this vaccine in pregnant women is from a study in which seven women receiving it in their eighth month of pregnancy all delivered healthy and apparently normal term babies. Unfortunately, these results offer no clues about the ability of measles vaccine to cause birth defects because exposure to the vaccine took place after the babies' organs were already developed (see the Second Principle of Teratology, page 33).

Reference:

[1] J. S. Remington and J. O. Klein (eds.), *Infectious Diseases of the Fetus and Newborn Infant,* 2d ed. (Philadelphia: W. B. Saunders, 1983), pp. 412–13.

GENERIC NAME: **MECLIZINE**

Brand Names: **(Antivert, Antrizine, Bonine, Dizmiss, Motion Cure, Wehvert)**

FDA Pregnancy Category: B

ESTIMATED RISK SUMMARY:
  Time of Exposure throughout pregnancy
  Risk No known risk*
  Pregnancy Outcome appears favorable
  Documentation inconclusive, based on minimal data

*above the 4% back ground risk

pre-conception	All or None		Organ Development – (in weeks)						Maturation – (in weeks)				
	1	2	3	4	5	6	7	8	9	10	12	20-36	38

conception ← Time of Greatest Risk → birth

Meclizine is used to treat and prevent nausea, vomiting, and the dizziness associated with motion sickness. This drug is similar to buclizine (see page 92) and cyclizine (see page 130).

A variety of case reports, published primarily during the 1960s and early 1970s, present conflicting opinions on the safe use of meclizine during pregnancy. But cause-and-effect is suspected only when individual reports reveal common malformation patterns among similarly exposed infants. Such was not the case here.

Three large studies (two prospective and one retrospective) evaluating meclizine have failed to associate its use during pregnancy with an increase in birth defects. The Collaborative Perinatal Project, a prospective study which evaluated pregnancy outcome in more than 50,000 mother-child pairs exposed to a wide variety of drugs, found no association between meclizine and large categories of major or minor malformations.[1] This study included 1,014 mothers who took meclizine during their first trimester of pregnancy. Another large prospective study that examined the pregnancy outcomes of 613 women who took meclizine as an antinauseant also found no adverse effects from its use.[2] The retrospective investigation compared drug consumption in pregnancies resulting in normal children and in malformed infants.[3] It found that signficantly fewer mothers of children with major malformations took antinausea drugs during their first three months of pregnancy. (Meclizine was the third most commonly consumed antinauseant by women in this study.) While each of these studies suffer from some shortcomings, their similar conclusions combined have more meaning.

Long-term follow-up studies of children exposed before birth have not been located.

References:

[1] O. P. Heinonen, D. Slone, and S. Shapiro, *Birth Defects and Drugs in Pregnancy* (Littleton, Mass.: Publishing Sciences Group, 1977).

[2] L. Milkovich and B. J. Van den Berg, An evaluation of the teratogenicity of certain antinauseant drugs, *American Journal of Obstetrics and Gynecology,* 125 (1976): 244–48.

[3] M. M. Nelson and J. O. Forfar, Associations between drugs administered during pregnancy and congenital abnormalities of the fetus, *British Medical Journal* 1 (1971): 523–27.

GENERIC NAME: **MEPERIDINE**

Brand Names: **(Demerol, Meperidine Hydrochloride, Pethadol)**

FDA Pregnancy Category: C

ESTIMATED RISK SUMMARY:

> *Time of Exposure* throughout most of pregnancy
> *Risk* Risk assessment for birth defects is not possible
> *Pregnancy Outcome* uncertain
> *Documentation* insufficient

> *Time of Exposure* particularly near delivery or during labor
> *Risk* Known risk* (related to dose and duration of the drug)
> *Pregnancy Outcome* adverse
> *Documentation* conclusive, based on current knowledge

← pre-conception ←		All or None		Organ Development – (in weeks)						Maturation – (in weeks)				
		1	2	3	4	5	6	7	8	9	10	12	20-36	38

conception   ←— Time of Greatest Risk —→   birth

Meperidine[1] is a narcotic derivative used to relieve moderate to severe pain. As a narcotic, meperidine can become habit-forming if used for prolonged periods, so the potential for its abuse does exist. Abuse of any narcotic during pregnancy always carries with it the risk of addiction in the mother as well as the unborn baby.

Like other narcotics, meperidine is not suspected of causing physical birth defects, although it is important to recognize that meperidine has not been extensively studied in early pregnancy, when structural development takes place. The majority of the experience with this drug during pregnancy relates to its use during labor and delivery.

The large doses of meperidine used during labor in the past have been associated with breathing difficulty (respiratory depression), low Apgar scores (numerical assessment of infant well-being at birth), and irregular brain waves (electroencephalogram—a method of evaluating the neurological condition) in the newborn. As with all narcotic pain relievers, effects of the drug are related to the dose used and the duration of the exposure. In fact, the results of some of the early studies on meperidine might have

*above the 4% background risk

been influenced by the use of high drug doses (which is no longer practiced) and the combined effects of other drugs administered together with meperidine.

A concern for altered neurobehavioral response in babies from even low-dose meperidine administration during labor has been raised. Observed differences in exposed newborns versus control groups, as measured by performance on the Brazelton Neonatal Behavioral Assessment Scale, were extremely subtle.[1] The influence of such subtle differences in the responses of newborns on later infant development is unknown.

It is reassuring to note the findings of a 1969 prospective study examining causes of brain damage (see prospective studies, page 42). At age 5 years, seventy children exposed before birth to meperidine during delivery were no different from children who had not been so exposed.[2] Evaluations during their third or fourth year of school supported earlier observations. All children were of mature birth weight. No other complications during pregnancy and labor were present, and adjustments were made for socioeconomic differences.

References:

[1]B. R. Kuhnert, P. L. Linn, M. J. Kennard, and P. M. Kuhnert, Effects of low doses of Meperidine on neonatal behavior, *Anesthesia and Analgesia* 64 (1985): 335–42.

[2]C. Buck, R. Gregg, K. Stavraky, et. al., The effect of single prenatal and natal complications upon the development of children of mature birthweight, *Pediatrics* 43 (1969): 942–55.

GENERIC NAME: **MEPROBAMATE**

Brand Names: **(Equanil, Mepriam, Meprospan, Miltown, Neuramate, Sedabamate)**

FDA Pregnancy Category:—

ESTIMATED RISK SUMMARY:

Time of Exposure throughout pregnancy

Risk Risk assessment is not possible

Pregnancy Outcome uncertain

Documentation insufficient

*above the 4% background risk

← pre-conception ←	All or None		Organ Development – (in weeks)						Maturation – (in weeks)				
	1	2	3	4	5	6	7	8	9	10	12	20-36	38

conception   ←—Time of Greatest Risk—→   birth

Meprobamate is used for the management of anxiety disorders or their symptoms.

Meprobamate use during pregnancy is noted in several case reports of children displaying a variety of birth defects.[1,2,3,4,5] Cause and effect cannot be determined by individual case reports, particularly since these defects are totally dissimilar (see case reports, page 44). This lack of recognizable pattern means that one specific cause was probably not responsible.

Large-scale studies investigating the relationship between meprobamate and birth defects have come to varying conclusions. A large retrospective study described an increase in serious birth defects when meprobamate was prescribed during the first forty-two days of gestation.[6] (The term *gestation* often is used to describe the time from the first day of the last menstrual period to birth, as opposed to, from conception to birth. Here the first forty-two days of gestation is equivalent to the first twenty-eight days of pregnancy.) It is interesting that five of the eight children with birth defects had congenital heart disease. However, other potential risk factors were not eliminated and the use of over-the-counter preparations was not assessed.

On the other hand, no increase in the frequency of stillbirths or birth defects was found in an investigation of the children of 735 women treated with meprobamate during pregnancy.[7] A similar result was also observed in a large prospective study in which meprobamate use any time during pregnancy was not associated with an increase in birth defects, death in childhood, or delayed mental development at 4 years of age.[8] Each of these studies has some shortcomings, so the negative findings cannot be interpreted as proof that meprobamate is safe. Similarly, finding an association in this case does not prove that meprobamate actually causes birth defects.

Certainly more information is needed on this drug's effect on a developing baby before any definitive conclusions can be reached. Until such a time, meprobamate should be avoided or used with great care during pregnancy.

Long-term follow-up studies of children exposed before birth have not been located.

References:

[1]C. A. D. Ringrose, The hazard of neurotropic drugs in the fertile years, *Canadian Medical Association Journal* 106 (1972): 1058.

[2]S. Vaage and J. Berezy, Drug-induced abnormalities, *Tidsskrift for den Norske Laegeforen* 18 (1962): 1202.

[3]J. R. Daube and S. M. Chow, Lissencephaly: Two cases, *Neurology* 16 (1966): 179–91.

[4]J. Gauthier, P. Monnet, and B. Salle, Malfaçons type ectromelie. Discussion sur le rôle teratolgene de médications au cours de la grossesse, *Pédiatrie* 20 (1965): 489.

[5]M. J. Adrian, The birth of a monster following ingestion of meprobamate by the mother: Cause or coincidence? *Bulletin de la Fédération des Sociétés de Gynécologie et d'Obstétrique de Langue Française* 15 (1963): 121.

[6]L. Milkovich and B. J. van den Berg, Effects of prenatal meprobamate and chlordiazepoxide hydrochloride on human embryonic and fetal development, *New England Journal of Medicine* 291 (1974): 1268–71.

[7]H. A. Belafsky, S. Breslow, L. M. Hirsch, J. E. Shangold, and M. B. Stahl, Meprobamate during pregnancy, *Obstetrics and Gynecology* 34 (1969): 378–86.

[8]S. C. Hartz, O. P. Heinonen, S. Shapiro, V. Siskind, and D. Slone, Antenatal exposure to meprobamate and chlordiazepoxide in relation to malformations, mental development and childhood mortality, *New England Journal of Medicine* 292 (1975): 726–28.

COMMON NAME: **MERCURY**

Chemical Names: **(elemental mercury, methlymercury)**

FDA Pregnancy Category: not applicable

ESTIMATED RISK SUMMARY:

> *Time of Exposure* throughout pregnancy
> *Risk* Known risk,* particularly for methylmercury
> (related to the dose and duration of the exposure)
> *Pregnancy Outcome* adverse
> *Documentation* conclusive, based on current knowledge

pre-conception	All or None	Organ Development – (in weeks)						Maturation – (in weeks)				
	1	2	3	4	5	6	7	8	9	10	12	20-36	38

conception   ←— Time of Greatest Risk —→   birth

Mercury[1,2,3] is a metallic element, whose most toxic form is the organic compound **methylmercury.** Methylmercury is absorbed through the skin, lungs, stomach, and intestines and it accumulates in body tissues. Pregnant women exposed to

*above the 4% background risk

large amounts of this compound have given birth to abnormal children. Investigations into the teratogenicity of mercury compounds have focused on methylmercury because in several epidemics of mercury poisoning around the world, it has been implicated as a cause of abnormal fetal development.

Methlylmercury-related birth defects were first observed in a small fishing village on Minamata Bay, Japan. The bay had become polluted by industrial wastes discharged by a nearby factory. Between 1953 and 1971, the consumption of contaminated fish resulted in 134 cases (78 adults and 56 children) of methylmercury poisoning and 25 malformed infants.

Damage to the developing baby commonly occurred without evidence of typical symptoms of methylmercury poisoning in the mother. Fetal methylmercury effects include growth deficiency, abnormally small head size (microcephaly), mental retardation, developmental delay, cerebral palsy, deafness, blindness, tremors, seizures, and jerky and involuntary muscle movements. Methlymercury is particularly teratogenic to the developing brain, so a theoretical risk exists for exposures throughout pregnancy.

Cases of fetal poisoning have also been reported elsewhere, the most widespread occurring in Iraq during the early 1970s among people eating bread made from contaminated wheat. This resulted in an epidemic of methylmercury poisoning that killed over 450 people and hospitalized 6,530 others. Ten cases of exposure before birth were associated with mental retardation, low birth weight, cerebral palsy, and decreased muscle tone.

To be on the safe side, women of childbearing age, particularly those who are actually pregnant, should totally avoid occupational exposure to methylmercury. They should also avoid exposure to dangerous amounts of methylmercury through the consumption of commercially caught fish, eating an average of no more than about 350 gm (three-quarters of a pound) per week. It is also wise for pregnant women to avoid eating large amounts of fish caught for sport in mercury-contaminated water, since these might contain higher amounts than are permitted commercially. The 350 gm weekly "limit" represents what is considered to be "reasonably safe" and is not a maximum "no effect" level.[1] Moreover, this amount applies to fish consumption over an indefinite period of time, so if you eat more some weeks, you should eat less during others.

Less toxic than methylmercury is the inorganic compound **elemental mercury**. Elemental mercury can be absorbed through the skin and its vapors are absorbed by the lungs, but the process is very slow. Thermometers contain elemental mercury, and dentists use this substance too.

The recommended safe level in air for elemental mercury vapor is conservatively 0.01 mg per cubic meter for pregnant women and 0.05 mg per cubic meters for all other individuals. (This scientific jargon is required for accuracy. If the language is confusing, ask your doctor for clarification.) Accidental exposure to elemental mercury from a broken thermometer results in almost no exposure, only 0.004 mg to 0.006 mg per cubic meter of mercury vapor is emitted into a room.

Mercury exposures in the dental environment do not increase the number of children born with abnormalities or the rate of miscarriages among women whose husbands are dentists or in women who are directly exposed to it at work.[4] These conclusions were made from a retrospective survey of more than 42,000 dental workers with high (more than forty mercury amalgams per week) or low (zero to forty mercury amalgams per week) exposures to this compound. The information was gathered from mailed questionnaires, so the results reflect the outcome of only those who responded—making it difficult to collect accurate data on who was actually exposed, for how long, and how often. No follow-up on the accuracy of the information was made. Although it is reassuring to know that no obvious problems were noted in this study, its many flaws make the results less meaningful (see retrospective studies, page 43). Well-conducted investigations on occupational expo-sures to elemental mercury and pregnancy outcome have not been located.

Even though there is a distinct margin of safety in the guidelines recommended for mercury, dental personnel should take the necessary precautions to insure that their working environment is free of risk from mercury toxicity. Working with encapsulated mercury, as opposed to using it in the bulk form, is one way to reduce the chances of mercury escaping into the environment.[5]

References:

[1]B. J. Koos and L. D. Longo, Mercury toxicity in the pregnant woman, fetus and newborn infant: A review, *American Journal of Obstetrics and Gynecology* 126 (1976): 390–409.

[2]D. Harris, J. J. Nicols, R. Stark, and K. Hill, The dental working environment and the risk of mercury exposure, *Journal of the American Dental Association* 97 (1978): 811–15.

[3]A. Wannag and J. Skæråsen, Mercury accumulation in placental and foetal membranes: A study of dental workers and their babies, *Environmental Physiology and Biochemistry* 5 (1975): 348–52.

[4]J. B. Brodsky, E. N. Cohen, C. Whitcher, B. W. Brown, and M. L. Wu, Occupational exposure to mercury in dentistry and pregnancy outcome, *Journal of the American Dental Association* 111 (1985): 779–80.

[5]D. Harris, J. J. Nicols, R. Stark, and K. Hill. The dental working environment and the risk of mercury exposure, *Journal of the American Dental Association* 97 (1978): 811–15.

GENERIC NAME: **METHADONE**

Brand Names: **(Dolophine)**

FDA Pregnancy Category: C

ESTIMATED RISK SUMMARY:

Time of Exposure throughout pregnancy
Risk No known risk for birth defects*
Pregnancy Outcome appears favorable
Documentation inconclusive

Time of Exposure consistent doses, primarily in the last trimester and up to
the time of delivery
Risk Known risk* for low birth weight and withdrawal syndrome
Pregnancy Outcome adverse
Documentation conclusive, based on current knowledge

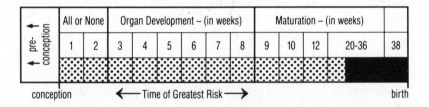

Methadone is a narcotic. It is used to relieve severe pain and also as a substitute
drug for people being detoxified for addictions to other narcotics. The use of
methadone during pregnancy decreases the incidence of problems such as obstetrical
complications, death of the baby just before or after birth, low birth weight, and
prematurity, which are often seen in heroin-addicted pregnancies. Prenatal care and
supervision during pregnancy further reduces the frequency of these problems.

Most treatment programs recommend that women stay on a maintenance dose of
methadone during pregnancy.[1] Dose reduction, if desired, should take place only
during the first two trimesters. Detoxification during the third trimester presents a
significant risk to fetal well-being.

Birth weight below 2,500 gms (5.5 pounds) is observed in approximately 35 percent
of infants born to methadone addicts.[2,3] Methadone-exposed babies also tend to have
smaller head sizes at birth, but examination at 7½ months revealed that head growth
compensated somewhat. This suggests that growth accelerates as withdrawal symptoms
disappear.[4] Similarly, the children of heroin and/or methadone users had subtle
differences in head size at birth, but no differences were seen three or four years later,

*above the 4% background risk

when compared to a matched but drug-free group.[5] The continued use of other drugs during pregnancy, particularly heroin, alcohol, and nicotine, also influences the size of these children at birth.

Birth defects are not reported with an increased frequency in the children of women maintained on methadone.

To date, studies have failed to show any major neurological abnormalities in infants born to either heroine- or methadone-addicted mothers. Most studies examining the behavior of methadone-exposed babies focus on the newborn period. Investigations into later motor and intellectual development are inadequate.[6] Some investigations reveal that methadone-addicted children score lower than comparison groups on infant tests (the Bayley Mental Developmental Index and the Bayley Motor Developmental Index). Still, their scores are often within the normal range.[7] Differences between exposed and nonexposed groups of children are less noticeable as prolonged withdrawal symptoms diminish. Symptoms of attention deficit disorder (also called minimal brain dysfunction), including short attention span, poor coordination, and hyperactivity, have been observed in methadone-addicted children.[8] Long-term follow-up and better controlled studies are needed before the significance of any of these findings are really known.

The onset and severity of withdrawal symptoms, referred to as neonatal abstinence syndrome, varies among individual infants. But 70–90 percent of infants born to narcotic addicts do experience some degree of withdrawal. Neonatal abstinence syndrome is characterized by disturbed nervous system function, which includes irritability, trembling, increased muscle tone, high-pitched crying, weak sucking, and frantic hand-to-mouth movements. Withdrawal symptoms usually appear within twenty-four to seventy-two hours after birth, but 5–10 percent of methadone-addicted infants have delayed symptoms, beginning from 2 to 4 weeks of age. Some infants will continue to display symptoms such as restlessness, tremors, agitation, and sleep disturbances for as long as three to four months after birth.[4] Although infrequent, seizures may accompany withdrawal. Symptoms are milder and occur less frequently in infants born to mothers maintained on less than 20 mg of methadone per day. The use of other narcotic agents at the same time as methadone is related to more severe withdrawal problems.

Reports of sudden infant death syndrome (SIDS) in a small number of infants exposed to methadone and, less frequently, to both methadone and heroin exist, but the relationship between SIDS and infant narcotic addiction remains unclear.[9]

Drug use is just one of a constellation of factors that affects the growth, development, and intellectual performance of the children born to methadone-dependent women. During pregnancy other risk factors include poor maternal health and nutritional habits, lack of prenatal care, obstetric complications (particularly infections), and the concomitant use of other drugs. After birth, the quality of the caretaking environment will ultimately influence the development of these children.

References:

[1] F. P. Zuspan, J. A. Gumpel, A. Mejia-Zelaya, J. Madden, R. Davis, M. Filer, and A. Tiamson, Fetal stress from methadone withdrawal, *American Journal of Obstetrics and Gynecology* 122 (1975): 43–46.

[2] R. G. Newman, S. Bashkow, and D. Calko, Results of 313 consecutive live births of infants delivered to New York City Methadone Maintenance Treatment Program, *American Journal of Obstetrics and Gynecology* 121 (1975): 233–37.

[3] G. Blink, E. Jerez, and R. Wallach, Methadone maintenance, pregnancy and progeny, *Journal of the American Medical Association* 225 (1973): 477–79.

[4] I. J. Chasnoff, R. Hatcher, and W. J. Burns, Early growth patterns of methadone-addicted infants, *American Journal of Diseases of Children* 134 (1980): 1049–51.

[5] M. H. Lifshitz, G. S. Wilson, E, Obrian-Smith, and M. M. Desmond, Factors affecting head growth and intellectual function in children of drug addicts, *Pediatrics* 75 (1985): 269–74.

[6] G. P. Aylward, Methadone outcome studies: Is it more than the methadone? *Journal of Pediatrics* 101 (1982): 214–15.

[7] K. Kaltenbach and L. P. Finnegan, Developmental outcome of children born to methadone maintained women: A review of longitudinal studies, *Neurobehavioral Teratology and Toxicology* 6 (1984): 271–75.

[8] S. L. Hans and J. Marcus, Motoric and attentional behavior in infants of methadone-maintained women, *NIDA Research Monograph* 43 (1983): 287–93.

[9] B. K. Rajegowda, S. R. Kandall, and H. Falciglia, Sudden unexpected death in infants of narcotic-dependent mothers, *Early Human Development* 2/3 (1978): 219–25.

GENERIC NAME: **METHYLDOPA**

Brand name: **(Aldomet)**

FDA Pregnancy Category:—

ESTIMATED RISK SUMMARY:

Time of Exposure before conception and throughout most of pregnancy
Risk No known risk*
Pregnancy Outcome appears favorable
Documentation inconclusive

Time of Exposure near the time of delivery
Risk Possible risk*
Pregnancy outcome uncertain: favorable and adverse outcomes observed
Documentation inconclusive, based on minimal data

*above the expected 4% background risk

pre-conception ← conception	All or None	Organ Development – (in weeks)						Maturation – (in weeks)				
	1	2	3	4	5	6	7	8	9	10	12	20-36	38

conception   ← Time of Greatest Risk →   birth

Methyldopa[1] is an antihypertensive—a drug used to treat high blood pressure (hypertension). Methyldopa has been more extensively studied than any other antihypertensive agent used by pregnant women. Many scientific sources consider it to be the drug of choice for long-term treatment of hypertension during pregnancy. Studies have revealed fewer miscarriages, a slight increase in birth weight over other babies born to hypertensive mothers, and a reduction in premature births in children born to mothers who have taken it. To date, an increased frequency of birth defects has not been reported from its use during pregnancy.

One study presented a questionable association between fetal growth retardation and the use of methyldopa during pregnancy. The study concluded that this finding could be a result of severe chronic maternal hypertension or perhaps the drug itself.[2]

Some studies have found a mild but temporary reduction in a newborn baby's blood pressure when methyldopa was used close to delivery, but this was not considered significant.

One study associated methyldopa taken during the sixteenth to twentieth weeks of pregnancy with slightly reduced head size in the infants. However, by age 4, the children exhibited normal physical and mental characteristics.[3]

References:

[1] A. L. Wilson and G. R. Matzke, The treatment of hypertension in pregnancy. *Drug Intelligence and Clinical Pharmacy* 15 (1981): 21–26.

[2] W. C. Mabie, M. L. Pernoll, and M. K. Biswas, Chronic hypertension in pregnancy, *Obstetrics and Gynecology* 67 (1986): 197–205.

[3] J. Cockburn, M. Ounsted, V.A. Moar, and C. W. G. Redman, Final report of study on hypertention during pregnancy: The effects of specific treatment on the growth and development of the children, *Lancet* 1 (1982): 647–49.

GENERIC NAME: **METOPROLOL**

Brand Name: **(Lopressor)**

FDA Pregnancy Category: C

ESTIMATED RISK SUMMARY
  Time of Exposure first 3 months
  Risk Risk assessment is not possible
  Pregnancy Outcome uncertain
  Documentation insufficient

  Time of Exposure last 6 months of pregnancy
  Risk No known risk*
  Pregnancy Outcome appears favorable
  Documentation inconclusive

pre-conception	All or None		Organ Development – (in weeks)						Maturation – (in weeks)				
	1	2	3	4	5	6	7	8	9	10	12	20-36	38

conception   ⟵ Time of Greatest Risk ⟶   birth

Metoprolol belongs to a group of drugs that are classified as beta-adrenergic blocking agents (beta blockers). It is used to treat high blood pressure (hypertension) and rapid heart rate (tachycardia). Metoprolol has been successfully used during pregnancy with no reported ill effects. However, information relative to the effects of its use during the first three months of pregnancy is lacking.

In comparison to hydralazine, another antihypertensive drug, metoprolol-exposed babies were less likely to be growth-retarded and fewer of them died in the period shortly before and after birth.[1]

While metoprolol has not been associated with slower than normal heartbeat (bradycardia) and/or low blood pressure (hypotension) in newborn babies; such effects have been reported with other beta-blocking agents. (see acebutolol, page 51, and atenolol, page 89). For this reason, prenatally exposed newborns should be observed for a couple of days for any evidence of these symptoms.

Long-term follow-up studies of children exposed before birth have not been located.

Reference:

[1]B. Sandstrom, Antihypertensive treatment with the adrenergic beta-receptor blocker metoprolol during pregnancy, *Gynecolic Investigations* 9 (1978): 195–204.

*above the 4% background risk

GENERIC NAME: **METRONIDAZOLE**

Brand Names: **(Flagyl, Metryl, Protostat, Sātric)**

FDA Pregnancy Category:—

ESTIMATED RISK SUMMARY:
   Time of Exposure throughout pregnancy
   Risk No known risk*
   Pregnancy Outcome appears favorable
   Documentation inconclusive

pre-conception	All or None		Organ Development – (in weeks)						Maturation – (in weeks)				
	1	2	3	4	5	6	7	8	9	10	12	20-36	38

conception   ←— Time of Greatest Risk —→   birth

Metronidazole is an anti-infective drug used to treat amoebic dysentery, trichomoniasis ("trich," a vaginal infection caused by the protozoan *Trichomonas vaginalis*), and certain vaginal and other bacterial infections (including those caused by *Hemophilus vaginalis*).

Five prospective studies examining the potential teratogenicity of metronidazole in 1,344 pregnancies treated for trichomoniasis have failed to demonstrate an increased risk for adverse pregnancy outcome, in terms of birth weight, premature birth, newborn deaths, malformations and Apgar scores (a numerical rating of the condition of the newborn).[1,2,3,4,5] In several cases patients received multiple courses of drug therapy; single-dose treatment was not evaluated.

Information on exposure times was available for 1,231 pregnant women, of whom 135 took the drug in the first trimester. Information on infant well-being was gathered in the best way possible—through clinical examinations rather than hospital records. Among the abnormalities observed, no specific type of defect or pattern of abnormality was identified, which means they probably weren't the result of a single cause. Most importantly, the time of exposure did not correspond with the described defects (see Second Principle of Teratology, page 33).

Two isolated cases of midline facial defects were reported in unrelated children

*above the 4% background risk

after metronidazole exposure during the first trimester.[6] The lack of any other corroborative data makes it impossible to determine cause-and-effect.

Animal studies evaluating *chronic* (not therapeutic) use of metronidazole found that it causes mutations in bacteria, and tumors and cancers in mice and rats. These results have caused great confusion over the drug's potential dangers to humans. Fortunately, human investigations on metronidazole use have failed to demonstrate a significant increased risk of cancer,[7,8] chromosomal defects,[8] or malformations in exposed children. [1-5] Despite the lack of evidence that metronidazole actually causes an increase in the frequency of birth defects, most still believe it prudent to defer treatment until after the first trimester of pregnancy.

Long-term follow-up studies of children exposed before birth have not been located.

References:

[1]S. C. Robinson and G. Mirchandani, Trichomona vaginalis. V. Further observations on metronidazole (Flagyl) (including infant follow-up), *American Journal of Obstetrics and Gynecology* 93 (1965): 502–5.
[2]W. F. Peterson, J. E. Stauch, and C. D. Ryder, Metronidazole in pregnancy, *American Journal of Obstetrics and Gynecology* 94 (1966): 343–49.
[3]I. Morgan, Metronidazole treatment in pregnancy, *International Journal of Obstetrics and Gynecology* 15 (1978):501–2.
[4]G. Pearl, Metronidazole treatment of trichomoniasis in pregnancy, *Obstetrics and Gynecology* 25 (1965): 273–76.
[5]R. X. Sands, Pregnancy, trichomoniasis and metronidazole, *American Journal of Obstetrics and Gynecology* 94 (1966): 350–53.
[6]J. M. Cantú and D. Garcia-Cruz, Midline facial defect as a teratogenic effect of metronidazole, *Birth Defects*, Original article series, 18 (1982): 85–88.
[7]C. M. Beard, K. L. Noller, W. M. O'Fallon, L. T. Kurland, and M. B. Dockerty, Lack of evidence for cancer due to use of metronidazole, *New England Journal of Medicine* 301 (1979): 519–22.
[8]G. D. Friedman and H. K. Ury, The initial screening for carcinogenicity of 53 commonly used drugs, *National Cancer Institute* 65 (1980): 723–31.

GENERIC NAME: **MICONAZOLE**

Brand Names: **(Monistat, Monistat 3, Monistat 7, Monistat-Derm, Micatin)**

FDA Pregnancy Category:—

ESTIMATED RISK SUMMARY:
 Time of Exposure throughout pregnancy
 Risk No known risk* for topical use
 Pregnancy Outcome appears favorable
 Documentation inconclusive, based on minimal data

*above the 4% background risk

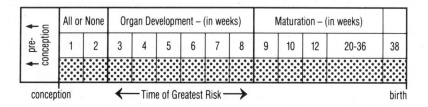

		All or None	Organ Development – (in weeks)						Maturation – (in weeks)				
pre-conception	1	2	3	4	5	6	7	8	9	10	12	20-36	38

conception ←—Time of Greatest Risk—→ birth

Miconazole is an antibiotic used to treat moniliasis, a fungal or "yeast" infection of the vagina. The infection is sometimes called candida, after the fungus *Candida albicans.*

Studies monitoring the topical use of this drug by pregnant women have not observed any birth defects caused by it.[1,2] A recent retrospective study raised some question about miconazole-related spontaneous abortions (miscarriages).[3] The authors cautioned that these results should not be interpreted as definitive, but rather they signal the need for further investigation. No investigations into the intravenous use of this drug by pregnant women have been conducted.

Long-term follow-up studies of children exposed before birth have not been located.

References:

[1]J. E. Davis, J. H. Frudenfeld, and J. L. Goddard, Comparative evaluation of Monistat and Mycostatin in the treatment of vulvovaginal candidiasis, *Obstetrics and Gynecology* 44 (1974): 403–6.

[2]H. C. S. Wallenburg and J. W. Wladimiroff, Recurrence of vulvovaginal candidiasis during pregnancy: Comparison of miconazole vs. nystatin treatment, *Obstetrics and Gynecology* 48 (1976): 491–94.

[3]F. W. Rosa, C. Baum, and M. Shaw, Pregnancy outcomes after first trimester vaginitis drug therapy, *Obstetrics and Gynecology* 69 (1987): 751–755.

COMMON NAME: **MICROWAVES**

Brand Name/Chemical Name: **not applicable**

FDA Pregnancy Category: not applicable

ESTIMATED RISK SUMMARY:

Time of Exposure throughout pregnancy

Risk No known risk*

Pregnancy Outcome appears favorable

Documentation inconclusive

*above the 4% background risk

← pre-conception ←	All or None		Organ Development – (in weeks)						Maturation – (in weeks)				
	1	2	3	4	5	6	7	8	9	10	12	20-36	38

conception   ←—Time of Greatest Risk—→   birth

Microwaves[1] are long electromagnetic waves that do not produce ionizing radiation (X rays). (See X rays, page 347.)

Exposure to microwaves from a microwave oven has not been studied for its effect on an unborn baby. However, unless you bypass several safety systems, there is really no way to be exposed to microwaves from a microwave oven. It is theoretically possible to be exposed by direct contact with a leaking oven door. But the dose could not even be measured unless the contact were maintained for several hours. Even if your microwave oven did leak, microwaves dissipate over a fairly short distance, so staying away from the oven would probably eliminate any possible exposure.

In general, it's probably a good practice to walk away from the oven while cooking. I should probably take my own advice here, since I tend to stare into the microwave oven when I'm melting butter, in an attempt not to overdo it! In short, commonsense precautions will protect you from even a remote risk of exposure.

Reference:

[1] R. L. Brent, The effects of embryonic and fetal exposure to X-Ray, microwaves and ultrasound, *Clinical Obstetrics and Gynecology* 26 (1983): 484–510.

MEDICATION CLASSIFICATION: **MINERALS**

GENERIC NAMES: **CALCIUM, COPPER, IODINE** (separate entry), **IRON, MAGNESIUM, PHOSPHORUS, ZINC, FLUORIDE**

Brand Names: **various**

FDA Pregnancy Category:—

ESTIMATED RISK SUMMARY:

  Time of Exposure throughout pregnancy

  Risk No measurable risk* when doses are within the RDA

*above the 4% background risk

Pregnancy Outcome favorable
Documentation conclusive, based on current knowledge

pre-conception	All or None		Organ Development – (in weeks)						Maturation – (in weeks)				
	1	2	3	4	5	6	7	8	9	10	12	20-36	38
	o o o	o o o	o o o	o o o	o o o	o o o	o o o	o o o	o o o	o o o	o o o	o o o o o o	o o
	o o o	o o o	o o o	o o o	o o o	o o o	o o o	o o o	o o o	o o o	o o o	o o o o o o	o o
	o o o	o o o	o o o	o o o	o o o	o o o	o o o	o o o	o o o	o o o	o o o	o o o o o o	o o

conception   ←—Time of Greatest Risk—→   birth

Minerals[1] are elements necessary in small or trace amounts for good metabolism. An unborn baby requires a steady supply of these, along with vitamins, for its optimal growth and development.

Calcium

The recommended dietary allowance (RDA) for calcium during pregnancy is 1,200 mg. per day for women 19 and older, and 1,600 mg. for those 18 and younger. Calcium is the main component of bone and teeth, and is particularly needed in pregnancy during the third trimester. However, the pregnant woman should begin storing this mineral in her body early in the pregnancy, both for use by the developing child and for nursing later. The principal source of calcium is dairy products. Women who take adequate amounts of these (one quart of milk = 1,200 mg. of calcium) might not need calcium supplements. Other sources of calcium include sardines and salmon (with the bones), and green vegetables, such as cabbage, bok choy, and broccoli.

Copper

The RDA is 2 mg. daily; additional supplements are usually not required during pregnancy. This mineral plays a role in the storage of iron and its transformation into hemoglobin. Good sources of copper are cereal grain, cocoa, shellfish, peas, and nuts.

Iodine

Iodine is necessary for normal functioning of the thyroid hormone. The RDA for pregnant women is 150 to 175 micrograms daily. Too much or too little of this mineral can be detrimental during pregnancy (see iodine, page 203).

Iron

The RDA for all women is 300 mg. per day. The National Research Council believes that the extra 30 to 60 mg. needed by pregnant women cannot be met by the usual

American diet, and recommends obtaining it from a supplement. Additional iron is not usually required until after the first three months of pregnancy. But there is some dispute over whether iron supplements should even be routinely given to women during pregnancy; some argue that not all pregnant women require it. Iron is present in red meats and liver, eggs, raisins, grains, and green leafy vegetables. It is necessary for maintaining the blood supply in the mother. It is also stored in the liver of the unborn child.

Current scientific evidence does not indicate that birth defects are associated with iron ingested during pregnancy.

Magnesium

The RDA for pregnant women of magnesium is 450 mg. per day. It is necessary for the growth of body tissues, proper functioning of every cell, working of the muscles, and for body metabolism. Good sources of magnesium are seafood, fruits, and vegetables.

Phosphorus

The RDA during pregnancy for phosphorus is 1,200 mg. per day for women 19 and older, and 1600 mg. daily for those 18 and younger. This mineral is found in dairy products and lean meats. It is necessary for formation of the child's bones and teeth, as well as increasing the pregnant woman's metabolism of calcium.

Zinc

The RDA for pregnant women is 175 micrograms per day. Zinc is necessary for tissue growth, for use of vitamin A, and for the metabolism of carbohydrates and protein. Seafood, dairy products, red meat, and eggs are good sources of this mineral. Women with a protein-deficient diet may require zinc supplements during pregnancy.

Low levels of zinc have been associated with pregnancy problems, including difficult labor, bleeding, and premature birth. Zinc has also been found to cause birth defects in laboratory animals.

Fluoride

Much controversy surrounds the efficacy of giving fluoride supplements to pregnant women in order to prevent future cavities (caries) in their children. A pediatric dentist whose research supports a caries-protective effect, concluded that prenatal fluoride supplementation acts like a ''vaccine'' for the primary teeth (baby teeth). Others argue that the benefits of prenatal fluoride supplementation have not been adequately demonstrated in clinical studies.

Women who reside in communities with fluoridated water probably do not need additional amounts of this mineral during pregnancy. If your water does not contain optimal amounts of fluoride (if you don't know, contact your local Public Health Department), a daily supplement of 1 to 2.2 mg. might have some benefits. Birth defects have not been associated with fluoride intake during pregnancy.

Reference:

[1] K. S. Moghassi, Risks and benefits of nutritional supplements during pregnancy, *Obstetrics and Gynecology* 58 (supplement) (1981): 68S–78S.

COMMON NAME: **MUMPS**

Brand Name/Chemical Name: **not applicable**

FDA Pregnancy Category: not applicable

ESTIMATED RISK SUMMARY:

Time of Exposure throughout pregnancy
Risk Risk assessment for birth defects is not possible
Pregnancy Outcome uncertain
Documentation insufficient

Time of Exposure first 3–4 months
Risk suspected risk* for miscarriage
Pregnancy Outcome uncertain: favorable and adverse outcomes observed
Documentation inconclusive, based on minimal data

← pre-conception ←	All or None		Organ Development – (in weeks)						Maturation – (in weeks)				
	1	2	3	4	5	6	7	8	9	10	12	20-36	38

conception   ←— Time of Greatest Risk —→   birth

Mumps[1] is an infectious disease whose name probably originally meant "to sulk" or "to speak indistinctly."

Women who contract mumps during the first three or four months of pregnancy appear to have an increased risk of miscarriage. Only isolated case reports have

*above the 4% background risk

described abnormalities in children of women who had mumps while pregnant. No association between birth defects and mumps was found in two investigative studies that evaluated a total of 618 pregnancies complicated by mumps. Only one of these studies indicated the number of women (twenty-four individuals) who had mumps during the first three months, the most vulnerable time for organ development. Because of the relatively small number of first trimester cases that have been followed, it would be premature to draw definitive conclusions about the teratogenicity of the mumps.

There are several reports of babies born with some clinical signs of mumps (inflammation of the glands situated near the ear). But scientists are not certain of how to interpret this, particularly when there is no evidence of mumps infection in the mother. Nevertheless, it is reassuring to know that cases of mumps that have been observed during the first year of life have been very mild.

Long-term follow-up studies of children exposed before birth have not been located.

Reference:

[1] J. S. Remington and J. O. Klein (ed.), *Infectious Diseases of the Fetus and Newborn Infant*, 2d ed. (Philadelphia: W. B. Saunders, 1983), pp. 415–22.

GENERIC NAME: **MUMPS VACCINE**

Brand Name: **(Mumpsvax)**

FDA Pregnancy Category:—

ESTIMATED RISK SUMMARY:
   Time of Exposure throughout pregnancy
   Risk Risk assessment is not possible
   Pregnancy Outcome uncertain
   Documentation insufficient

pre-conception	All or None		Organ Development – (in weeks)						Maturation – (in weeks)				
	1	2	3	4	5	6	7	8	9	10	12	20-36	38

conception   ←—Time of Greatest Risk—→   birth

Mumps vaccine[1] protects against mumps infection (see mumps, page 245). Mumps vaccine contains the live virus, which has been made noninfectious—what is called a live attenuated vaccine. Even so, some evidence exists that the vaccine can infect the placenta, though there is no proof that fetal infection actually occurs. Because of this largely theoretical concern for infection before birth, mumps vaccine should not be used during pregnancy. In addition, the vaccine offers no protection from the infection if the recipient has already been exposed to the mumps virus.

Reference:

[1] J. D. Blanco and R. S. Gibbs, Immunizations in pregnancy, *Clinical Obstetrics and Gynecology* 25 (1982): 611–17.

GENERIC NAME: **NADOLOL**

Brand Name: **(Corgard)**

FDA Pregnancy Category: C

ESTIMATED RISK SUMMARY:
Time of Exposure throughout pregnancy
Risk Risk assessment is not possible
Pregnancy Outcome uncertain
Documentation insufficient

← pre-conception ←	All or None		Organ Development – (in weeks)						Maturation – (in weeks)				
	1	2	3	4	5	6	7	8	9	10	12	20-36	38

conception   ←—Time of Greatest Risk—→   birth

Nadolol belongs to a group of drugs that are classified as beta-adrenergic blocking agents (beta blockers). It is used to treat high blood pressure (hypertension) and for the management of a heart condition that causes pain and a feeling of suffocation (angina).

Currently there are no controlled studies of the effects of this drug on a developing baby. Only one case report has been located that described an infant with a series of complications, including: growth retardation, quick shallow breathing,. mild low blood sugar, slowed heart rate, and lowered body temperature.[1] The child's problems were attributed in part to nadolol, in part to the mother's illness, and in part to other medicines the mother was taking.

Long-term follow-up studies of children exposed before birth have not been located.

Reference:

[1]R. E. Fox, C. Marx, A. R. Strak, Neonatal effects of maternal nadolol therapy, *American Journal of Obstetrics and Gynecology* 152 (1985): 1045–46.

GENERIC NAME: **NALIDIXIC ACID**

Brand Name: **(NegGram)**

FDA Pregnancy Category: —

ESTIMATED RISK SUMMARY:
   Time of Exposure throughout pregnancy
   Risk Risk assessment is not possible
   Pregnancy Outcome uncertain
   Documentation insufficient

pre-conception	All or None	Organ Development – (in weeks)						Maturation – (in weeks)				
	1	2	3	4	5	6	7	8	9	10	12	20-36	38

conception   ←——Time of Greatest Risk——→   birth

Nalidixic acid is an antibiotic used to treat urinary tract infections. For more information about this infection, see page 331. Its effects during pregnancy have not been systematically evaluated. One researcher has suggested a relationship between exposure to this drug and hydrocephalus (enlargement of the cerebral ventricles related to the accumulation of fluid within the baby's brain).[1] However, a study evaluating the children of sixty-three women who used nalidixic acid at various times during pregnancy found no adverse effects.[2]

Long-term follow-up studies of children exposed before birth have not been located.

References:

[1]A. W. Asscher, Diseases of the urinary system: Urinary tract infections, *British Medical Journal* 1 (1977): 1332.
[2]E. D. S. Murray, Nalidixic acid in pregnancy, *British Medical Journal* 282 (1981): 224.

GENERIC NAME: **NITROFURANTOIN**

Brand Names: **(Furadantin, Furalan, Furan, Furanite, Furatoin, Ivadantin, Macrodantin, Nitrofan, Nitrofuran)**

FDA Pregnancy Category:—

ESTIMATED RISK SUMMARY

> *Time of Exposure* throughout pregnancy*
> *Risk* No known risk**
> *Pregnancy Outcome* appears favorable
> *Documentation* inconclusive, based on minimal data

← pre-conception	All or None	Organ Development – (in weeks)						Maturation – (in weeks)				
	1	2	3	4	5	6	7	8	9	10	12	20-36	38

conception   ←—Time of Greatest Risk—→   birth

Nitrofurantoin[1] is prescribed for the treatment of urinary tract infections. For more information about this type of infection, see page 331. Birth defects have not been associated with the use of this drug by pregnant women. But there is concern about a *theoretical* risk for hemolytic anemia in newborn babies exposed to nitrofurantoin shortly before birth. Hemolytic anemia results from the shortened survival of red blood cells. The use of nitrofurantoin during pregnancy has never caused hemolytic anemia in a newborn baby. But it can produce the disorder in individuals with the inherited condition glucose-6-phosphate dehydrogenase (G6PD) deficiency[2] and in people whose red blood cells lack enough of what is called reduced glutathione. Newborn babies happen to be deficient in reduced glutathione. For these reasons the drug manufacturer too warns against the use of nitrofurantoin near the time of delivery.

Long-term follow-up studies of children exposed before birth have not been located.

References:

[1] A. W. Chow and P. J. Jewesson, Pharmacokinetics and safety of antimicrobial agents during pregnancy, *Reviews of Infectious Diseases,* 7 (1985): 287–313.

*theoretical but unproven risk when used near the time of delivery
**above the 4% background risk

[2]R. D. Powell, R. L. DeGowin, and A. S. Alving, Nitrofurantoin-induced hemolysis, *Journal of Laboratory and Clinical Medicine* 62 (1963): 1002–3.

MEDICATION CLASSIFICATION: NONSTEROIDAL ANTI-INFLAMMATORY DRUGS

GENERIC NAMES: FENOPROFEN, IBUPROFEN, INDOME-THACIN, KETOPROFEN, MECLOFENAMATE, NAP-ROXEN, OXYPHENBUTAZONE, PHENYLBUTAZONE, SULINDAC, SUPROFEN, TOLMETIN

Brand Names: (*Advil, Anaprox, Azolid, Butagen, Buta-zolidin, Clinoril, ◊ Indameth, ◊ Indocin, ◊ Indo-Lemmon, ◊ Indomed, *Motrin, Nalfon, Naprosyn, *Nuprin, Orudis, Oxalid, Ponstel, *Rufen, Suprol)

FDA Pregnancy Category: KETOPROFEN, NAPROXEN, SUPROFEN: B; OXYPHENBUTAZONE, PHENYLBUTAZONE, TOLMETIN: C; FENOPROFEN, IBUPROFEN, INDOMETHACIN, MECLOFENAMATE, SULINDAC —

ESTIMATED RISK SUMMARY:

Time of Exposure throughout pregnancy
Risk Risk assessment for birth defects is not possible
Pregnancy Outcome uncertain
Documentation insufficient (for the most part unavailable)

Time of Exposure primarily after the thirty-fourth or thirty-fifth week of pregnancy
Risk suspected risk**
Pregnancy Outcome uncertain: favorable and adverse outcomes observed
Documentation inconclusive

← pre-conception ←		All or None		Organ Development – (in weeks)						Maturation – (in weeks)				
		1	2	3	4	5	6	7	8	9	10	12	20-36	38
													▒▒	

conception   ←—— Time of Greatest Risk ——→   birth

*contains ibuprofen
◊ contains indomethacin
**above the 4% background risk

Nonsteroidal anti-inflammatory drugs (NSAIDs) relieve pain and reduce inflammation and fever. As such, they are prescribed for a variety of reasons: joint and muscle pain and inflammation, menstrual discomfort, sprains and other athletic injuries, and relief from tooth extractions and other dental surgeries. Aspirin, another NSAID, is discussed separately (see salicylates, page 293).

NSAIDs are commonly used, and even more so since 1984, when **ibuprofen** (Motrin) became available without a prescription. Women with rheumatic diseases, such as rheumatoid arthritis, have used these drugs under prescription (especially **aspirin, phenylbutazone**, and **indomethacin**) for decades, with no reported teratogenic effects.[1] However, I should stress that this is the result of clinical experience with these drugs, not of scientific investigations conducted in pregnant women. With the exception of a few isolated reports, published accounts of the effects of NSAIDs during pregnancy are limited to their use near or at the time of delivery.

Isolated instances of birth defects appearing in case reports are known for **indomethacin** and **phenylbutazone**.[2,3] Because these two drugs have been so frequently used, it is likely that their use by the mothers of the few children with birth defects was just a chance occurrence. There is no indication that either of these drugs actually caused the abnormalities. The observed malformations were all different, suggesting that a single environmental cause was probably not responsible. All known teratogens display a recognizable pattern of malformation that was not apparent among these children.

NSAIDs slow the body's ability to make prostaglandins (PGs)—hormone-like substances that play several important roles during pregnancy. For example, since PGs are necessary to produce uterine contractions, some NSAIDs have been used to delay premature labor. Theoretically, then, all NSAIDs could prolong the pregnancy and/or labor. For this reason, these drugs should not be taken near the time of delivery unless indicated by a physician.

PGs are also important for normal blood circulation in the *unborn* baby. While the baby is still in the womb, it extracts oxygen from the blood. A valve in the baby's heart, the ductus arteriosus, facilitates the process by diverting blood from the baby's not-yet-used lungs to the arteries in the umbilical cord. The umbilical arteries supply blood to the unborn child's lower body and then send it to the placenta to pick up a new supply of oxygen. At birth the ductus arteriosus closes, permitting the newborn baby's lungs to provide oxygen to its system. All this is important to know, because PGs are necessary to keep the ductus arteriosus open before birth. If NSAIDs inhibit PGs, the result can be the premature closing of the ductus arteriosus, meaning lessening of the amount of oxygen the unborn baby receives. A further complication is that NSAIDs can interfere with the adjustments necessary for the baby to breathe freely once it is born, resulting in a condition called persistent pulmonary hypertension. The use of some NSAIDs near the time of delivery, particularly after the thirty-fourth or thirty-fifth week of pregnancy,[4] has been linked to these problems by some researchers[5,6,7] but not by others.[8,9] Since **Indomethacin** has been used specifically to treat premature labor, most of the reported problems have involved its use.

Long-term follow-up studies of children exposed before birth have not been located.

References:

[1]M. Østensen and G. Husby, Antirheumatic drug treatment during pregnancy and lactation, *Scandinavian Journal of Rheumatology* 14 (1985): 1–7.

[2]C. Di Battista, L. Landizi, and G. Tamborino, Focomelia ed agenesia del pene in neonato, *Minerva Pediatrica* 27 (1975): 675.

[3]H. Tuchmann-Duplesis, Medication in the course of pregnancy and teratogenic malformation, *Concours. Medical* 89 (1967): 2119–20.

[4]J. R. Niebyl, Prostaglandin synthesis inhibitors, *Seminars in Perinatology*, 5 (1981): 274–87.

[5]H. Zuckerman, U. Reiss and I. Rubenstein Inhibition of human premature labor by indomethacin, *British Journal of Obstetrics and Gynecology* 44 (1974): 787–92.

[6]U. Reiss, J. Atad, I. Rubenstein, et al., The effect of indomethacin in labour at term, *International Journal of Obstetrics and Gynecology* 14 (1976): 369–74.

[7]D. L. Levin, L. J. Mills, and A. G. Weinberg, Hemodynamic, pulmonary vascular, and myocardial abnormalities secondary to pharmacologic constriction of the fetal ductus arteriosus: A possible mechanism for persistent pulmonary hypertension and transient tricuspid insufficiency in the newborn infant, *Circulation* 60 (1979): 360–64.

[8]N. Wiqvist, V. Lundström, and K. Green, Premature labor and indomethacin, *Prostaglandins* 10 (1975): 515–26.

[9]K. M. Kumor, R. D. White, D. A. Blake, et al., Indomethacin as a treatment for premature labor: Neonatal outcome, *Pediatric Research* 13 (1979): 370.

GENERIC NAME: **NYSTATIN**

Brand Names: **(Mycostatin, Nilstat, Nystex, O-V Statin)**

FDA Pregnancy Category:—

ESTIMATED RISK SUMMARY:

Time of Exposure throughout pregnancy

Risk No known risk*

Pregnancy Outcome appears favorable

Documentation inconclusive, based on minimal data

*above the 4% background risk

← pre-conception	All or None		Organ Development – (in weeks)						Maturation – (in weeks)				
	1	2	3	4	5	6	7	8	9	10	12	20-36	38

conception   ←——Time of Greatest Risk——→   birth

Nystatin is an antibiotic used to treat moniliasis, a fungal or "yeast" infection of the vagina. The infection is sometimes called candida, after the fungus *Candida albicans*. It is reassuring to know that the body absorbs nystatin very poorly. Even after oral administration there are no detectable levels of the drug in the blood.

Studies monitoring nystatin's use by pregnant women have not observed an increase in birth defects in their children.[1,2]

Long-term follow-up studies of children exposed before birth have not been located.

References:

[1] J. E. Davis, J. H. Frudenfeld, and J. L. Goddard, Comparative evaluation of Monistat and Mycostatin in the treatment of vulvovaginal candidiasis, *Obstetrics and Gynecology* 44 (1974): 403–6.

[2] H. C. S. Wallenburg and J. W. Wladimiroff, Recurrence of vulvovaginal candidiasis during pregnancy: Comparison of miconazole vs nystatin treatment, *Obstetrics and Gynecology* 48 (1976): 491–94.

GENERIC NAME: **OXYCODONE**

Brand Names: (**Percocet, ◇ Percodan*)

FDA Pregnancy Category: C

ESTIMATED RISK SUMMARY:

Time of Exposure throughout pregnancy
Risk Risk assessment is not possible
Pregnancy Outcome uncertain
Documentation unavailable

*also contains acetaminophen
◇ also contains aspirin

pre-conception	All or None		Organ Development – (in weeks)						Maturation – (in weeks)				
	1	2	3	4	5	6	7	8	9	10	12	20-36	38

conception　　　←——Time of Greatest Risk——→　　　birth

Oxycodone is a semisynthetic narcotic used to treat moderate and moderately severe pain. As with other narcotics, prolonged use of oxycodone can result in physical and psychological dependence.

Oxycodone has not been evaluated for any possible effects it might have on the unborn baby. Theoretically, the consistent use of any narcotic agent near birth could cause addiction and withdrawal symptoms in the newborn.

Long-term follow-up studies of children exposed before birth have not been located.

COMMON NAME: **PAINT**

Chemical Names: **too many to list**

FDA Pregnancy Category: not applicable

ESTIMATED RISK SUMMARY:

Time of Exposure throughout pregnancy
Risk Risk assessment is not possible
Pregnancy Outcome uncertain
Documentation unavailable

pre-conception	All or None		Organ Development – (in weeks)						Maturation – (in weeks)				
	1	2	3	4	5	6	7	8	9	10	12	20-36	38

conception　　　←——Time of Greatest Risk——→　　　birth

There is a well-established popular belief claiming that women who *paint* their house walls during pregnancy are engaging in a dangerous practice. This belief is not really true, and probably is based on the fact that at one time interior house paint contained lead. Lead has been observed to cause an increased frequency in the number of miscarriages in pregnant women who were exposed to high levels of the compound (see lead, page 214). Lead is also responsible for causing mental retardation in some children who consumed paint chips from the walls of *old* buildings. Lead has not been an ingredient in paint for more than thirty years now. But if you happen to live in an older house, you could be exposed to lead if you scraped the paint from the walls.

There are, of course, various chemicals in paint, whether the paint is latex (water-based), oil-based, or enamel. There are also various chemicals and solvents in lacquer and furniture stripper (see chemicals, page 101). The very little information that is available on these substances during pregnancy is related to large doses and longtime exposures, as experienced by those who *work* with these substances.

Women who work as painters should read the entry on chemicals. This is very different from the temporary and brief exposure from painting a room in the house. These more common exposures encountered by women during pregnancy have not been studied for effects on the unborn.

Certainly it would be better to have someone else do the painting while you're pregnant, but this is not always possible. If you do choose to paint during pregnancy, minimize your exposure by working in a *very well ventilated* room.

COMMON NAME: **PCP**

Chemical Name: **(phencyclidine)**

FDA Pregnancy Category: not applicable

ESTIMATED RISK SUMMARY:

  Time of Exposure throughout pregnancy
  Risk Risk assessment is not possible
  Pregnancy Outcome uncertain
  Documentation insufficient

  Time of Exposure theoretically, near the time of delivery
  Risk Known risk* for withdrawal symptoms
  Pregnancy Outcome adverse
  Documentation conclusive, based on current knowledge

---

*above the 4% background risk

← pre-conception ←	All or None		Organ Development – (in weeks)						Maturation – (in weeks)				
	1	2	3	4	5	6	7	8	9	10	12	20-36	38

conception   ←——Time of Greatest Risk——→   birth

Phencyclidine (PCP) is an illicit chemical that is inexpensively manufactured and widely available. Usually smoked with tobacco or marijuana, PCP is used for its hallucinogenic effects. While many of the dangers from the use of this drug are understood, the effect of PCP on an unborn baby remains largely a mystery.

The majority of exposures to PCP before birth have occurred in conjunction with other drugs, including marijuana, alcohol, nicotine, Valium (diazepam), cocaine, and LSD. In evaluating the effect of PCP on the unborn baby, the additional influence of these other drugs must be considered.

Scientific studies have been able to demonstrate that PCP can enter into fetal circulation. However worrisome, this information alone does not reveal whether or not PCP causes birth defects. In order to determine the effects of PCP on a developing baby, studies that evaluate a large number of infants exposed before birth are badly needed.

One case report of a PCP-exposed child with abnormalities has appeared in the medical literature. This report described a child born to a woman who smoked PCP throughout her pregnancy (six phencyclidine-laced marijuana cigarettes per day).[1] The child's facial appearance was unusual. He displayed a variety of abnormal neurological signs, including increased muscle tone, and even the slightest sound or touch caused coarse movements of his arms and legs. Some of his symptoms were characteristic of drug withdrawal. At the age of five he was noted to be severely retarded.[2] In the absence of other reported birth defects in similarly exposed children, cause-and-effect cannot be implied from this single observation. Nevertheless, the lack of knowledge about the drug, plus the variation in its quality and strength, make it prudent for pregnant women to avoid it entirely.

Withdrawal-like symptoms have been reported in many newborns of women who used PCP during pregnancy.[1,2,3,4] To affect the newborn in this manner, the drug was probably taken close to the time of delivery. The symptoms are a little different from those observed in narcotic-addicted infants. Characteristic of PCP "withdrawal" is lethargy, contrasted with coarse, flappy tremors after stimulation. These babies have also exhibited irritability, jitteriness, poor feeding, poor attention, increased muscle tone (hypertonia), and depressed neonatal reflexes (grasp and rotating).

At 3 months of age, infant development tests (Bayley scale) were administered to seven children who displayed signs of PCP withdrawal at birth. No differences were seen between the exposed and nonexposed groups.[3] Long-term follow-up of these infants is required before the true consequences of their prenatal drug exposures can be predicted.

References:

[1]N. L. Golden, R. J. Sokol, and I. L. Rubin, Angel dust: Possible effects on the fetus, *Pediatrics* 65 (1980): 18–20.

[2]N. L. Golden, B. R. Kuhmert, R. J. Sokol, S. Martier, and T. Williams, Neonatal manifestations of maternal phencyclidine exposure, *Journal of Perinatal Medicine* 15 (1987): 185–191.

[3]I. J. Chasnoff, W. J. Burns, R. P. Hatcher, and K. A. Burns, Phencyclidine: Effects on the fetus and neonate, *Developmental Pharmacology and Therapeutics* 6 (1983): 404–8.

[4]A. A. Strauss, H. D. Modanlou, and S. K. Bosu, Neonatal manifestations of maternal phencyclidine (PCP) abuse, *Pediatrics* 69 (1981): 550–52.

MEDICATION CLASSIFICATION: **PENICILLINS**

GENERIC NAMES: **AMOXICILLIN, AMPICILLIN, BACAMPICILLIN, CARBENICILLIN, CLOXACILLIN, CYCLACILLIN, DICLOXACILLIN, HETACILLIN, METHICILLIN, NAFCILLIN, OXACILLIN, PENICILLIN G BENZATHINE, PENICILLIN V, PENICILLIN VK, TICARCILLIN**

Brand Names: **Amcap, Amcill, Amoxil, Bactocill, Beepen-VK, Betapen-VK, Bicillin, Celbenin, Cloxapen, Cyclapen-W, D-Amp, Deltapen-VK, Dycill, Dynapen, Geocillin, Geopen, Larotid, Ledercillin VK, M-Cillin B-400, Nafcil, Omnipen, Pathocil, Penapar VK, Penicillin GK, Penicillin V, Pentids, Pen-Vee K, Pfizerpen A, Pfizerpen G, Pfizerpen VK, Polycillin, Polymox, Principen, Prostaphlin, Pyopen, Repen-VK, Robicillin VK, SK-Ampicillin, SK-Penicillin G, SK-Penicillin VK, Spectrobid, Staphcillin, Sumox, Supen, Tegopen, Ticar, Totacillin, Trimox, Unipen, Utimox, Uticillin VK, V-Cillin K, Veetids, Veracillin, Versapen, Wymox**

FDA Pregnancy Category: B

ESTIMATED RISK SUMMARY:
   Time of Exposure throughout pregnancy

Risk No measurable risk*
Pregnancy Outcome favorable
Documentation conclusive, based on current knowledge

pre-conception	All or None		Organ Development – (in weeks)						Maturation – (in weeks)				
	1	2	3	4	5	6	7	8	9	10	12	20-36	38

conception   ← Time of Greatest Risk →   birth

Penicillins[1] are antibiotics, available in both natural forms and semisynthetic derivatives. Both types are routinely prescribed for pregnant women. These antibiotics are sometimes used to treat urinary tract infections during pregnancy. For more information about this type of infection, see page 331. Penicillins destroy bacteria by weakening their cell walls. Human cells do not have walls, so the process affects only bacteria.

There is no evidence that penicillin antibiotics are teratogenic when used at any time during pregnancy. Much of the information on their effects on the unborn has come from years of clinical experience, rather than well-controlled investigations. But the fact that no suspicion of human teratogenicity has appeared in the widespread use of penicillins over almost sixty years is quite remarkable and very reassuring.

Ampicillin may reduce the efficacy of oral contraceptives (birth control pills), leading to unplanned pregnancies, but this has not been confirmed.

If a pregnancy woman has gonorrhea or syphilis, she should receive treatment, so that both she and her unborn child will benefit from it. Penicillins cross the placenta and therapeutic drug levels reach the fetus, so these drugs are often used during pregnancy to treat venereal disease (see gonorrhea, page 169 and syphilis, page 308).

In summary, penicillins are considered safe for use in pregnancy, because of both the way they act on cells and the lack of evidence against them.

Long-term follow-up studies of children exposed before birth have not been located.

Reference:
[1]D. V. Landers, J. R. Green, and R. L. Sweet, Antibiotic use during pregnancy and the postpartum period, *Clinics in Obstetrics and Gynecology* 26 (1983): 391–406.

*above the 4% b ckground risk

GENERIC NAME: **PENICILLAMINE**

Brand Names: **(Cuprimine, Depen Titratabs)**

FDA Pregnancy Category:—

ESTIMATED RISK SUMMARY:

Time of Exposure difficult to specify, possibly throughout pregnancy
Risk Suspected risk*
Pregnancy Outcome uncertain: favorable and adverse outcomes observed
Documentation inconclusive

pre-conception	All or None		Organ Development – (in weeks)						Maturation – (in weeks)				
	1	2	3	4	5	6	7	8	9	10	12	20-36	38

conception   ←—Time of Greatest Risk—→   birth

Penicillamine[1] is used to treat rheumatoid arthritis, cystinuria (excessive urinary excretion of cystine, an amino acid), and Wilson's disease (an abnormality in copper metabolism).

Of children born to eighty-nine women who were treated with penicillamine for one of these three conditions (forty-six of them throughout pregnancy), three had defects of the connective tissue, including unusually lax and wrinkled skin. Two of the infants had additional complications and died. Whether the adverse effects are related to drug dosage is suspected but has not yet been proven.

In order to reduce the potential teratogenic effects, penicillamine dosage in pregnant women with cystinuria or Wilson's disease is usually kept as low as possible and perhaps even discontinued in those with cystinuria. Complete avoidance of the drug is recommended in the case of rheumatoid arthritis.[2]

Long-term follow-up studies of children exposed before birth have not been located.

References:

[1]J. H. Lewis, A. B. Weingold, and the committee on FDA-related matters, American College of Gastroenterology, The use of gastrointestinal drugs during pregnancy and lactation. *American Journal of Gastroenterology* 80 (1985): 912–23.
[2]W. Endres, D-penicillamine in pregnancy—to ban or not to ban? *Klinische Wochenschrift*, 59 (1981): 535–37.

*above the 4% background risk

GENERIC NAME: **PENTAZOCINE**

Brand Name: †**Talacen, Talwin, ***Talwin Compound,** ◇**Talwin NX**

FDA Pregnancy Category: C

ESTIMATED RISK SUMMARY

Time of Exposure throughout pregnancy
Risk Risk assessment for birth defects not possible
Pregnancy Outcome uncertain
Documentation insufficient

Time of Exposure in the latter part of pregnancy
Risk Possible risk** for low birth weight
Pregnancy Outcome uncertain; favorable and adverse outcomes observed
Documentation inconclusive, based on minimal data

Time of Exposure particularly near the time of delivery
Risk Known risk** for withdrawal symptoms
Pregnancy Outcome adverse
Documentation conclusive, based on current knowledge

← pre-conception	All or None		Organ Development – (in weeks)						Maturation – (in weeks)				
	1	2	3	4	5	6	7	8	9	10	12	20-36	38
												▓▓▓	███

conception   ←——Time of Greatest Risk——→   birth

Pentazocine is a narcotic analgesic, used to relieve moderate to severe pain.

Pentazocine has been abused in conjunction with the drug tripelenannamine, (an antihistamine). The combination is known as T's and Blues and it first became popular during the 1970s as a heroin substitute. (*T's* comes from the *T* in Talwin, the brand name for pentazocine. *Blues* comes from the blue color of the tripelennamine tablet.) Abuse of this combination has declined since pentazocine was reformulated to contain the drug **naloxone** (brand name Talwin NX). Naloxone prevents the effect of pentazocine if the product is injected intravenously.

†also contains acetaminophen
*also contains aspirin
◇ also contains naloxone
**above the 4% background risk

Although birth defects have not been reported from pentazocine use during pregnancy, withdrawal symptoms and low birth weight have been observed. Birth weights below 2,500 gms (5½ pounds) were observed in eleven of twenty-four infants exposed before birth to pentazocine and tripelennamine.[1] Nine of these babies were also premature. Another investigation also noted lower birth weights (below 2,800 gms) in seven of nine infants born to mothers who abused T's and Blues.[2] One baby whose mother used pentazocine for back pain was small at birth and died at 3 months of age from sudden infant death syndrome.[3] A causal relationship between the infant's death and pentazocine was *not* suspected.

Case reports have described withdrawal symptoms similar to those reported in babies born to heroin and methadone addicts, in newborns whose mothers used pentazocine throughout pregnancy for back pain.[3,4] The same symptoms have been observed in babies born to women who chronically abused pentazocine combined with tripelennamine.[1,2] The withdrawals begin approximately twenty-four hours after birth and usually disappear within three to eleven days. Such symptoms usually result from *consistent* use of the drug in the latter part of pregnancy, particularly near the time of delivery. The withdrawal symptoms are characterized by jitteriness, irritability, hyperactivity, feeding difficulties (vomiting and weak suck), increased muscle tone, and a loud shrill cry. These problems are most likely attributed to pentazocine, although additional or additive effects from tripelennamine are certainly possible.

Pentazocine has caused breathing problems in newborns whose mothers received the drug to relieve pain during labor.[5]

Long-term follow-up studies of children exposed before birth have not been located.

References:

[1]D. W. Dunn and J. Reynolds, Neonatal withdrawal symptoms associated with "T's and Blues" (pentazocine and tripelennamine), *American Journal of Diseases of Children* 136(1982): 644–45.

[2]R. J. Wapner, R. D. Ross, J. M. Fitsdimmons, et al., Fetal growth in drug dependent women: Quantitative assessments, abstracted, *Pediatric Research* 15 (1981): 1222.

[3]R. L. Geetz and R. V. Balm, Neonatal withdrawal symptoms associated with material use of pentazocine, *Journal of Pediatrics* 84 (1974): 887–88.

[4]A. E. Kopelman, Fetal addiction to pentazocine, *Pediatrics* 55 (1975): 888–89.

[5]S. O. Refstad and E. Lindback, Ventilatory depression of the newborn of women receiving pethadine or pentazocine, *British Journal of Aneasthesia,* 52 (1980): 265–70.

COMMON NAME: **PESTICIDES**

Chemical names: **(carbamates, organochlorines [chlorinated hydrocarbons], organophosphates, pyrethroids)**

FDA Pregnancy Category: Not applicable

ESTIMATED RISK SUMMARY:

Time of Exposure throughout pregnancy
Risk Risk assessment is not possible
Pregnancy Outcome uncertain
Documentation insufficient

pre-conception	All or None		Organ Development – (in weeks)						Maturation – (in weeks)				
	1	2	3	4	5	6	7	8	9	10	12	20-36	38

conception   ←—Time of Greatest Risk—→   birth

Pesticides[1] are poisons used to destroy household pests and to control insect damage to agricultural crops. The basic groups are **organochlorines** (also called chlorinated hydrocarbons), **organophosphates, carbamates,** and **pyrethroids.** Pesticides, which are difficult to generalize about, are discussed together here only because of the very limited amount of information available regarding their effect on the unborn child.

Many animal studies of pesticides have found no adverse effects on the unborn, but others have shown evidence of impaired fetal survival, birth defects, and sterility in adult animals. Often the chemical dose required to detect an effect was high enough to poison the pregnant animal, sometimes causing death—both circumstances that may have caused or contributed to the abnormalities.

The animal studies imply that high dosage of pesticides over a long period of time has the most adverse effect on pregnancy outcome. Along that line, the only reports describing malformations in humans involved toxic doses of pesticides. In Japan, a few cases of fetal death and abnormalities were attributed to pregnant women's poisoning from **organophosphate** pesticides sprinkled in agricultural fields. Important things to remember here are (1) large doses administered directly to pregnant animals cannot be compared to most human exposures, (2) cause-and-effect cannot be determined from case reports, more studies are needed, and (3) such intensive doses are not comparable to low-level exposures.

Unfortunately, there have been very few studies of pesticides exposures in human pregnancy. Researchers have suggested that higher levels of **organochlorine** in the mother's blood might be related to an increase in pregnancy loss and premature delivery. This information was derived from a very small population. In addition, the pesticide levels in the "control" group and in the study group overlapped, so the significance of these findings is difficult to determine.

To my knowledge there is no information available on the teratogenicity of **carbamate** pesticides in humans. High doses of **carbaryl** (brand name Sevin) have been found to cause birth defects in guinea pigs, but for most species no significant incidence of abnormalities has been found.

Pyrethroids are derived from chrysanthemum flowers, but their organic origin cannot be equated with safety. The most commonly used pyrethroid is **pyrethrum.** Pyrethrum is less toxic than are the other pesticides, but many people are allergic to it. The lack of evaluation of this compound in human pregnancy means that it should be approached with the same amount of caution used with all pesticides.

Long-term follow-up studies of children exposed before birth have not been located.

Care should always be taken when using either herbicides or pesticides. Direct contact with the chemical should be avoided, and when necessary, protective gear and clothing should be selected, a disposable face mask and gloves are the basics.

Many women are concerned about how to rid their homes of fleas during pregnancy. Here are a few tips:

The flea problem:

1. Try vacuuming thoroughly and avoid using pesticides.

2. Vacuum thoroughly. Put fresh eucalyptus leaves under and behind furniture, using as many as possible. If possible, close up the house for three to five days. Revacuum. Leaves can be left in inconspicuous places for further protection.

3. Vacuum thoroughly. Sprinkle table salt on floor and carpet, especially around the base of walls and corners. (Fleas lay their eggs in the lint and dust in corners.) Leave salt on the floor for about four days. Vacuum thoroughly. Salt tends to clog the holes of the vacuum cleaner bag, so you may use several bags in the process.

4. If you choose to use pyrethrum, it can be used in the same way recommended for table salt. Instead of leaving the product on the floor for four days, only twenty-four hours is necessary. Avoid contact with this pesticide.

CAUTION: Pyrethrum is highly allergenic and high dose exposures can cause toxic symptoms.

5. While I'm not recommending their use, as a last resort some people choose flea "bombs."

If you use flea bombs, store and protect all food products safely away from being sprayed. The refrigerator is a good place, as it does not draw air from the room. Remember to close closet doors to avoid spraying your clothing. Preferably have someone else do the spraying and remain out of the house during the process and, ideally, for twenty-four hours afterward. The home should be aired out and the eating surfaces washed down by someone other than you, if you are pregnant.

Reference:

[1]Reproductive Toxicology, a medical letter on Environmental Hazards to Reproduction, Insecticides, Reproductive Toxicology Center, Washington, D. C. 4(2) (1985): 5–9.

GENERIC NAME: **PHENOBARBITAL**

Brand Names: **(Barbita, Luminal Ovoids, PBR/12, Sedadrops, Solfoton)**

FDA Pregnancy Category:—

ESTIMATED RISK SUMMARY:
    Time of Exposure throughout pregnancy
    Risk Possible risk*
    Pregnancy Outcome uncertain: favorable and adverse outcomes observed
    Documentation inconclusive

    Time of Exposure near the time of delivery
    Risk Known risk*
    Pregnancy Outcome adverse (withdrawal symptoms and bleeding problems)
    Documentation conclusive, based on current knowledge

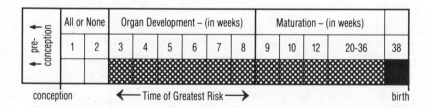

pre-conception	All or None		Organ Development – (in weeks)						Maturation – (in weeks)				
	1	2	3	4	5	6	7	8	9	10	12	20-36	38

conception   ⟵ Time of Greatest Risk ⟶   birth

    Phenobarbital is a barbiturate, and has several medical uses:
• pre-anesthetic for sedation,
• hypnotic for the short-term treatment of insomnia,

*above the 4% background risk

• long-term anticonvulsant in the treatment of seizures and epilepsy, and
• emergency treatment of acute convulsive episodes.

The relationship between the use of phenobarbital and birth defects remains unclear. One reason is that few studies consider phenobarbital by itself. Most evaluate it as a long-term anticonvulsant together with other medications, particularly hydantoins, which are known teratogens (see hydantoins, page 191). Also, most of the studies are not directly comparable, because they are designed so differently.

Opinions differ about the specific risk of anticonvulsants. Many experts believe there is two to three times the risk of major malformations in the children of epileptic women as in the general population. Some think the underlying disease is the cause. Others believe it results from exposure to anticonvulsant medications that are teratogens. This difference of opinion arises, in part, from the variation in types of defect, and in their incidence. The best explanation of this variation is the way the genetics of the mother and fetus influence drug reaction[1] (First Principle of Teratology).

Many investigations of phenobarbital fail to reveal an increased incidence of a clear pattern of abnormality resulting from exposure to phenobarbital.[2,3] Others have concluded that it causes malformations similar to those in the fetal hydantoin syndrome, whether taken alone or with another barbiturate (see primadone, page 271).[4,5,6] One study says that when taken with hydantoins, phenobarbital increases the risk of "hydantoin-like" malformations.[7]

Extremely large doses of phenobarbital may be teratogenic, though the evidence is limited—the result of observing a brother and a sister born to a woman who took such doses.[8] Both children displayed growth retardation and a peculiar facial appearance, along with some minor malformations. One child also experienced delayed psychomotor development. So far, only one human study of the levels of anticonvulsants in the blood has related the frequency of abnormalities to the dose.[9] Further research must be conducted before the severity of risk can be predicted from such measurements. In the meantime, physicians usually prescribe the lowest dose possible during pregnancy.

There are reports of tumors in ten children exposed before birth to a barbiturate (phenobarbital or methylphenobarbitone) and phenytoin (plus alcohol in 2 cases).[10] From this evidence, some experts suspect that prenatal exposure to the drugs may cause cancer. But the number of cases is too small to allow a definitive conclusion.

Withdrawal symptoms often occur in babies born to women using barbiturates. These symptoms include tremors, irritability, restlessness, high-pitched cry, voracious appetite, spitting up, and overreaction to cold, hunger, household noises, and other environmental effects. Withdrawal symptoms usually start when the baby is a week old, and can continue for 2 to 4 months.

Barbiturates are associated with a blood coagulation defect in newborns that can cause severe bleeding (usually within the first twenty-four hours). To help prevent this, your physician will usually administer vitamin K_1 to you some weeks before delivery, and during labor. (Vitamin K_1 is required for normal blood clotting.) At birth, your baby will also receive vitamin K_1.

Using phenobarbital might reduce your level of one of the B-complex vitamins, folic acid or folate. The need for folate increases greatly during pregnancy, as it is required for fetal growth and development. Some suggest that taking folic acid during pregnancy might reduce the risk of abnormalities.[11]

Most women continue taking anticonvulsant medication during pregnancy, unless they have been seizure-free for many years. *Under no circumstances should you ever discontinue your anticonvulsant medication, unless under the direction and supervision of the prescribing physician.* Sudden withdrawal could cause a seizure. And while seizures are not known to cause malformations, they do present a possible risk to both you and your unborn baby.

Many women question how epilepsy or anticonvulsant medication in the father might affect their baby. Although not all scientists agree, most experts think this presents no increased risk. They believe that children fathered by men taking these drugs have the same chance of being normal and healthy as anyone else's, and well-conducted animal research confirms this belief.[12] (For more information on this see Risks from Exposures in the Baby's Father, page 14.)

References:

[1]R. H. Finnell and G. F. Chernoff, Genetic background: The elusive component of the Fetal Hydantoin Syndrome, *American Journal of Medical Genetics* 19 (1984): 459–62.

[2]O. P. Heinonen, D. Slone, and S. Shapiro, *Birth Defects and Drugs in Pregnancy*. (Littleton, Mass.: Publishing Sciences Group, 1977), pp. 336–39.

[3]C. R. Lowe, Congenital malformations among infants born to epileptic women, *Lancet* 1 (1973): 9.

[4]F. E. Berkowitz, Fetal malformation due to phenobarbitone: A case report, *South African Medical Journal* 55 (1979): 100–101.

[5]L. J. Ptacek, A new syndrome: Multiple congenital anomalies with spastic diplegia, in offspring of epileptic mothers on anticonvulsant therapy, read before the Wisconsin Neurological Society meeting, Green Lake, Wisc., November 16, 1974.

[6]B. D. Speidel and S. R. Medow, Maternal epilepsy and abnormalities of the fetus and newborn, *Lancet* 2 (1972): 839.

[7]J. Fedrick, Epilepsy and pregnancy: A report from the Oxford Record Linkage Study, *British Medical Journal* 2 (1973): 442.

[8]M. Seip, Growth retardation, dysmorphic facies and minor malformations following massive exposure to phenobarbitone in utero, *Acta Pediatrica Scandinavica* 65 (1976): 617–21.

[9]L. Dansky, E. Andermann, F. Andermann, A. L. Sherwin, and R. A. Kinch, Maternal epilepsy and congenital malformations: correlations with maternal plasma anticonvulsant levels during pregnancy, in Janz et al. (eds.) *Epilepsy, Pregnancy and the Child* (New York: Raven Press, 1982), pp. 251–58.

[10]A. Lipson and P. Bale, Ependymoblastoma associated with prenatal exposure to Diphenylhydantoin and methylphenobarbitone, *Cancer* 55 (1985): 1859–62.

[11]Y. Biale and H. Lewenthal, Effect of folic acid supplementation on congenital malformations due to anticonvulsive drugs, *European Journal of Obstetrics, Gynecology, and Reproductive Biology* 18 (1984): 211–16.

[12]R. H. Finnell and J. F. Baer, Congenital defects among the offspring of epileptic fathers: Role of the genotype and phenytoin therapy in a mouse model, *Epilepsia* 25 (1986): 697–705.

MEDICATION CLASSIFICATION: **PHENOTHIAZINES**

GENERIC NAMES: **ACETOPHENAZINE, MALEATE, CHLORPROMAZINE, FLUPHENAZINE, MESORIDAZINE, PERPHENAZINE, PROCHLORPERAZINE, PROMAZINE, PROMETHAZINE, THIORIDAZINE, TRIFLUOPERAZINE, TRIFLUOPROMAZINE, TRIMEPRAZINE**

Brand Names: **(Baymethazine, Chlorazine, Compazine, Mellaril, Millazine, Permitil, Phenergan, Phenazine 25, Prolixin, Promapar, Prozine, Serentil, SK-Thioridazine, Sonazine, Sparine, Stelazine, Suprazine, Temaril, Thorazine, Thor-Prom, Tindal, Trilafon, Vesprin)**

FDA Pregnancy Category: —

ESTIMATED RISK SUMMARY:

Time of Exposure throughout pregnancy
Risk No known risk*
Pregnancy Outcome appears favorable
Documentation inconclusive, based on minimal data

Time of Exposure near the time of delivery
Risk Suspected risk* for adverse effects in the newborn
Pregnancy Outcome uncertain: favorable and adverse outcomes observed
Documentation inconclusive, based on minimal data

*above the 4% background risk

pre-conception	All or None		Organ Development – (in weeks)						Maturation – (in weeks)				
	1	2	3	4	5	6	7	8	9	10	12	20-36	38

conception   ←——Time of Greatest Risk——→   birth

Phenothiazines[1] are major tranquilizers belonging to a therapeutic class of drugs known as antipsychotics. Their primary use is to treat psychiatric illness (psychosis). These drugs also act as sedatives, antiemetics (antinauseants), and antihistamines (**promethazine** and **trimeprazine**). As a result, some of them are used for these purposes in addition to, or instead of, being used as antipsychotics. **Chlorpromazine** and **prochlorperazine** have been used for years, throughout pregnancy, to treat nausea and vomiting.

Most research concludes that phenothiazines are not teratogenic. However, a few reports have linked them to birth defects.

A large prospective investigation observed a 3.5 percent malformation rate for phenothiazines as a group as opposed to 1.6 percent in the control population.[2] The study linked **chlorpromazine** to an increase in *nonspecific* malformations, but some of the abnormalities could not have resulted from the drug because the time of exposure did not correspond with the described defects (see Second Principle of Teratology, page 33). So cause-and-effect cannot be implied. In one instance, a child with microcephaly (abnormally small head size) was born to a woman who had two previous children with the same defect, raising suspicion that the cause was genetic and not from the drug. Since other possible causes were not accounted for, the significance of all these findings is further reduced.

Results from the Collaborative Perinatal Project, which evaluated pregnancy outcome in more than 50,000 mother-child pairs exposed to a wide variety of drugs revealed no birth defects in 1,209 children exposed to phenothiazines (142 of them to **chlorpromazine**).[3] In fact, these children's birth weight, mortality rate soon after birth, and IQs at 4 years of age were apparently unaffected by the exposure. However, the value of this study in teratogen risk counseling has been questioned primarily for two reasons: Other possible causes were not eliminated, and a critical issue, the time of exposure, was not specified. Also, because of frequent multiproduct use during pregnancy, difficulty exists in determining which drug, if any, could have caused birth defects.

An investigation that compared drug consumption in pregnancies resulting in normal children and in malformed infants found that fewer mothers of infants with major and minor abnormalities took antihistamines in the first trimester[4] (see also antihistamines, page 81). **Promethazine** was the most frequently taken product. **Trimeprazine** was also included in the list of commonly consumed antihistamines. This study was conducted after the babies were born, so its findings are not as reliable as they could be. Gathered information was based on a mother's recall of events during pregnancy. The most significant problem with this approach is the difficulty in accurately documenting exactly what drugs were used and specifically when during pregnancy the drug was taken (see retrospective studies, page 43). Nevertheless, this investigation lends some additional support to the apparent lack of teratogenic effects with drugs of this class.

Other studies have also failed to link the use of phenothiazines during pregnancy with an increased incidence of malformations. One expert summarized the issue by stating controlled studies have proven that phenothiazines are not teratogens, despite the isolated reports of possible harmful effects.[5]

Regular use of phenothizaines near the time of delivery has resulted in adverse side effects in some newborn babies. Still, many investigations have also reported infants with no apparent symptoms. The adverse effects include increased muscle tone (hypertonicity) with tremors and abnormal muscle movements (hyperreflexia). In some infants, symptoms have persisted for six to nine months. While discontinuing the drug before delivery would reduce the likelihood of such adverse effects, the mother's psychiatric condition may worsen. Therefore, the decision to continue or to discontinue antipsychotic medication before delivery or when labor begins must be made by the physician on an individual basis.

One clinician found no abnormalities and normal subsequent development among his patients' twenty children (ages not stated) exposed before birth to **thioridazine** during at least the first trimester.[6] The value of such an informal survey, however, is very limited. A small study of fifty-two children born to women taking **chlorpromazine** throughout pregnancy also revealed normal development through ages 4–5[7]. Formal, large-scale, long-term follow-up studies on phenothiazines are still needed before their effect on later development can be predicted.

References:

[1]J. R. Calabrese and A. D. Gulledge, Psychotropics during pregnancy and lactation: A review, *Psychosomatics* 26 (1985): 413–26.

[2]C. Rumeau-Roiquette, J. Goujard, and G. Huel, Possible teratogenic effect of phenothiazines in human beings, *Teratology* 15 (1976): 57–64.

[3]O. P. Heinonen, D. Slone, and S. Shapiro *Birth Defects and Drugs in Pregnancy* (Littleton, Mass.: Publishing Sciences Group, 1977).

[4]M. M. Nelson and J. O. Forfar, Associations between drugs administered during pregnancy and congenital abnormalities of the fetus, *British Medical Journal* 1 (1971): 523–27.

[5]J. Anath, Congenital malformations with psychopharmacologic agents, *Comprehensive Psychiatry* 16 (1975): 437–45.

[6]F. J. Scanlan, The use of thioridazine (Melleril) during the first trimester, *Medical Journal of Australia* 1 (1972): 1271–72.

[7]E. B. Kris, Children of mothers maintained on pharmacotherapy during pregnancy and postpartum, *Current Therapeutic Research* 7 (1965): 785–89.

GENERIC NAME: **PINDOLOL**

Brand Name: **(Visken)**

FDA Pregnancy Category: B

ESTIMATED RISK SUMMARY:

Time of Exposure throughout pregnancy

Risk Risk assessment is not possible

Pregnancy Outcome uncertain

Documentation insufficient

pre-conception	All or None		Organ Development – (in weeks)						Maturation – (in weeks)				
	1	2	3	4	5	6	7	8	9	10	12	20-36	38

conception   ←——Time of Greatest Risk——→   birth

Pindolol belongs to a group of drugs that are classified as beta-adrenergic blocking agents (beta blockers). It is used to treat high blood pressure (hypertension).

Pindolol has not been associated with causing birth defects, but information relative to its use during the first three months of pregnancy is lacking. Some studies have reported that pindolol has an adverse effect on birth weight;[1] others have found higher birth weights when pindolol-exposed babies were compared to infants exposed to other antihypertensive drugs.[2] Further investigation is warranted before any conclusions about the effect this drug has on birth weight can be determined.

While pindolol has not been associated with slower than normal heartbeat (bradycardia) and/or low blood pressure (hypotension) in newborn babies; such effects have been reported with other beta-blocking agents (see acebutolol, page 50 and atenolol, page 89). For this reason, prenatally exposed newborns should be observed for a couple of days for any evidence of these symptoms.

Long-term follow-up studies of children exposed before birth have not been located.

References:

[1]E. Sukerman-Voldman, Pindolol therapy in pregnant hypertensive patients, *British Journal of Clinical Pharmacology* 13 (suppl.) 1982: 379S.

[2]D. Dubois, J. Petitcolas, B. Temperville, A. Klepper, and P. H. Catherine, Treatment of hypertension in pregnancy with B-adrenoceptor antagonists, *British Journal of Clinical Pharmacology* 13 (suppl.) (1982): 375S–78S.

GENERIC NAME: **PRIMIDONE**

Brand Name: **(Myidone, Mysoline)**

FDA Pregnancy Category:—

ESTIMATED RISK SUMMARY:

Time of Exposure throughout most of pregnancy
Risk Risk assessment is not possible
Pregnancy Outcome uncertain
Documentation insufficient; available information is insufficient

Time of Exposure near the time of delivery
Risk Known risk*
Pregnancy Outcome adverse (withdrawal symptoms and bleeding problems)
Documentation conclusive, based on current knowledge

pre-conception	All or None		Organ Development – (in weeks)						Maturation – (in weeks)				
	1	2	3	4	5	6	7	8	9	10	12	20-36	38

conception　　←—Time of Greatest Risk—→　　birth

Primidone is an anticonvulsant—a drug that inhibits seizures or epilepsy. It is chemically related to a group of drugs known as barbiturates. In fact, when in the human body, primidone breaks down into two products, one of which is the barbiturate phenobarbital (see phenobarbital, page 264).

*above the 4% background risk

Opinions differ about the specific risk of anticonvulsants. Many experts say there is two to three times the risk of major malformations in the children of epileptic women as in the general population. Some think the underlying disease is the cause. Others believe this statistic reflects a population of women who are exposed more often to anticonvulsant drugs, particularly hydantoins (see hydantoins, page 191), which are known teratogens.

Most studies evaluate primidone used with other anticonvulsants, mainly phenytoin, which is one of the hydantoins. So the relationship between birth defects and primidone alone is difficult to discern. Many babies exposed before birth to a combination of primidone and phenytoin have exhibited the fetal hydantoin syndrome. Whether these effects are due to the phenytoin alone, or to its use along with primidone, remains unclear.

Case reports and one small prospective study have observed abnormalities in the children of women *using only* primidone.[1,2,3,4,5,6] But there was no specific pattern of malformation. Interestingly, many of the descriptions resembled those of children exposed to hydantoins:

- *head and facial* alterations: short nose, bowed upper lip, broad nose bridge, eyes spaced wider than normal;
- *heart defects;* and
- *growth retardation.*

Some of these children also had:

- *underdeveloped fingertips,* with small or flat nails (a defect some think only associated with hydantoins);
- *hernias,* and
- *hypospadias* (abnormal placement of the urethral opening of the penis).

Further study is needed to determine the significance of these findings.

Several studies of primidone alone[1,5,6] and with other anticonvulsants[2,7] have occasionally found children exhibiting growth retardation and abnormally small head size (microcephaly). Normal intelligence but some delay in motor skills,[4] or complete developmental delay[8] have also been observed. Developmental examinations revealed slight retardation in the first year only in two children exposed to primidone.[5] In this same study, two children reported to have small heads, performed normally. The significance of these findings is unknown.

One study of the levels of anticonvulsants in the blood has related the frequency of abnormalities to the dose.[9] But further research must be conducted before the severity of risk can be predicted from such measurements. In a few cases, the most noticeably affected children were exposed to the highest doses of primidone, phenobarbital, or both. In some cases the dose exceeded the usual therapeutic range, suggesting that high doses may cause the birth defects.[1,5,7] Physicians usually prescribe the lowest dose possible during pregnancy.

There are case reports of tumors in ten children exposed before birth to barbiturates and phenytoin (a hydantoin), plus alcohol in two cases.[10] From this evidence, some experts suspect that prenatal exposure to the drugs may have caused the cancer. To date, none of these cases have involved the use of primidone.

Barbiturates are associated with a blood coagulation defect in newborns, which can cause severe bleeding (usually within the first twenty-four hours). To help prevent this your physician will usually administer vitamin K_1 to you some weeks before delivery, and during labor. (Vitamin K_1 is required for normal blood clotting.) At birth, your baby will also receive vitamin K_1.

Using primidone might reduce your levels of one of the B-complex vitamins, folic acid or folate. The need for folate increases greatly during pregnancy, as it is required for fetal growth and development. Some suggest that taking folic acid supplements during pregnancy might reduce the risk of abnormal babies.[8]

Withdrawal symptoms often occur in babies born to women using barbiturates. These symptoms incude tremors, irritability, restlessness, high-pitched cry, voracious appetite, spitting up, and overreaction to cold, hunger, household noises, and other environmental effects. These symptoms usually start when the baby is a week old, and continue for two to four months.[11]

Most women continue taking anticonvulsant medication during pregnancy, unless they have been seizure-free for many years. *Under no circumstances should you ever discontinue your anticonvulsant medication, unless this action is under the direction and supervision of the prescribing physician.* Sudden withdrawal could cause a seizure. And while seizures are not known to cause malformations, they do present a possible risk to both you and your unborn baby.

Many women question how epilepsy or anticonvulsant medication in the father might affect their baby. Although not all scientists agree, most experts think this presents no increased risk. They believe that children fathered by men taking these drugs have the same chance of being normal and healthy as anyone else's and well-conducted animal research confirms this belief.[12] (For more information on this, see Risks From Exposures in the Baby's Father, page 14)

References:

[1]N. L. Rudd and R. M. Freedom, A possible primadone embryopathy, *Journal of Pediatrics* 94 (1979): 835–37.
[2]C. Krauss, L. B. Holmes, Q. N. Vanlang, and D. A. Keith, Four siblings with similar malformations after exposure to phenytoin and primidone, *Journal of Pediatrics* 105 (1984): 750–55.

[5]R. M. Goodman, M. B. M. Katznelson, M. Hertz, D. Katznelson, and Y. Rotem, Congenital malformations in four siblings of a mother taking anticonvulsants, *American Journal of Diseases of Children* 130 (1976): 884–87.

[6]S. A. Myhre and R. Williams, Teratogenic effects associated with maternal primidone therapy, *Journal of Pediatrics* 99 (1981): 160–62.

[5]D. Rating, H. Nau, E. Jäger-Roman, I. Göpfert-Geyer, S. Koch, G. Beck-Mannagetta, D. Schmidt, and H. Helge, Teratogenic and pharmokenetic studies of primidone during pregnancy and in the offspring of epileptic women, *Acta Pædiatrica Scandinavica* 71 (1982): 301–11.

[6]S. Shapiro, S. C. Hartz, V. Suskind, A. A. Mitchell, D. Slone, L. Rosenberg, R. R. Monson, O. P. Heinonen, J. Idänpän-Heikkilä, S. Härö, and L. Saxen, Anticonvulsants and parental epilepsy in the development of birth defects, *Lancet* 1 (1976): 272–75.

[7]M. Seip, Growth retardation, dysmorphic facies and minor malformations following massive exposure to phenobarbitone in utero, *Acta Pædiatrica Scandinavica* 65 (1976): 617–21.

[8]Y. Biale and H. Lewenthal, Effect of folic acid supplementation on congenital malformations due to anticonvulsive drugs, *Europeon Journal of Obstetrics, Gynecology, and Reproductive Biology* 18 (1984): 211–16.

[9]L. Dansky, E. Andermann, F. Andermann, A. L. Sherwin, and R. A. Kinch, Maternal epilepsy and congenital malformations: Correlations with maternal plasma anticonvulsant levels during pregnancy, in Janz et al. (eds.), *Epilepsy, Pregnancy and the Child* (New York: Raven Press, 1982), pp. 251–58.

[10]A. Lipson and P. Bale, Ependymoblastoma associated with prenatal exposure to Diphenylhydantoin and methylphenobarbitone, *Cancer* 55 (1985): 1859–62.

[11]M. M. Desmond, R. P. Schwanecke, G. S. Wilson, S. Yasunaga, and I. Burgdorff, Maternal barbiturate utilization and neonatal withdrawal symptomology, *Journal of Pediatrics* 80 (1972): 190–97.

[12]R. H. Finnell and J. F. Baer, Congenital defects among the offspring of epileptic fathers: Role of the genotype and phenytoin therapy in a mouse model, *Epilepsia* 25 (1986): 697–705.

GENERIC NAME: **PRIMAQUINE PHOSPHATE**

Brand Name: **(Primaquine Phosphate)**

FDA Pregnancy Category:—

ESTIMATED RISK SUMMARY:

Time of Exposure throughout pregnancy

Risk Risk assessment is not possible

Pregnancy Outcome uncertain

Documentation insufficient: no information is available

◄── pre-conception	All or None		Organ Development – (in weeks)						Maturation – (in weeks)				
	1	2	3	4	5	6	7	8	9	10	12	20-36	38

conception   ◄─── Time of Greatest Risk ───►   birth

Primaquine is used to treat and prevent malaria. Little is known about its potential teratogenicity, and to date no reports of primaquine-caused birth defects have appeared. Definitive conclusions about the safety of the use of this drug during pregnancy await further study.

A complication called hemolytic anemia may arise from the use of primaquine in patients with the inherited condition glucose-6-phosphate dehydrogenase (G6PD) deficiency. Hemolytic anemia results from the shortened survival of red blood cells. G6PD deficiency should be ruled out before initiating primaquine therapy during pregnancy.

Malaria during pregnancy is associated with miscarriages, growth retardation before birth, and rarely, congenital infection. The incidence of prematurity and stillbirth may also increase, but more studies must be performed to confirm this belief. It is important to realize that the risks from malaria infection to both the mother and unborn child are significantly greater than are any remote risks from preventative drug therapy. In addition, treatment for acute malaria during pregnancy requires higher doses of antimalarial drugs than are needed to prevent it. Therefore, pregnant women who are not immune to malaria should not travel to areas with a high incidence of malaria without consulting a physician and beginning antimalarial drug therapy. Therapy usually begins one or two weeks before departure and is continued after returning for another six to eight weeks. Commonsense precautions to help avoid bites by infected insects include sensible clothing, screens, nets, and topical insect-repellents.

GENERIC NAME: **PROCAINAMIDE**

Brand Names: **(Procan SR, Promine, Pronestyl)**

FDA Pregnancy Category: C

ESTIMATED RISK SUMMARY:

> *Time of Exposure* throughout pregnancy
> *Risk* Risk assessment is not possible
> *Pregnancy Outcome* uncertain
> *Documentation* insufficient

← pre- conception	All or None		Organ Development – (in weeks)						Maturation – (in weeks)				
	1	2	3	4	5	6	7	8	9	10	12	20-36	38

conception   ←——Time of Greatest Risk——→   birth

Procainamide[1] is used to treat abnormal heart rate and rhythm. There have been no controlled studies of its effect on pregnancy outcome. But it is reassuring to note that clinical experience with procainamide during pregnancy has not shown any adverse effects on the developing child. Nevertheless, formal investigations are required before its teratogenicity can be determined.

Procainamide crosses the placenta and enters the unborn child's bloodstream. Because of this, it has been administered to a pregnant woman to return her child's rapid heartbeat (tachycardia) to normal.

Long-term follow-up studies of children exposed before birth have not been located.

Reference:

[1]H. H. Rotmensch, U. Elkayam, and W. Frishman, Antiarrhythmic drug therapy during pregnancy, *Annals of Internal Medicine* 98 (1983): 487–97.

GENERIC NAME: **PROPOXYPHENE**

Brand Names: (◊ **Bexophene, Darvon,** ◊ **Darvon Compound, Dolene,** ◊ **Dolene Compound,** *Dolene A–65, Doxaphene, ◊ **Doxaphene Compound, Profene, SK–65 APAP,** ◊ **SK-65 Compound,** *Wygesic)

FDA Pregnancy Category:—

ESTIMATED RISK SUMMARY:

Time of Exposure throughout pregnancy
Risk Risk of assessment for birth defects is not possible
Pregnancy Outcome uncertain
Documentation insufficient

Time of Exposure particularly near delivery or during labor
Risk Known risk** (related to dose and duration of the drug)
Pregnancy Outcome adverse
Documentation conclusive, based on current knowledge

*also contains acetaminophen
◊ also contains aspirin and caffeine
**above the 4% background risk

← pre-conception ←		All or None		Organ Development – (in weeks)						Maturation – (in weeks)				
		1	2	3	4	5	6	7	8	9	10	12	20-36	38

conception　　　　←—Time of Greatest Risk —→　　　　birth

Propoxyphene is a narcotic analgesic, or pain reliever, chemically related to methadone. It is used to relieve mild to moderate pain and as a suppressant in cough syrups. Although propoxyphene is a mild narcotic, it can become habit-forming if used for prolonged periods, and the potential for its abuse does exist. Abuse of any narcotic during pregnancy always carries with it the risk of addiction in the mother, as well as the unborn child.

Limited information is available on the effects of this drug on a developing baby. The only study that actually looked at propoxyphene exposure in pregnancy is the Collaborative Perinatal Project, which evaluated pregnancy outcome in more than 50,000 mother-child pairs, exposed to a wide variety of drugs.[1] This large prospective investigation has a variety of shortcomings and its conclusions are by no means definitive. But it is reassuring to know that among 686 first trimester exposures to propoxyphene studied, no increased frequency of birth defects was observed.

Four isolated instances of birth defects have been reported in children whose mothers used propoxyphene while pregnant.[2,3,4] In each case, the mother also used other drugs, including the known teratogen diphenylhydantoin (see hydantoins, page 191). So the other drug, their combination, or chance alone, may have been responsible for the defects. The fact that the malformations were all different suggests that a single environmental cause was probably not responsible. All known teratogens display a recognizable pattern of malformation, which was not apparent in these children. In conclusion, cause-and-effect cannot be determined from the limited information currently available.

Withdrawal symptoms have been observed in a number of newborns whose mothers used large amounts of this drug near the time of delivery. Often severe, these symptoms included tremors, irritability, vomiting, diarrhea, fever, and seizures. Withdrawal in these babies usually resolves without the need of medical assistance.

Long-term follow-up studies of children exposed before birth have not been located.

References:

[1] O. P. Heinonen, D. Slone, and S. Shapiro, *Birth Defects and Drugs in Pregnancy* (Littleton, Mass.: Publishing Sciences Group, 1977).

[2]M. V. Barrow and D. E. Souder, Propoxyphene and congenital malformations, *Journal of the American Medical Association* 217 (1971): 1551–52.

[3]C. A. D. Ringrose, The hazard of neurotrophic drugs in the fertile years. *Canadian Medical Association Journal* 106 (1972): 1058.

[4]N. L. Golden, K. C. King, and R. J. Sokol, Propoxyphene and acetaminophen, *Clinical Pediatrics* 21 (1982): 752–54.

GENERIC NAME: **PROPANOLOL**

Brand Name: **(Inderal)**

FDA Pregnancy Category: C

ESTIMATED RISK SUMMARY:

Time of Exposure throughout the first 6 or 7 months of pregnancy
Risk No known risk*
Pregnancy Outcome appears favorable
Documentation inconclusive

Time of Exposure last few weeks of pregnancy, particularly near the time of delivery
Risk Suspected risk*
Pregnancy Outcome uncertain: favorable and adverse outcomes observed
Documentation inconclusive, based on minimal data

← pre-conception	All or None		Organ Development – (in weeks)						Maturation – (in weeks)				
	1	2	3	4	5	6	7	8	9	10	12	20-36	38

conception   ← Time of Greatest Risk →   birth

Propranolol[1] belongs to a group of drugs classified as beta-adrenergic blocking agents (beta blockers). Propranolol is indicated for the treatment of hypertension, angina, cardiac arrhythmias (abnormal heartbeat rhythms), and in the prevention of migraine headaches.

Propranolol has frequently been used in pregnancy, and only three isolated case reports describing nonrelated birth defects in babies born to mothers taking propranolol have been located. (These include an abnormality of the trachea and esophagus

*above the expected 4% background risk

[tracheoesophageal fistula], of the hip [crepitus of the hip], and constriction in the stomach's outlet [pyloric stenosis].) It is notable that the abnormalities cited among the children were all very different, meaning that they probably were not the result of one specific cause. The widespread use of this drug and the fact that similar findings have not appeared in other children born to mothers taking it, makes it even more unlikely that the drug caused the defects.

Several adverse effects, which may be related to the size of the dose, have been observed in the fetus and newborn after prenatal exposure to this drug. Complications include growth retardation, slower than normal heartbeat (bradycardia), breathing problems (respiratory depression), and severe hypoglycemia (abnormally low blood sugar). These problems are usually associated with drug use late in the third trimester, particularly near the time of delivery.

It is also important to be aware that the mother's illness and the other medications she's taking might contribute to the problems observed in propranolol-treated pregnancies.

Long-term follow-up studies of children exposed before birth have not been located.

Reference:

[1] A. L. Wilson and G. R. Matzke, The treatment of hypertension in pregnancy, *Drug Intelligence and Clinical Pharmacy* 15 (1981): 21–26.

GENERIC NAME: **PYRIMETHAMINE**

Brand Names: **(Daraprim, ◇ Fansidar)**

FDA Pregnancy Category: C

ESTIMATED RISK SUMMARY:

Time of Exposure throughout pregnancy

Risk No known risk,* although judicious use is recommended, particularly in the first trimester

Pregnancy Outcome appears favorable

Documentation inconclusive, based on minimal data

◇ contains sulfadoxine
*above the 4% background risk

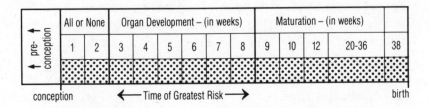

pre-conception	All or None		Organ Development – (in weeks)						Maturation – (in weeks)				
	1	2	3	4	5	6	7	8	9	10	12	20-36	38

conception   ←——Time of Greatest Risk——→   birth

Pyrimethamine,[1] an anti-infective drug, is used to prevent contracting malaria. It is also combined with a sulfonamide (sulfadoxine), another anti-infective, to both prevent and treat malaria as well as to treat toxoplasmosis (see sulfonamides, page 305.)

Malaria and toxoplasmosis are caused by organisms called protozoa. Pyrimethamine, a folic acid antagonist drug, kills protozoa by blocking their use of folic acid, one of the B vitamins. It *does not* have this effect on human cells. But when used in higher doses to treat disease, as opposed to the doses used for disease prevention, pyrimethamine can cause folic acid deficiency. For this reason, physicians often recommend taking folic acid supplements when the drug is used during pregnancy.

The entire group of folic acid antagonist drugs became suspect when the drug aminopterin was identified as a human teratogen (see also chemotherapeutic drugs, page 103). *Unlike* pyrimethamine, aminopterin can interfere with the growth of certain rapidly dividing *human* cells: cancer cells, fetal cells, and bone marrow. For these reasons, pyrimethamine and other folic acid antagonists often carry a warning about usage during pregnancy, particularly in the first trimester.

Another concern over the use of pyrimethamine in pregnancy stems from its teratogenic effects when given in high doses to pregnant rats. It is important to keep in mind that no abnormalities directly attributable to pyrimethamine have been reported in children whose mothers took the drug during pregnancy. So the results of the animal studies have no apparent bearing on human risk.

The most widely used antimalarial drug is chloroquine. The Centers for Disease Control (CDC) recommends Fansidar (pyrimethamine and sulfadoxine) for travelers to chloroquine-resistant areas.[2] In 1985, this was revised as several cases of adverse reactions to this drug combination were reported.[3] Now the CDC recommends that the use of Fansidar be limited to people traveling to areas where there is a very high risk of encountering chloroquine-resistent malaria parasites.

Malaria during pregnancy is associated with miscarriages, growth retardation before birth, and, rarely, congenital infection. The incidence of prematurity and still birth may also increase, but more studies must be performed to confirm this belief. It is important to realize that the risks from malarial infection to both the mother and unborn child are significantly greater than are any remote risks from preventative drug therapy. In addition, treatment for acute malaria during pregnancy requires higher doses of antimalarial drugs than are needed to prevent it. Therefore, pregnant women who are not immune to malaria are advised not to travel to areas with a high incidence of malaria without consulting a physician and beginning antimalarial drug therapy. Therapy usually begins one or two weeks before departure and is continued after returning for another six to eight weeks. Commonsense precautions to help avoid bites by infected insects include sensible clothing, screens, nets and topical insect-repellents.

Long-term follow-up studies of children exposed before birth have not been located.

References:

[1]Editorial. Pyrimethamine Combinations in Pregnancy. Lancet 2 (1983): 1005–1007.

[2]Centers for Disease Control. Prevention of malaria in travellers, 1982, *Morbidity and Mortality Weekly Report* 31(No.1S)(1982): 1–28S.

[3]Centers for Disease Control, Revised recommendations for preventing malaria in travelers to area with cloroquine-resistant P falciparum, *Morbidity and Mortality Weekly Report* 34 (1985): 185–90.

GENERIC NAME: **QUINIDINE**

Brand Names: **(Cardioquin, Cin-Quin, Duraquin, Quin-Release, Quinaglute Dura-Tabs, Quinatime, Quinidex, Quinora)**

FDA Pregnancy Category: C

ESTIMATED RISK SUMMARY:

Time of Exposure throughout pregnancy

Risk No known risk*

Pregnancy Outcome appears favorable

Documentation inconclusive

← pre-conception	All or None		Organ Development – (in weeks)						Maturation – (in weeks)				
	1	2	3	4	5	6	7	8	9	10	12	20-36	38

conception ← Time of Greatest Risk → birth

*above the 4% background risk

Quinidine,[1,2] a quinine derivative, has been regularly used to treat abnormal heartbeat rhythms (arrhythmias) since 1918. Its use during pregnancy dates from the early 1930s. Quinidine freely crosses the placenta, achieving therapeutic drug levels in the fetus. A review of the scientific literature indicates that it is without apparent teratogenic effects.

There is a report of thrombocytopenia (a decrease in blood platelets, which are essential for blood coagulation) in a baby whose mother took quinidine during pregnancy. Another study found that minimal uterine contractions were associated with the use of quinidine, but this was usually after spontaneous contractions had already begun. No other reports of adverse effects have been located.

Quinine derivatives as a group are known to cause damage to the auditory (hearing) nerve, but only in doses significantly higher than those used to treat heart ailments. Some sources,[3] misquoting a research article, suggest that very high doses of quinidine caused damage to the auditory nerve of an unborn child. In fact, the original report implicated *quinine*, not quinidine[4] (see quinine, page 282). Also, the original article supports the notion that exposure to quinidine before birth does not cause similar problems.

Long-term follow-up studies of children exposed before birth have not been located.

References:

[1]K. Ueland, J. H. McAnulty, F. R. Ueland, and J. Metcalfe. Special considerations in the use of cardiovascular drugs, *Clinical Obstetrics and Gynecology* 24 (1981): 809–23.

[2]H. H. Rotmensch, U. Elkayam, and W. Frishman, Antiarrhythmic drug therapy during pregnancy, *Annals of Internal Medicine* 98 (1983): 487–97.

[3]R. L. Berkowitz, D. R. Coustoan, T. K. Mochizuke, *Handbook of Prescribing Medications During Pregnancy* (Boston: Little, Brown, 1981), p. 191.

[4]C. L. Mendelson, Disorders of the heartbeat during pregnancy, *American Journal of Obstetrics and Gynecology* 72 (1956): 1268–1301.

GENERIC NAME: **QUININE**

Brand Names: **(Quin-260, Quinamm, Quine, Quinine Sulfate, Quinite, Quiphile, Strema)**

FDA Pregnancy Category: X

ESTIMATED RISK SUMMARY:

Time of Exposure difficult to determine: problems reported from first and second trimester exposures

Risk Known risk*, when taken in very large doses

*above the 4% background risk

Pregnancy Outcome adverse
Documentation conclusive, based on current knowledge

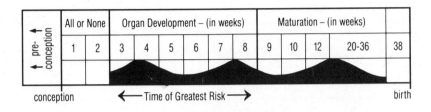

	All or None	Organ Development – (in weeks)						Maturation – (in weeks)				
pre-conception ← →	1	2	3	4	5	6	7	8	9	10	12	20-36	38

conception   ← Time of Greatest Risk →   birth

Quinine[1] has been used for two very different purposes. Once it was the only drug used for the treatment of malaria. Now it has been replaced by more effective and less toxic drugs. Quinine has also been used as a "folk remedy" for inducing abortions, though not an effective one. A variety of teratogenic effects are associated with quinine's use as an abortion inducer. But when it was used against malaria, no effects were observed. This may be related to the smaller doses used to treat malaria, as opposed to the large and often fatal doses used in abortion attempts. Quinine is usually fatal in adults when 8 grams are ingested, but death has been reported after a 1-gram dose. A 4-gram dose produces poisonous effects.

A review of seventy quinine-attempted abortions in known or suspected pregnancies revealed that the mother died in eleven cases, forty-one children had birth defects, and in only three cases where abortion was successful did the mother survive.[1] Abnormalities frequently seen in children exposed to quinine before birth include damage to the central nervous system, defects of the arms and legs, blindness, underdeveloped eye nerve (hypoplasia optic nerve), deafness, and hearing impairments.

Long-term follow-up studies of children exposed before birth have not been located.

Reference:

[1]A. L. Dannenberg, S. F. Dorfman, and J. Johnson. Use of quinine for self-induced abortion, *Southern Medical Journal* 76 (1983): 846–49.

GENERIC NAME: **RABIES VACCINE**

Brand Names: **(Imovax Rabies Vaccine, WYVAC Rabies Vaccine)**

FDA Pregnancy Category: C

ESTIMATED RISK SUMMARY:

Time of Exposure throughout pregnancy

Risk Risk assessment is not possible
Pregnancy Outcome uncertain
Documentation insufficient

← pre-conception →	All or None		Organ Development – (in weeks)						Maturation – (in weeks)				
	1	2	3	4	5	6	7	8	9	10	12	20-36	38

conception   ← Time of Greatest Risk →   birth

Rabies, when contracted, is always fatal. For this reason, pregnancy is not a contraindication for vaccination in those who have been exposed to the disease.

There are two types of *rabies vaccine*,[1] duck embryo vaccine and human diploid cell vaccine. Use of the duck embryo vaccine has been replaced by the human diploid cell vaccine, which was approved for use in the United States in 1980. Both vaccines contain the inactivated virus, so theroetically they should pose no increased risk during pregnancy. Only a few reports of rabies vaccination in pregnancy exist. While no serious adverse effects in the mother or unborn baby have appeared, there are still too few cases to conclude that rabies vaccine is absolutely safe during pregnancy.

Reference:

[1]M. W. Varner, G. A. McGuiness, and R. P. Galask, Rabies vaccination in pregnancy, *American Journal of Obstetrics and Gynecology* 143 (1982): 717–78.

MEDICATION CLASSIFICATION: **RADIOACTIVE IODINE**

GENERIC NAMES: **SODIUM IODINE I^{125}, SODIUM IODIDE I^{131}**

Brand Names: (**Iodotope Therapeutic, Sodium Iodide I^{131} Therapeutic**)

FDA Pregnancy Category:—

ESTIMATED RISK SUMMARY:

Time of Exposure prior to conception

Risk No known risk*

*above the 4% background risk

Pregnancy Outcome appears favorable
Documentation inconclusive, based on very minimal data

Time of Exposure potentially from 10 weeks on
Risk Known risk*
Pregnancy Outcome adverse
Documentation conclusive, based on current knowledge

pre-conception	All or None	Organ Development – (in weeks)						Maturation – (in weeks)				
	1	2	3	4	5	6	7	8	9	10	12	20-36	38

conception   ⟵ Time of Greatest Risk ⟶   birth

Radioactive iodine[1] is used to diagnose thyroid problems and is used therapeutically to destroy thyroid tissue.

There are two potential concerns regarding radioactive iodine exposures during pregnancy. One involves the possible risks from the radiation, the other relates to the iodine itself. Risk assessment for both of these issues involves evaluating the time of the exposure and the amount or dose received. Exposures involving therapeutic doses of radioactive iodine are of greatest concern. This is because they are approximately one thousand times greater than diagnostic doses. If you have been treated with radioactive iodine not realizing you were pregnant, your physician or a radiation physicist can calculate the amount of radiation you received (see also X rays, page 347; and iodine, page 203).

Radioactive iodine does cross the placenta. But like other iodines, this compound will not likely affect fetal thyroid development until after it begins to function, at about ten weeks of pregnancy. After this time the gland takes up increasing amounts of iodine. Too much iodine during pregnancy can severely damage the fetal thyroid gland and cause mental and physical retardation in the exposed baby.

Hypothyroidism (underactive thyroid gland), accompanied by mental and physical retardation, has been reported in several children born to pregnant women who received therapeutic doses of radioactive iodine.[2] How much radioactive iodine is needed to produce these problems is not known, although as expected, the effects of this drug appear to be related to the amount received (dose).

*above the 4% background risk

No increase in birth defects or in chromosomal abnormalities have been observed in the children of women who received high doses of radioactive iodine *prior* to becoming pregnant.[3]

References:

[1]J. H. Mestman, Diagnosis and management of hyperthyroidism in pregnancy, *Current Problems in Obstetrics and Gynecology* 4 (1981): 1–51.

[2]H. G. Green, F. J. Garesis, T. H. Shepard, and V. C. Kelley, Cretinism associated with maternal sodium iodide I[131] therapy during pregnancy, *American Journal of Diseases of Children* 122 (1971): 247–49.

[3]J. Einhorn, M. Hulten, J. Lindsten, H. Wicklund, and P. Zetterqvist, *Acta Radiologica* 2 (1972): 193–208.

GENERIC NAME: **RESERPINE**

Brand names: **(Releserp-5, Sandril, Serpalan, Serpasil, Serpate, Zepine)**

FDA Pregnancy Category: D

ESTIMATED RISK SUMMARY:

Time of Exposure throughout most of pregnancy

Risk Risk assessment is not possible

Pregnancy Outcome uncertain

Documentation insufficient

Time of Exposure near the time of delivery, particularly within 48 hours of birth

Risk Known risk*

Pregnancy Outcome adverse

Documentation conclusive, based on current data

← pre-conception		All or None		Organ Development – (in weeks)						Maturation – (in weeks)				
		1	2	3	4	5	6	7	8	9	10	12	20-36	38

conception   ←— Time of Greatest Risk —→   birth

*above the expected 4% background risk

Reserpine[1] is used to treat hypertension and in some cases to relieve symptoms in psychiatric disorders.

Three human studies testing reserpine have not associated it with birth defects.[2,3,4] In contrast, the Collaborative Perinatal Project which evaluated pregnancy outcome in more than 50,000 mother-child pairs exposed to a wide variety of drugs, reported an increased frequency of birth defects in those exposed to reserpine.[5] The value of the information from this study for use in teratogen risk counseling has been questioned for several reasons: There are few controls for other possible causes. The critical issue of medication timing was not specified. Because of frequent multiproduct use during pregnancy, difficulty exists in determining which drugs, if any, could have caused the birth defects. When several substances are examined together, as they were in this study, an association between any of the drugs and birth defects may simply be a chance occurrence. It is notable that the abnormalities cited among the children exposed to reserpine were not similar, meaning they probably were not the result of one specific cause. Last, even if there was an association, it does not prove that the substance actually caused the defect. In summary, further investigation is required before the significance of the associations disclosed in this study can be determined.

Newborn children whose mothers have been given reserpine within forty-eight hours of birth have exhibited a temporary nasal discharge. Because newborns breathe through their noses, this complication can be a problem. Other side effects from near-term exposures are slow fetal heartbeat (bradycardia), lethargy, and poor appetite. These problems might be avoided if drug use were discontinued at least a few days before delivery.

Long-term follow-up studies of children exposed before birth have not been located.

References:

[1] A. L. Wilson and G. R. Matzke, The treatment of hypertension in pregnancy, *Drug Intelligence and Clinical Pharmacy* 15 (1981): 21–26.

[2] D. E. Sobel, Fetal damage due to ECT, insulin coma, chlorpromazine or reserpine, *Archives of General Psychiatry* 2 (1960): 606–11.

[3] J. H. Ravina, Les thérapeutiques dangereuses chez la femme enceinte, *Presse Médicale* 72 (1964): 3057.

[4] R. Gaunt, A. A. Renzi, N. Antonchak, G. J. Miller, and M. Gillman. Endocrine aspects of the pharmacology of reserpine, *Annals of the New York Academy of Science* 59 (1959): 22–35.

[5] O. P. Heinonen, D. Slone, and S. Shapiro, *Birth Defects and Drugs in Pregnancy* (Littleton, Mass.: Publishing Sciences Group, 1977).

GENERIC NAME: **RIFAMPIN**

Brand Names: **(Rifadin, Rimactane)**

FDA Pregnancy Category:—

ESTIMATED RISK SUMMARY:
Time of Exposure throughout pregnancy
Risk No known risk* for birth defects
Pregnancy Outcome appears favorable
Documentation inconclusive, based on minimal data

Time of Exposure near term
Risk assessment for bleeding tendencies is not possible
Pregnancy Outcome uncertain
Documentation insufficient

pre-conception ←		All or None		Organ Development – (in weeks)						Maturation – (in weeks)				
		1	2	3	4	5	6	7	8	9	10	12	20-36	38

conception   ←——Time of Greatest Risk——→   birth

Rifampin is used to treat tuberculosis. An extensive review of the medical literature on pregnant women treated with various antitubercular medications was conducted in an effort to discover the effect of these drugs on the developing baby.[1] The investigators located information on the pregnancies of 2,787 women and found that 94 percent of them had full-term infants who appeared normal at birth. Approximately 3 percent of the pregnancies resulted in miscarriages, stillbirths, or premature births, while 2.89 percent resulted in birth defects. The reported frequency of problems is within the expected range. As abnormalities are likely to be overrepresented in the literature, the small incidence of adverse pregnancy outcomes is particularly reassuring.

Of the entire number of pregnant women in this literature review, 446 took rifampin. From this population there were 386 normal term infants (86.5%), 7 miscarriages (1.56%), 9 stillbirths (2%), 2 premature births (.44%), and 13 birth defects (2.9%), of which most were minor.

While the overall risk for birth defects is not higher in unborn children exposed to rifampin, thirteen infants did have bleeding tendencies (hypoprothrombinemia). This observation raises some concern, particularly when the drug is used near term. Further experience with rifampin in pregnancy is required before its potential adverse effects can truly be assessed.

*above the 4% background risk

Rifampin may interfere with the efficacy of birth control pills, leading to unplanned pregnancies.

Long-term follow-up studies of children exposed before birth have not been located.

Reference:

[1]D. E. Snider, P. M. Layde, M. W. Johnson, and M. A. Lyle, Treatment of tuberculosis during pregnancy, *American Review of Respiratory Diseases* 122 (1980): 65–79.

COMMON NAME: **RUBELLA (German measles)**

Brand name/Chemical Name: **not applicable**

FDA Pregnancy Category: not applicable

ESTIMATED RISK SUMMARY:

Time of Exposure throughout pregnancy

Risk Known risk*

Pregnancy Outcome adverse

Documentation conclusive, based on current knowledge

← pre-conception	All or None		Organ Development – (in weeks)						Maturation – (in weeks)				
	1	2	3	4	5	6	7	8	9	10	12	20-36	38

conception   ←—Time of Greatest Risk—→   birth

Rubella,[1] also called German measles, is a viral infection that can be transmitted from the mother to her developing baby.

A variety of information indicates that rubella infection during any stage of pregnancy carries some risk for the unborn baby. Both the degree of risk and the type of complications depend on the time the infection occurs. During the first eight weeks, as many as 85 percent will have detectable defects. During weeks nine to twelve, the rate is 52 percent. The rate decreases to approximately 16 percent during weeks thirteen to twenty. And the percentage has not been determined for twenty weeks and beyond. The reason the incidence of defects declines as pregnancy advances is that the

*above the 4% background risk

embryo becomes more and more able to withstand environmental influences (teratogenesis). This examplifies one of the principles of teratology—that the potential for a substance to interfere with a baby's development depends on the stage of pregnancy (see Second Principle of Teratology, page 33).

The consequences of rubella infection vary. It can cause death of the baby before birth (miscarriage or stillbirth) or result in severe multiple birth defects (heart abnormalities, eye defects [cataracts], deafness, growth retardation, and mental retardation). Or it may have no obvious effect, resulting in the delivery of normal-appearing newborn infants. Long-term observation is partiuclarly important for babies in this last category, as many do develop some evidence of disease before 5 years of age.

The risk for all defects is definitely highest during the critical time of organ formation, primarily from three to eight weeks. Abnormalities of the heart are very common when infection coincides with cardiac development (the first eight weeks). Hearing loss is the most common of the rubella defects and the one most likely to occur by itself. The risk for hearing impairment exists throughout pregnancy. Growth retardation also could occur from infection at any time in pregnancy, but this persists beyond birth only after a first trimester infection.

The saddest thing today about rubella infection is that its existence is unnecessary. In 1969 a vaccine was developed that created the opportunity to eliminate rubella as a disease and *prevent* rubella-caused birth defects (see rubella vaccine, below). Unfortunately, a percentage of our population have not yet had either the infection or the vaccination, and they remain susceptible. *It is therefore imperative that all nonpregnant women of childbearing age be screened for rubella and that all susceptible persons be vaccinated.*

Reference:

[1] J. S. Remington and J. O. Klein (eds.), *Infectious Diseases of the Fetus and Newborn Infant*, 2d ed. (Philadelphia: W. B. Saunders, 1983), pp. 69–103.

GENERIC NAME: **RUBELLA (German Measles) VACCINE**

Brand name: **(Meruvax II)**

FDA Pregnancy Category:—

ESTIMATED RISK SUMMARY:

Time of Exposure before conception and throughout pregnancy

Risk No measurable risk*
Pregnancy Outcome favorable
Documentation conclusive, based on current knowledge

pre-conception	All or None	Organ Development – (in weeks)						Maturation – (in weeks)				
	1	2	3	4	5	6	7	8	9	10	12	20-36	38

conception   ⟵——Time of Greatest Risk——⟶   birth

Rubella vaccine[1] is used to prevent rubella or German measles. During 1964–65 an epidemic of rubella resulted in approximatedly 20,000 malformed infants and 30,000 stillbirths in the United States. The introduction of rubella vaccine in 1969 provided the opportunity to prevent similar tragedies.

Rubella vaccine contains the live virus, which has been made noninfectious. It is what is called a live attenuated vaccine. Since 1979 only one type of rubella vaccine has been used, RA 27/3. Prior to this time both Cendehill and HPV-77 vaccines were available. Even though rubella vaccine cannot cause rubella, it was once feared to have the same teratogenic potential as the infection itself (see rubella virus, page 289). Those fears are not founded. In fact, inadvertent vaccination either shortly before or during pregnancy (in women who didn't expect to become pregnant or who didn't know they were) has an observed risk of *zero,* meaning that there is no evidence of rubella vaccine–related birth defects.[2,3] This finding is based on hundreds of cases of normal children following inadvertent vaccination of their mothers. Long-term follow-up of these children (extending from 17 months to 9 years) continues to be reassuring, with normal growth and development.[4]

Despite all the reassuring evidence, a very small *theoretical* risk of prenatal infection must be considered. For this reason, intentional rubella vaccination during pregnancy is prohibited. The United States Public Health Service recommends that women avoid conception for three months after vaccination, which I believe is a wise precautionary measure.

If you should accidentally be vaccinated during pregnancy, an expert has summed up by stating that "fetal exposure to the vaccine should not in itself constitute a reason to terminate the pregnancy."[4]

*above the 4% background risk

Jennifer's Story

Last September I found out I was pregnant. During my first exam with a local midwife I volunteered information of my recent vaccination of German measles, three days before I was married in July. She then asked if the person who gave me the vaccination had told me to wait three months before conceiving. I said, "No." She then stated that the vaccination used the live virus itself and went on to tell me the effects German measles has on an unborn during the first trimester. I had studied all this in high school, so I knew and understood what the chances were. She asked me my views on abortion, which were negative. I refused to do anything drastic until I knew exactly what my child's chances were.

I had lost a child just three months prior to this. Now I was eight weeks along. I decided to fight for this one. Two days later I contacted a place twenty miles from my hometown. They were involved in amniocentesis testing and told me to contact you.

I was greatly relieved after hearing the research on this particular topic. No effects were being found in any of the unborn babies in mothers that had the vaccination close to conception or during the first trimester. I went back to the midwife to tell her what I had been told. She refused to agree and said my baby's chances were less than 50–50. I decided to see my out-of-town doctor and explained what happened at the midwife's. He was stunned and said he had to agree with the midwife, but would contact an associate at the University of California to find out more. When he returned, he was astonished that I had been telling him something he should have already known. He said he was glad it came up and that from now on he would no longer have to tell his patients in this predicament to consider an abortion.

Today I have a new son who is 7 months old. He was born a hefty eight pounds nine and one-half ounces and I'm glad to say he is in perfect health. I fought for his life and he won!

References:

[1]J. D. Blanco and R. S. Gibbs, Immunizations in pregnancy, *Clinical Obstetrics and Gynecology* 1982; 25: 611–7.

[2]Centers for Disease Control, Rubella vaccination during pregnancy—United States, 1971–83 *Morbidity and Mortality Weekly Report* 33 (1984): 365.

[3]G. Enders, Rubella antibody titers in vaccinated and nonvaccinated women and results of vaccination during pregnancy, *Reviews of Infectious Diseases* 7 (1985): S103–S107.

[4]S. R. Preblud, Some current issues relating to rubella vaccine, *Journal of the American Medical Association* 254 (1985): 253–56.

MEDICATION CLASSIFICATION: **SALICYLATES**

GENERIC NAMES: **ASPIRIN, CHOLINE SALICYLATE, MAGNESIUM SALICYLATE, SALSALATE, SODIUM SALICYLATE**

Brand Names: (◇ **Artha-G**, ◇ **Arthritis Pain Formula, Arthropan, A. S. A., Asperbuf, Aspergum, Bayer,** ◇ **Buffaprin,** ◇ **Bufferin,** ◇ **Buffex,** ◇ **Buf-Tabs, Cosprin, Disalcid, Doan's Pills, Ecotrin, Empirin, Encaprin, Magan, Mobidin, Mono-Gesic, Uracel)**
[most, but not all brand names are listed]

FDA Pregnancy Category:
aspirin: D; salicylate, magnesium salicylate: C; all others:—

ESTIMATED RISK SUMMARY:
Time of Exposure throughout pregnancy
Risk No known risk* for birth defects
Pregnancy Outcome appears favorable
Documentation inconclusive, based on minimal data

Time of Exposure the last month of pregnancy
Risk Known risk* particularly for bleeding tendencies
Pregnancy Outcome adverse
Documentation conclusive, based on current knowledge

pre-conception	All or None		Organ Development – (in weeks)						Maturation – (in weeks)				
	1	2	3	4	5	6	7	8	9	10	12	20-36	38

conception   ←——Time of Greatest Risk——→   birth

Salicylates[1,2] are used to relieve moderate pain, reduce fever, and control inflammation.

Salicylates have been studied more than any other pain reliever used by pregnant women; this is due in part to their wide use. Commonly used drugs, such as aspirin,

◇ buffered aspirin
*above the 4% background risk

can be erroneously associated with an increase in problems. This is particularly true if only the mothers of malformed children are surveyed, and if the study is performed some years after the pregnancy. In these circumstances, memories are not always accurate about what drug was used and when during the pregnancy. In addition, mothers of babies with birth defects recall the events during their pregnancy much differently than do mothers of normal children. Some retrospective studies of this type have raised questions about the safety of salicylate use during pregnancy.[3,4,5] However, cause-and-effect is doubtful, because of these flaws and the failure to exclude other potential causes, including the use of additional drugs (see retrospective studies, page 43).

In contrast, several investigations have consistently failed to associate aspirin use during pregnancy with an increase in birth defects. Among these studies are the findings from the Collaborative Perinatal Project, which evaluated pregnancy outcome in more than 50,000 mother-child pairs exposed to a wide variety of drugs.[6] In this large prospective study, up to 64 percent of the women reported using salicylates sometime during pregnancy. While this study does have some flaws, it is reassuring to know that an increased risk was not detected among so many exposures. It is also noteworthy that a recognizable pattern of malformation, which all known teratogens display, has not been described in salicylate-exposed children (see prospective studies, page 42).

Studies have shown that continuous high doses of aspirin are associated with prolonged pregnancy, prolonged labor, and an increase in blood loss at delivery.[7] The risk of bleeding is one of the primary reasons that these drugs are contraindicted during the latter part of pregnancy. Salicylates interfere with the ability of the blood to clot (aggregation of platelets), and this prolongs bleeding time. (This is also why we tend to bruise when aspirin is taken on a regular basis.) Bleeding inside the baby's head (intracranial hemorrhage) has occurred more often in premature infants whose mothers took aspirin within one week of delivery.[8] This complication also occurs more often in premature babies in general.

Some researchers have observed an increase in the frequency of death shortly before or after birth, when salicylates are taken on a regular basis.[9] Causes have been attributed to excessive bleeding and the possibility of closure of the ductus arteriosus prior to birth. This is a passageway in the fetal heart that must remain open in order for the unborn to receive the oxygen it needs. It closes at birth, when the newborn begins to breathe. These findings have not been confirmed by the Collaborative Perinatal Project, which reported no increase in the incidence of perinatal deaths among women ingesting salicylates. The differences could be related to the amount and duration of drug use by women in the two studies.

While there is no convincing evidence that salicylates cause birth defects, some problems have been observed when these drugs were used near or at the time of delivery. For this reason women are advised to avoid salicylate-containing products in the latter part of their pregnancy, particularly in the last month.

Long-term follow-up studies of children exposed before birth have not been located.

*Natural Remedies for Headaches:**

The bodily changes and emotional stress of pregnancy may cause headaches. While an occasional headache might be anticipated, if you have frequent or severe headaches, consult your health care provider. And do not take *any* headache medications, either prescription or over-the-counter, without the approval of your health care provider.

The better-safe-than-sorry approach to dealing with headache would be to avoid any kind of medication. Here are some alternative methods[10] of dealing with headache and with the stress that may cause it:

Avoidance. If you can determine which situations or substances—such as eyestrain, fluorescent light, and stuffy rooms—cause your headache, make an effort to avoid them.

Empty stomach. Eat often during the day, but be certain not to overeat.

Fluids. Don't allow yourself to become dehydrated. Drink adequate amounts of fluid.

Fresh air. Try to spend part of each day outside if the air is fresh.

Stress reduction. Rest during the day and get enough sleep at night.

Massage. Muscle relaxation is a good way to avoid or reduce headaches. Massage (or have someone else massage) your scalp, face, neck, and shoulders.

References:

[1]A. M. Rudolph, Effects of aspirin and acetaminophen in pregnancy and in the newborn, *Archives of Internal Medicine* 141 (1981): 358–63.

[2]E. Collins, Maternal and fetal effects of acetaminophen and salicyclates in pregnancy, *Obstetrics and Gynecology* 58(suppl.) (1981): 57S–62S.

[3]I. D. Richards, Congenital malformations and environmental influences in pregnancy, *British Journal of Preventive and Social Medicine* 23 (1969): 218–25.

[4]M. M. Nelson and J. O. Forfar, Associations between drugs administered during pregnancy and congenital abnormalities of the fetus, *British Medical Journal* 1 (1971): 523–27.

[5]I. Saxen, Association between oral clefts and drugs taken during pregnancy, *International Journal of Epidimiology.* 4 (1975): 37–44.

[6]O. P. Heinonen, D. Slone, and S. Shapiro, *Birth Defects and Drugs in Pregnancy* (Littleton, Mass.: Publishing Sciences Group, 1977).

[7]R. B. Lewis and J. D. Shulman, Influence of acetylsalicylic acid, an inhibitor of prostaglandin synthesis, on the duration of human gestation and labour, *Lancet* 2 (1973): 1159–61.

[8]C. M. Rumack, M. A. Guggenheim, R. H. Rumack, R. G. Peterson, M. L. Johnson, and W. R. Braithwaite, Neonatal intracranial hemorrhage and maternal use of aspirin, *Obstetrics and Gynecology* 58 (1981): 52S–56S.

*None of these commonsense remedies have been medically proven. They are listed here because I have found them useful.

[9]E. Collins and G. Turner, Maternal effects of regular salicylate ingestion in pregnancy, *Lancet* 2 (1975): 335–38.

[10]The Over-The-Counter-Drug Committee of the Coalition for the Medical Rights of Women, *Safe and Natural Remedies for Discomforts of Pregnancy* (San Francisco, Calif. January 1981; rev. 1982.)

COMMON NAME: **SCUBA DIVING**

Brand Name/Chemical name: **not applicable**

FDA Pregnancy Category: not applicable

ESTIMATED RISK SUMMARY:
   Time of Exposure throughout pregnancy
   Risk Risk assessment is not possible
   Pregnancy Outcome uncertain
   Documentation insufficient

pre-conception	All or None		Organ Development – (in weeks)						Maturation – (in weeks)				
	1	2	3	4	5	6	7	8	9	10	12	20-36	38

conception   ←—Time of Greatest Risk—→   birth

The safety of *scuba diving* during pregnancy has not yet been fully evaluated. Several theoretical concerns for the pregnant diver do, however, exist.

The reduction of atmospheric pressure causes the release of nitrogen bubbles in the blood. When this happens too rapidly, it results in decompression sickness, or "the bends." Bubbles can also be present in the blood without causing overt symptoms of the bends. Under normal circumstances these "silent" bubbles should pose no problems for the diver because they are filtered out of the blood in the lungs. However, blood circulates quite uniquely in the unborn baby, and whether the unborn is free from risk of these silent bubbles is not known.

An increase in fluid, or "water retention," often occurs during pregnancy. Theoretically, this could alter the mother's ability to get rid of excess nitrogen that dissolves in the body fluids when she is submerged, thus increasing her risk of getting the bends.

Two medical reports, one isolated case and one retrospective survey, have raised the question of the safety of diving during pregnancy. A case report described one child with multiple malformations born to a woman who made twenty dives during fifteen days early in her pregnancy.[1] And a survey of pregnant divers detected a slight increase in birth defects among their children.[2] All of this information was gathered after the pregnancy outcome was known and presents no proof that the problems were actually caused by scuba diving (see Evaluating Scientific Information, page 41). It does, however, caution pregnant women about the possible risks of diving during pregnancy.

The risk for decompression sickness, or the bends, increases for any one diving below thirty feet (9 m). The rather-safe-than-sorry approach would be to consider not diving below thirty feet or, even more conservatively, to postpone diving until after the baby is born.

Long-term follow-up studies of children exposed before birth have not been located.

References:

[1] G. Turner and I. Unsworth, Intrauterine bends? *Lancet,* 1, 1982, p. 905.
[2] M. E. Bolton, Scuba diving and fetal well-being: A survey of 208 women, *Undersea Biomedical Research* 7 (1980): 183–89.

GENERIC NAME: SMALLPOX VACCINE

Brand name/Chemical name: **not applicable**

FDA pregnancy Category: X

ESTIMATED RISK SUMMARY:
   Time of Exposure potentially throughout pregnancy, particularly 3 to 24 weeks
   Risk Suspected risk*
   Pregnancy Outcome uncertain: favorable and adverse outcomes observed
   Documentation inconclusive, based on minimal data

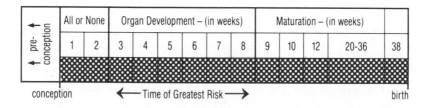

← pre-conception	All or None		Organ Development – (in weeks)						Maturation – (in weeks)				
	1	2	3	4	5	6	7	8	9	10	12	20-36	38

conception   ← Time of Greatest Risk →   birth

Smallpox vaccine[1] is used to prevent smallpox. Fortunately, the world is now considered free of this disease. In the United States, vaccination is recommended

*above the 4% background risk

only for those individuals working with smallpox or with related viruses.

Smallpox vaccine contains the live virus, which has been made noninfectious—what is called a live attenuated vaccine. Even so, there have been rare reports of fetal infection from vaccination during pregnancy. More commonly, the developing baby has died following vaccination of the mother.

Reference:

[1] J. D. Blanco and R. S. Gibbs, Immunizations in pregnancy, *Clinical Obstetrics and Gynecology* 25 (1982): 611–17.

GENERIC NAME: **SPECTINOMYCIN**

Brand Name: **(Trobicin)**

FDA Pregnancy Category:—

ESTIMATED RISK SUMMARY:
   Time of Exposure throughout pregnancy
   Risk No known risk*
   Pregnancy Outcome appears favorable
   Documentation inconclusive, based on minimal data

pre-conception	All or None		Organ Development – (in weeks)						Maturation – (in weeks)				
	1	2	3	4	5	6	7	8	9	10	12	20-36	38

conception   ←—Time of Greatest Risk—→   birth

Spectinomycin[1] is an antibiotic often used to treat gonorrhea during pregnancy in patients allergic to penicillin (see gonorrhea, page 169). Spectinomycin is related to streptomycin and other aminoglycosides, but is structurally different from them (see aminoglycosides, page 70). This is important because streptomycin has been associated with birth defects in the eighth cranial nerve, which is responsible for hearing and balance (see streptomycin, page 302). However, there is absolutely no evidence that spectinomycin causes such damage. To date there is no indication that spectinomycin will harm either a pregnant woman or her unborn child.

*above the 4% background risk

Long-term follow-up studies of children exposed before birth have not been located.

Reference:

[1]W. M. McCormick and M. Finland, Spectinomycin, *Annals of Internal Medicine* 84 (1976): 712–16.

MEDICATION CLASSIFICATION: **SPERMICIDES (creams, foams, jellies, suppositories, and sponges)**
GENERIC NAMES: **NONOXYNOL 9, OCTOXYNOL**

Brand names: **(Because, Conceptrol Birth Control, Conceptrol Disposable Contraceptive, Delfen Contraceptive, Emko, Emko Pre-Fil, Encare, Gynol II Contraceptive, Intercept Contraceptive Inserts, Koromex, Koromex II-A, Ortho-Creme Contraceptive, Ortho-Gynol Contraceptive, Ramses, Semicid, Shur-Seal Gel, Today)**

FDA Pregnancy Category:—

ESTIMATED RISK SUMMARY:

Time of Exposure before conception or during an unspecified time in early pregnancy

Risk no known risk*

Pregnancy Outcome appears favorable

Documentation inconclusive

	All or None	Organ Development – (in weeks)						Maturation – (in weeks)				
pre-conception	1	2	3	4	5	6	7	8	9	10	12	20-36	38

conception   ←—Time of Greatest Risk—→   birth

Spermicides are used to prevent pregnancy by disrupting the mobility of sperm. Spermicides are available as creams, foams, jellies, suppositories, and sponges. These products can be used as the only method of contraception or together with a condom

*above the 4% background risk

or vaginal diaphragm. The most commonly used spermicides are nonoxynol 9 and the related compound, octoxynol.

In 1981, a research paper published in the Journal of the American Medical Association reported an increased incidence of birth defects in the children of women who had prescriptions for a vaginal spermicide within ten months before they conceived.[1] This well-publicized report created a high level of anxiety. In less than two weeks, warnings on the possibility of spermicide-related birth defects appeared in news magazines and newspapers, and on radio and television.[2]

People tended to interpret the results of the 1981 investigation as definitive, probably due to the amount of attention this study received. But even the authors of the paper acknowledged that the study had shortcomings. They also clearly stated that their results did not prove that spermicides caused the observed birth defects. In fact, one of the authors has recently stated that there really was not enough data even to warrant publishing the article and that overall, this particular paper has done more harm than good.[3] If the findings of this study were truly representative, then perhaps the extreme anxiety it created could be justified, but this was not the case.

What was wrong with the 1981 study? The greatest criticism is the manner in which the "exposed" and "unexposed" groups were selected. Women who filled a spermicide prescription through the pharmacy within *10 months* of conception were considered "exposed." But this definition did not prove that those who had the prescription actually used the spermicide. Nor did it reveal whether spermicides were used close to the time of conception. It is possible that some of the women who purchased spermicides discontinued using them months prior to a planned pregnancy. In fact, it was later revealed that this was the case: Four of the eight mothers who gave birth to children with abnormalities had planned pregnancies![4] Women who did not obtain a spermicide through the pharmacy served as the "unexposed" group. Therefore there was no way of knowing whether some women in the "unexposed" group used spermicides obtained through other means.

A second criticism is that the investigation only looked for major birth defects, but teratogens more often cause a subtle pattern of malformation. In addition, the abnormalities cited among the "exposed" children were not similar, meaning they were probably not the result of one specific cause. (The abnormalities included Down syndrome, limb defects, hypospadias.) Finally, the incidence of defects observed among the group who filled a spermicide prescription (2.2%) and those not filling a spermicide prescription (1%) were both *well below* the *expected* 4 percent rate of birth defects in our population.

Since these initial findings, other researchers have investigated the possibility of spermicide-related complications. In general they have found no association between vaginal spermicides and birth defects, miscarriage rates, or the incidence of low-birth-weight infants.[5,6]

The question of spermicide-induced chromosome abnormalities, specifically trisomies like Down syndrome, has also been explored, and a statistically significant relationship has not been found.[7]

Despite the overwhelming scientific evidence that spermicides do not cause birth defects, there has been at least one court case against a spermicide manufacturer claiming an association with the birth of a malformed child. The publicity generated by this decision has once again instilled fear in the minds of pregnant women. Regardless of how the judicial system perceived the information, the criticisms of the study remain unchanged. It is very important to understand that legal decisions have no bearing on scientific facts.

References:

[1]H. Jick, A. M. Walker, K. J. Rothman, J. R. Hunter, L. B. Holmes, R. N. Watkins, D. C. D'Ewart, A. Danford, and S. Madsen, Vaginal spermicides and congenital disorders, *Journal of the American Medical Association* 245 (1981): 1329–32.

[2]J. Seligmann, Warning on spermicides, *Newsweek*, April 13, 1981, p. 84.

[3]L. B. Holmes, Vaginal spermicides and congenital disorders: The validity of a study, *Journal of the American Medical Association* 256 (1986): 3096.

[4]R. N. Watkins, Vaginal spermicides and congenital disorders: The validity of a study, *Journal of the American Medical Association* 256 (1986): 3095.

[5]M. B. Braken, Spermicidal contraceptives and poor reproductive outcomes: The epidemiologic evidence against an association, *American Journal of Obstetrics and Gynecology* 151 (1985): 552–56.

[6]C. Louik, A. A. Mitchell, M. M. Werler, J. W. Hanson, and S. Shapiro, Maternal exposure to spermicides in relation to certain birth defects, *New England Journal of Medicine* 317 (1987): 474–78.

[7]D. Warburton, R. Hindin Newgut, A. Lustenberger, A. Giullo Nicholas, and J. Kline, Lack of Association between spermicide use and trisomy, *New England Journal of Medicine* 317 (1987): 478–82.

GENERIC NAME: **SPIRONOLACTONE**

Brand Names: **(Alatone, Aldactone)**

FDA Pregnancy Category:—

ESTIMATED RISK SUMMARY:

Time of Exposure throughout pregnancy

Risk Risk assessment is not possible

Pregnancy Outcome uncertain

Documentation unavailable

← pre- conception	All or None		Organ Development – (in weeks)						Maturation – (in weeks)				
	1	2	3	4	5	6	7	8	9	10	12	20-36	38

conception   ←—Time of Greatest Risk—→   birth

Spironolactone[1] is a diuretic—a drug used to promote urine excretion. The effects of this drug on human prenatal development have not been determined. Animal studies have revealed that spironolactone has a feminizing effect on male rat fetuses. At this time there is no evidence to support this finding in humans.

Long-term follow-up studies of children exposed before birth have not been located.

Refer to thiazides for a brief discussion on the use of diuretics during pregnancy and a natural remedy for discomfort relief, page 315.

Reference:

[1]A. L. Wilson and G. R. Matzke, The treatment of hypertension in pregnancy, *Drug Intelligence and Clinical Pharmacy* 15 (1981): 21–26.

GENERIC NAME: **STREPTOMYCIN**

Brand Name: (Streptomycin Sulfate)

FDA Pregnancy Category:—

ESTIMATED RISK SUMMARY:

   Time of Exposure the first 2 weeks of pregnancy

   Risk Risk assessment is not possible

   Pregnancy Outcome uncertain

   Documentation insufficient; no information available

   Time of Exposure cannot specify, information is insufficient

   Risk Highly suspected risk,*

   Pregnancy Outcome uncertain: favorable and adverse outcomes observed

   Documentation inconclusive

*above the expected 4% background risk

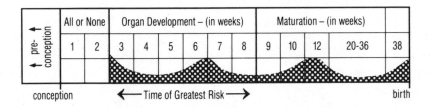

	pre-conception	All or None	Organ Development – (in weeks)						Maturation – (in weeks)				
		1	2	3	4	5	6	7	8	9	10	12	20-36	38

conception   ←— Time of Greatest Risk —→   birth

Streptomycin is used to treat tuberculosis.

An extensive review of the medical literature on pregnant women treated with various antitubercular medications was conducted in an effort to discover the effect of these drugs on the developing baby.[1] The investigators located information on the pregnancies of 2,787 women and found that 94 percent of them had full-term infants who appeared normal at birth. Approximately 3 percent of the pregnancies resulted in miscarriages, stillbirths, or premature births, while 2.89 percent resulted in birth defects. The reported frequency of problems is within the expected range. However, nearly half of the recorded abnormalities were associated with the use of streptomycin.

In this study, 206 of the women took streptomycin. While the majority of the babies exposed to this drug were apparently normal (82%), thirty-five children (16.5%) had damage to the eighth cranial nerve, which is responsible for hearing and balance. This resulted in hearing deficits that ranged in severity from minor high-frequency losses of little importance to total deafness. Although many reports did not specify when during pregnancy the streptomycin was taken, damage has been reported when the exposure occurred either early or late in the pregnancy. This lack of specific information on the timing of streptomycin exposures during pregnancy makes risk during the first two weeks (the usual "all or none" time of lethal damage or no effect) impossible to calculate (see page 34).

Reference:

[1] D. E. Snider, P. M. Layde, M. W. Johnson, and M. A. Lyle. Treatment of tuberculosis during pregnancy, *American Review of Respiratory Diseases* 122 (1980): 65–79.

GENERIC NAME: **SULFASALAZINE**

Brand Names: **(Azaline, Azulfidine, S.A.S.-500)**

FDA Pregnancy Category: B

ESTIMATED RISK SUMMARY:

Time of Exposure throughout pregnancy*
Risk No known risk**
Pregnancy Outcome appears favorable
Documentation inconclusive

pre-conception	All or None		Organ Development – (in weeks)						Maturation – (in weeks)				
	1	2	3	4	5	6	7	8	9	10	12	20-36	38

conception   ← Time of Greatest Risk →   birth

Sulfasalazine[1] is an anti-infective drug used primarily for the treatment of ulcerative colitis. It has also been used in the management of rheumatoid arthritis and Crohn's disease.

Sulfasalazine belongs to the class of medications known as sulfonamides. Concern over the use of sulfasalazine during pregnancy stems from its relationship to these drugs. These worries originated from *animal* studies, which have implicated sulfonamides as a cause of birth defects. (This is explained in detail in the sulfonamides entry; see page 305). Additional concerns over the use of sulfonamides are related to the theoretical risk for kernicterus. When these drugs are administered to newborn babies, particularly those born prematurely, they can raise the amount of biliruben (a bile pigment) in the blood. This condition can result in an increased risk for kernicterus, a severe disorder which can cause brain damage.

There have been isolated reports of birth defects in human pregnancies treated with sulfasalazine. But without any other evidence of abnormalities, the significance of these findings is unknown. It is possible that the defects were just a chance occurrence. Several hundred exposures to sulfasalazine before birth have been recorded without any reported increase in the frequency of fetal complications. In fact, a large retrospective study across the United States found the incidence of low birth weight, prematurity, pregnancy losses, and developmental defects to be lower than what is expected in the general population.[2] This study is not without its flaws, but the results confirm the observations of others (see retrospective studies, page 43).

---

*theoretical but unproven risk when used near the time of delivery
**above the 4% background risk

Although the actual risk for kernicterus from sulfasalazine seems negligible,[3] warnings against the use of sulfonamides in the third trimester are based on the fear of this problem occurring. Fortunately, scientific studies have consistently failed to show any relationship between the use of these drugs *during* pregnancy and kernicterus in the newborn.[2,4,5] Despite this lack of evidence, most sources still advocate cautious use of sulfonamides near the time of delivery.

Long-term follow-up studies of children exposed before birth have not been located.

References:

[1]J. H. Lewis, A. B. Weingold, and the committee on FDA-related matters, American College of Gastroenterology, The use of gastrointestinal drugs during pregnancy and lactation. *American Journal of Gastroenterology* 80 (1985): 912–923.

[2]M. Mogadam, W. O. Dobbins III, B. I. Korelitz, et al., Pregnancy in inflammatory bowel disease: effect of sulfasalazine and corticosteroids on fetal outcome, *Gastroenterology* 80 (1981): 72–76.

[3]G. Janerot, M. B. Into-Malmberg, and E. Esbjorner, Placental transfer of sulfasalazine and sulphapyridine and some of its metabolites, *Scandinavian Journal of Gastroenterology* 16 (1981): 693–97.

[4]C. G. Baskin, S. Law, and N. K. Wenger, Sulfadiazine rheumatic fever prophylaxis during pregnancy: Does it increase the risk of kernicterus in the newborn? *Cardiology* 65 (1980): 222–25.

[5]I. M. Hanan and J. B. Kirsner, Inflammatory bowel disease in the pregnant woman, *Clinics in Perinatology* 12 (1985): 669–83.

MEDICATION CLASSIFICATION: SULFONAMIDES

GENERIC NAMES: SULFACETAMIDE, SULFACYTINE, SULFADIAZINE, SULFADOXINE (with PYRIMETHAMINE), SULFAMETHIZOLE, SULFAMETHOXAZOLE (also with TRIMETHOPRIM), SULFAPYRIDINE, SULFASALAZINE, SULFISOXAZOLE

Brand names: **(Bactrim, Bethaprim, Cotrim, Fansidar, Gamazole, Gantanol, Gantrisin, Gulfasin, Lipo Gantrisin, Microsulfon, Proklar, Renoquid, Sebizon, Septra, SK-Soxazole, Sulfatrim, Thiosulfil, Thiosulfil Forte, Urobak)**

FDA Pregnancy Category: B

ESTIMATED RISK SUMMARY:
Time of Exposure throughout pregnancy*
Risk No known risk**

*theoretical but unproven risk when used near the time of delivery
**above the expected 4% background risk

Pregnancy Outcome appears favorable
Documentation inconclusive

← pre- ← conception	All or None		Organ Development – (in weeks)						Maturation – (in weeks)				
	1	2	3	4	5	6	7	8	9	10	12	20-36	38

conception   ← Time of Greatest Risk →   birth

Sulfonamides are anti-infective drugs, used to treat rheumatic fever, taken for inflammatory bowel disease (ulcerative colitis and Crohn's disease), sometimes used in the management of rheumatoid arthritis, commonly prescribed for the treatment of urinary tract infections, and combined with other anti-infective agents to treat various illnesses (see also pyrimethamine, page 279; trimethoprim, page 327; and urinary tract infections, page 331).

Initial concern over the use of these drugs during pregnancy came from animal studies that revealed an increased incidence of cleft palate and bone abnormalities. Conversely, investigations into the use of sulfonamides by pregnant women have failed to demonstrate that they cause cleft lip, cleft palate, or any other birth defect. Despite such reassurances, pregnant women may still encounter outdated warnings of the potential danger of these drugs to an unborn baby.

Controversy regarding sulfonamides and oral clefts has been perpetuated by an often quoted Finnish study.[1] This investigation compared drug consumption in pregnancies resulting in normal children and in infants with oral clefts (cleft lip with or without cleft palate or cleft palate alone). The information for this study was gathered both before and after delivery. The study discovered that the intake of sulfonamides during the first and second trimesters occurred only slightly more often in mothers of children with oral clefts. But it occurred *only* when other malformations were present. In other words, if there were no other malformations, oral clefts alone were not more frequent among the children born to mothers using sulfonamides.

There are further reasons that these findings do not prove that sulfonamides actually cause the defects. Since oral clefts occur only during very specific times in an unborn baby's development, recording exact medication timing is critical to accurately determine cause-and-effect. The lip is formed by thirty-five days after conception and the palate begins to develop at the end of the fifth week and is complete, for the most part, by seven weeks. Therefore, exposures beyond the first trimester cannot cause oral clefts. But this study included children with oral clefts whose mothers took the drug after the defect had occurred.

When several substances are statistically examined together, as they were in this study, an association observed between any of the drugs and birth defects may simply be a chance occurrence. For example, cleft lip and cleft palate are fairly common in our population, occurring in about 1 in every 1,000 births. Because some of the information was collected after the babies were born, the researchers had to depend on the mother's memory to record what drug was used and specifically when during pregnancy the drug was taken.

It is a well-known fact that people seldom remember even recent historical events accurately. Mothers of babies with birth defects recall the events during their pregnancies much differently than do mothers of normal children. Therefore, relying on mothers' memories can, in many ways, affect the reliability of the study's conclusions.

Sulfonamide drugs administered *directly to newborn babies,* particularly those born prematurely, may raise the amount of bilirubin (a bile pigment) in the blood. This condition can result in an increased risk for kernicterus, a severe disorder which can cause brain damage. The warnings against the use of sulfonamides in the third trimester are based on the fear of these same problems occurring. Fortunately, scientific studies have consistently failed to show any relationship between the use of these drugs *during pregnancy* and kernicterus in the newborn.[2,3,4] Despite this lack of evidence, most sources still advocate cautious use of sulfonamides near the time of delivery.

A complication called hemolytic anemia has been reported after exposure to a sulfonamide in two infants with the inherited condition glucose-6-phosphate dehydrogenase (G6PD) deficiency. Hemolytic anemia results from the shortened survival of red blood cells. The risk of hemolytic anemia occurring would be highest when sulfonamides are used by susceptible individuals (those with G6PD deficiency) near the time of delivery.

Long-term follow-up studies of children exposed before birth have not been located.

References:

[1]I. Saxen, Associations between oral clefts and drugs taken during pregnancy, *International Journal of Epidemiology* 4 (1975): 37–44.

[2]C. G. Baskin, S. Law, and N. K. Wenger, Sulfadiazine rheumatic fever prophylaxis during pregnancy: Does it increase the risk of kernicterus in the newborn? *Cardiology* 65 (1980): 222–25.

[3]M. Mogadam, W. O. Dobbins, B. I. Korelitz, and S. W. Ahmed, Pregnancy in inflammatory bowel disease: Effect of sulfasalazine and corticosteroids on fetal outcome, *Gastroenterology* 80 (1981): 72–76.

[4] I. M. Hanan and J. B. Kirsner, Inflammatory bowel disease in the pregnant woman, *Clinics in Perinatology* 12 (1985): 669–83.

COMMON NAME: **SYPHILIS**

Brand Name/Chemical Name: **not applicable**

FDA Pregnancy Category: not applicable

ESTIMATED RISK SUMMARY:

Time of Exposure possibly the 4th month, but most likely after the 6th month of pregnancy and during delivery

Risk Known risk*

Pregnancy Outcome adverse

Documentation conclusive, based on current knowledge

pre-conception	All or None		Organ Development – (in weeks)						Maturation – (in weeks)				
	1	2	3	4	5	6	7	8	9	10	12	20-36	38

conception   ←— Time of Greatest Risk —→   birth

Syphilis[1] is caused by a bacterium called *Treponema pallidum.* It is usually transmitted through sexual contact, but is easily passed from mother to infant during pregnancy or birth.

Syphilis begins as a hard, painless sore on the skin called a chancre. In women, this initial sign of infection may go unnoticed due to its hidden location on the cervix or within the vagina and because it produces no pain. When the chancres disappear, within a matter of three to eight weeks, the primary stage of syphilis is over. The secondary stage of syphilis is marked by the appearance of a rash, although other symptoms such as enlarged lymph nodes, headache, fever, weakness, and muscle and bone aches can also be present. This stage usually occurs within three months after the chancres heal, but it might not happen for months or even years later. The final stage, tertiary syphilis, begins three to ten years after the infection first appeared. At this point the disease is devastating and causes damage to nearly every organ and tissue in the body, including the heart, brain, eyes, skin, bones, and joints.

*above the 4% background risk

Traditionally, it is believed that the unborn baby cannot be infected with syphilis early in pregnancy because a layer of cells present in the placenta (Langhans' layer), prevents the infection from passing from the mother's bloodstream to the baby's. This layer of cells breaks down during the fourth month of pregnancy, and while a risk of infection exists at that time, it is not likely to occur until after the sixth month, when Langhans' cell layer completely disappears.

The risk to the developing baby depends on what stage of untreated syphilis the mother has. Observations from a variety of scientific sources give some indication of pregnancy outcome in syphilitic mothers:

• Untreated syphilis of less than two years: about half the babies are liveborn and do not have the infection.
• Untreated syphilis in the primary or secondary stage; about half of the babies are premature, stillborn, or die within four weeks after birth.
• Untreated syphilis in the early part of the tertiary stage: about 20–60 percent of the babies are normal, 40 percent have congenital syphilis, 20 percent are born prematurely, 16 percent are stillborn and die within four weeks after birth.
• Untreated syphilis in the late part of the tertiary stage: 75 percent of the babies are healthy, 10 percent have congenital syphilis, 9 percent are born prematurely, 10 percent are stillborn, and 1 percent die within four weeks after birth.

Congenital is a term used to refer to conditions that are present at birth. Although it exists at birth, congenital syphilis is usually not immediately apparent; most often, physical signs and symptoms are expressed months or years later. When congenital syphilis is obvious at birth, the prognosis for the baby is very poor.

Congenital syphilis is broken into two stages; early and late. Signs of infection appearing before the child is 2 years of age are termed early congenital syphilis. Late congenital syphilis is when symptoms manifest after this time. Infants with early congenital syphilis have a variety of problems including bony lesions, skin rash, enlarged liver and spleen (with or without jaundice), "snuffles" (a mucus discharge from the nose and throat), and anemia. Late congenital syphilis is characterized by eye defects (glaucoma, inflamed cornea), deafness, "saddle nose," teeth abnormalities, bone and joint defects, skin fissures, and central nervous system problems (including mental retardation).

Treatment can stop or even cure syphilis, but this depends on how extensive the damage was prior to the treatment. During pregnancy. adequate treatment can result in minimal effects in the baby, although if the damage is severe, it might not prevent a miscarriage or a stillbirth. In the absence of obvious signs of infection at a birth, treating the baby can prevent the symptoms of syphilis from appearing.

Penicillin is the drug of choice for treating syphilis. This antibiotic can be safely administered during the pregnancy and it poses no threat to newborns or small children (see penicillins, page 257). Some people are allergic to penicillin and this creates some problems for treating syphilis in pregnant women and young children. Tetracycline is an effective treatment, but it is not recommended during pregnancy or in children under 8 years of age (see tetracyclines, page 311). Erythromycin is also an alternative. Unfortunately, the levels of erythromycin that reach the fetus are low and unpredictable, so it is not the ideal drug for treating syphilis during pregnancy (see erythromycin, page 154).

The many problems posed by syphilis during pregnancy can be avoided if pregnant women routinely receive a blood test to detect the infection. Ideally, the test should be performed during the first three months and again at the end of pregnancy or at the time of delivery.

Reference:

J. S. Remington and J. O. Klein (eds.), *Infectious Diseases of the Fetus and Newborn Infant,* 2d ed. (Philadelphia: W. B. Saunders, 1983), pp. 335–74.

COMMON NAME: **TANNING BOOTHS**

Brand Name/Chemical Name: **not applicable**

FDA Pregnancy Category: not applicable

ESTIMATED RISK SUMMARY:
Time of Exposure throughout pregnancy
Risk Risk assessment is not possible
Pregnancy Outcome uncertain
Documentation unavailable

← pre-conception	All or None		Organ Development – (in weeks)						Maturation – (in weeks)				
	1	2	3	4	5	6	7	8	9	10	12	20-36	38

conception   ← Time of Greatest Risk →   birth

Tanning booths use ultraviolet rays, which are non-ionizing radiation, similar to microwaves and radio waves. These are all very different from the high-energy radiation emitted from X rays (ionizing radiation). Ultraviolet rays would not be expected to cause birth defects, but this issue has not actually been evaluated in pregnant women. The amount of heat produced from a tanning booth is minimal and it is doubtful that the small rise it might cause in your body temperature would be reason for concern (see hyperthermia, page 197).

However, using a tanning booth, just like being in the sun, will intensify chloasma. Chloasma, or "the mask of pregnancy," is the appearance of darkened areas on the face, which are caused by hormonal changes. (Birth control pills can also cause chloasma.) Using a sun screen, which is always a good idea anyway, will reduce these pigment changes.

MEDICATION CLASSIFICATION: **TETRACYCLINES**

GENERIC NAMES: **CHLORTETRACYCLINE, DEMECLO-CYCLINE, DOXYCYCLINE, METHACYCLINE, MINO-CYCLINE, OXYTETRACYCLINE, TETRACYLINE**

Brand Names: **(Achromycin, Aureomycin, Cycline-250, Cyclopar, Declomycin, Deltamycin, Doxy-Caps, Doxychel Hyclate, Doxy-Lemmon, E. P. Mycin, Minocin, Nor-Tet, Oxymycin, Panmycin, Retet, Robitet "250" Robicaps, Rondomycin, SK-Tetracycline, Sumycin, Terramycin, Tetra C, Tetracap, Tetracycline, Tetracyn, Tetralan, Tetram, Tettrex, Uri-Tet, Vibra-Tabs, Vibramycin)**

FDA Pregnancy Category: D

ESTIMATED RISK SUMMARY:
  Time of Exposure after the 4th month
  Risk Known risk*
  Pregnancy Outcome adverse
  Documentation conclusive, based on current knowledge

*above the 4% background risk

← pre-conception →	All or None		Organ Development – (in weeks)						Maturation – (in weeks)				
	1	2	3	4	5	6	7	8	9	10	12	20-36	38

conception   ←—Time of Greatest Risk—→   birth

Tetracyclines are antibiotics used to treat a variety of bacterial infections.
Tetracyclines are incorporated into calcifying bone and teeth.

The most consistently documented effect from tetracycline exposure before birth is its staining effect on developing teeth. Although it is initially yellow in color, exposure to light causes this pigment to become brown or grayish-brown. An association between this effect and teeth that are more susceptible to decay has been suspected,[1,2] but has not been confirmed by controlled studies.[3,4]

The critical period for staining of the baby's (deciduous) teeth begins in the fourth month, when the teeth start to calcify, and continues throughout pregnancy. The risk for discoloration increases with dose, duration and advancing pregnancy. Tetracycline administration during the third trimester may affect one-half to two-thirds of those exposed.[4,5]

The type and severity of the staining produced by different tetracycline compounds has been the focus of several investigations. Studies have demonstrated only minimal staining with **oxytetracycline**,[2] although other investigations have shown no differences between the various types of this drug.[6]

Studies of tetracycline administered before birth to chicks, mice, and rats in doses above the human therapeutic range, have reported slowing of bone growth and also skeleton defects. These problems, however, appear to be limited to animals. In human studies, including one of children aged 4–5, no skeleton or developmental defects have been observed from tetracycline use during pregnancy. Only in premature infants receiving tetracycline *directly* has a temporary slowing of bone growth been reported.[7]

Two isolated instances of physical birth defects have been reported with tetracycline use during the first trimester. One involved the hands,[8] while the other involved multiple malformations.[9] Since there is no corroborative evidence, these events appear to be coincidental.

A retrospective survey examined prenatal drug exposures in children with cataracts of unknown origin.[10] While four cases of exposures to either **tetracycline** or **oxytetracycline** were discovered, the significance of these findings is unknown.

The mother's liver is more susceptable to damage from intravenous (IV) administration of tetracycline during pregnancy, and although it is rare, high doses of IV therapy have led to death secondary to liver failure.

Breakthrough bleeding and failure of oral contraceptives (birth control pills) resulting in pregnancy have also been attributed to tetracycline therapy.[11]

References:

[1]C. J. Witkop and R. O. Wolf, Hypoplasia and intrinsic staining of enamel following tetracycline therapy, *Journal of the American Medical Association* 185 (1963): 1008.

[2]I. S. Wallman and H. B. Hilton, Teeth pigmented by tetracycline, *Lancet* 1(1962): 827–29.

[3]P. J. Porter, E. A. Sweeney, H. Golan, and E. H. Kass, Controlled study of the effect of prenatal tetracycline on primary dentition, *Antimicrobial Agents and Chemotherapy* 6(1965): 668–71.

[4]M. T. Genot, H. P. Golan, P. J. Porter, and E. H. Kass, Effect of administration of tetracycline in pregnancy on the primary dentition of the offspring, *Journal of Oral Medicine* 25 (1970): 75–79.

[5]R. Toaff and R. Ravid, Tetracyclines and the teeth, *Lancet* 2(1966): 281.

[6]J. N. Swallow, D. E. Haller, and W. F. Young, Side-effects to antibiotics in cystic fibrosis: Dental changes in relation to antibiotic administration, *Archives of Disease in Childhood* 42 (1967): 311–18.

[7]S. Q. Cohlan, G. Bevelander, and T. Tiamsic, Growth inhibition of prematures receiving tetracycline, *American Journal of Diseases in Children* 105(1963): 453–61.

[8]F. Wilson, Congenital defects in the newborn, *British Medical Journal* 2 (1962): 255.

[9]R. Corcoran and J. M. Castles, Tetracycline for acne vulgaris and possible teratogensis, *British Medical Journal* 2 (1977): 807– 8.

[10]J. D. Harley, J. F. Farrar, J. B. Gray, and I. C. Dunlop, Aromatic drugs and congenital cataracts, *Lancet* 1 (1964): 472–73.

[11]J. E. Bacon and G. M. Shenfield, Pregnancy attributable to interaction between tetracycline and oral contraceptives, *British Medical Journal* 1 (1980): 283.

GENERIC NAME: **THEOPHYLLINE**

Brand names: **(Accurbron, Aerolate, Aerolate Capsules, ◇ Amoline, Aquaphyllin, Asmalix, Bronkodyl, Bronkodyl Capsules, □Choledyl, Constant-T, Duraphyl, Elixicon, Elixomin, Elixophyllin, Elixophyllin SR, LāBID, Lanophyllin, Liquophylline, Lixolin, Lodrane, ◇ Phyllocontin, Quibron-T, Quibron-T/SR Dividose, Respbid, Slo-Bid, Gyrocaps, Slo-Phyllin Gyrocaps, ◇ Somophyllin, Somophyllin-CRT, Somophyllin-T, Sustaire, Theobid Duracaps, Theobid Jr. Duracaps, Theobron SR, Theoclear, Theoclear L. C. Centules, Theodur, Theo-Dur Sprinkle, Theolain-SR, Theolair, Theophyl, Theophyl-SR, Theospan-SR, Theostat, Theo-Time, Theo-24, Theovent, ◇ Truphylline, Uniphyl)**

□ = generic name OXTRIPHYLLINE
◇ = generic name AMINOPHYLLINE

FDA Pregnancy Category: C

ESTIMATED RISK SUMMARY:

Time of Exposure throughout most of pregnancy
Risk No known risk*
Pregnancy Outcome appears favorable
Documentation inconclusive, based on minimal data

Time of Exposure near the time of delivery
Risk Possible risk* (when doses are high)
Pregnancy outcome uncertain: favorable and adverse outcomes observed
Documentation inconclusive, knowledge gained through clinical experience, more research is needed

pre-conception	All or None		Organ Development – (in weeks)						Maturation – (in weeks)				
	1	2	3	4	5	6	7	8	9	10	12	20-36	38

conception   ⟵—Time of Greatest Risk—⟶   birth

Theophylline is a bronchodilator—a medication that helps constricted air passages become wider. It is used in the treatment of bronchial asthma, emphysema, bronchitis, and other lung problems. Theophylline is a xanthine derivative, as is caffeine. **Aminophylline** and **oxtriphylline**, both drugs related to theophylline, are also bronchodilators.

The clinical experience with this drug used in pregnancy is extensive, and I am not aware of any evidence linking theophylline to birth defects. Consistent with clinical observations are results from the Collaborative Perinatal Project, which evaluated pregnancy outcome in more than 50,000 mother-child pairs, exposed to a wide variety of drugs.[1] No increased risk was associated with the use of either theophylline (117 exposures) or with aminophylline (76 exposures) during the first three months of pregnancy. However, the number of exposures are relatively small and this large prospective study does have several shortcomings. For this reason, definitive conclusions about the drug's teratogenicity cannot be reached.

Women taking theophylline up to the time of delivery have given birth to babies

*above the 4% background risk

who had evidence of the drug in their systems.[2] Such newborns have rapid heart rates (tachycardia) and tend to be more irritable than expected.[3] These drug effects are temporary and appear to be dose-related, since they occurred more often in babies whose mothers took large amounts of the drug.

Theophylline and its related compounds do have the ability to inhibit uterine contractions, but they are not effective in actually treating and preventing premature labor.

Long-term follow-up studies of children exposed before birth have not been located.

References:

[1] O. P. Heinonen, D. Slone, and S. Shapiro, *Birth Defects and Drugs in Pregnancy* (Littleton, Mass.: Publishing Science Group, 1977).

[2] E. Labovitz and S. Spector, Placental theophylline transfer in pregnant asthmatics, *Journal of the American Medical Association* 247 (1982): 786–88.

[3] L. L. Arwood, J. F. Dasta, and C. Friedman, Placental transfer of theophylline: Two case reports, *Pediatrics* 63 (1979): 844–46.

MEDICATION CLASSIFICATION: **THIAZIDES**

GENERIC NAMES: **BENDROFLUMETHIAZIDE, BENZTHIAZIDE, CHLOROTHIAZIDE, CYCLOTHIAZIDE, HYDROCHLOROTHIAZIDE, HYDROFLUMETHIAZIDE, METHYCLOTHIAZIDE, POLYTHIAZIDE, TRICHLORMETHIAZIDE**

Brand Names: **(Anhydron, Aquatensen, Aquatag, Aquazide, Aquazides H, Chlorzide, Diachlor, Diaqua, Diu-Scrip, Diucardin, Diurese, Diuril, Enduron, Esidrix, Ethon, Exna, Fluidil, Hydrex, Hydro-T, HydroDiuril, Hydromal, Marazide, Metahydrin, Mono-Press, Naqua, Naturetin, Niazide, Oretic, Proaqua, Renese, Saluron, Thiuretic, Trichlorex)**

FDA Pregnancy Category: B

ESTIMATED RISK SUMMARY:

Time of Exposure throughout the first 6 or 7 months of pregnancy

Risk No known risk* for birth defects

---

*above the expected 4% background risk

Pregnancy Outcome appears favorable
Documentation inconclusive

Time of Exposure last trimester, particularly near the delivery date
Risk Suspected risk*
Pregnancy Outcome uncertain: favorable and adverse outcomes observed
Documentation inconclusive

pre-conception	All or None		Organ Development – (in weeks)						Maturation – (in weeks)				
	1	2	3	4	5	6	7	8	9	10	12	20-36	38

conception   ← Time of Greatest Risk →   birth

Thiazides[1,2] are diuretics (substances that cause fluid loss through urination). Much of the information available on diuretics in pregnancy, particularly thiazide diuretics, relates to their past use against a complication of pregnancy called pre-eclampsia. Preeclampsia usually occurs later in pregnancy and is characterized by high blood pressure (hypertension), protein in the urine (proteinuria), and swelling due to fluid retention (edema). Today, physicians recognize that preventive use of diuretics does not reduce the incidence of preeclampsia. Diuretics can also impair blood flow between the placenta and uterus, potentially compromising the health of the unborn baby. These realizations have limited the use of diuretics during pregnancy primarily to the prevention and treatment of congestive heart failure. Some sources do, however, recommend continuing thiazides in hypertensive patients who were already receiving them in early pregnancy.[3]

To date, thiazides have not been associated with an increased frequency of birth defects.

While many studies report normal pregnancy outcomes, the use of these drugs in late pregnancy can cause a variety of temporary problems in the fetus and newborn. These include: low blood sugars (hypoglycemia); salt depletion (hyponatremia); decrease in potassium (hypokalemia), which could slow down the baby's heartbeat; and decrease in blood platelets (thrombocytopenia), which are essential for blood coagulation.

*above the expected 4% background risk

On occasion, thiazide-associated complications *in the mother* have harmed or even caused the death of the fetus. These maternal health complications include severe decrease in potassium, bleeding of the pancreas, high blood sugars, and excess uric acid. Anticipating these medical complications will reduce the health risk to newborns exposed to thiazide diuretics before birth.

Long-term follow-up studies of children exposed before birth have not been located.

Natural Remedies:*

Uncomplicated edema (swelling caused by too much fluid in body tissues) is normal during pregnancy. As diuretics and other drugs are not recommended to treat this condition, here are some tips[4] to help you feel more comfortable.

• Try lying down for a while on your left side.
• Wear support stockings.
• Avoid standing for long periods of time.
• Keep your feet elevated whenever you have the chance.

References:

[1]A. L. Wilson and G. R. Matzke, The treatment of hypertension in pregnancy, *Drug Intelligence and Clinical Pharmacy*, 15 (1981): 21–26.

[2]B. M. Sibai, R. A. Grossman, and H. G. Grossman, Effects of diuretics on plasma volume in pregnancies with long-term hypertension, *American Journal of Obstetrics and Gynecology* 150 (1984): 831–35.

[3]R. L. Berkowitz, Antihypertensive drugs in the pregnant patient, *Obstetrical and Gynecological Survey* 35 (1980): 191–204.

[4]The Over-the-Counter-Drug Committee of the Coalition for the Medical Rights of Women, *Safe and Natural Remedies for Discomforts of Pregnancy*. (San Francisco, Calif., January 1981; rev. 1982).

MEDICATION CLASSIFICATION: THYROID HORMONES

GENERIC NAMES: LEVOTHYROXINE, LIOTHYRONINE, LIOTRIX, THYROGLOBULIN, THYROID

Brand Names: **Cyronine, Cytomel, Euthroid, Levothroid, Proloid, S-P-T, Synthroid, Synthrox, Syroxine, Thyrar, Thyroid Strong, Thyroid USP, Thyrolar**

FDA Pregnancy Category: A

ESTIMATED RISK SUMMARY:

Time of Exposure before conception and throughout pregnancy

---

*None of these commonsense remedies have been medically proven. They are listed here because I have found them useful.

Risk No measurable risk*
Pregnancy Outcome favorable
Documentation conclusive, based on current knowledge

pre-conception	All or None	Organ Development – (in weeks)						Maturation – (in weeks)				
		1	2	3	4	5	6	7	8	9	10	12	20-36	38

conception   ←—— Time of Greatest Risk ——→   birth

Thyroid hormones[1] are given as supplemental or replacement therapy in people with low thyroid activity (hypothyroidism) or for those who no longer have a thyroid gland.

In normal concentrations, little or no thyroid hormones cross the placenta, so taking them throughout pregnancy is considered safe.

Women with hypothyroidism are often infertile, because they do not ovulate. Past reports have raised the question of an association between hypothyroidism in the mother and an increased frequency of poor pregnancy outcome (miscarriages, infant death shortly before or after birth, and occasionally birth defects). However, these early observations might not be completely representative, because they failed to prove that the mothers actually were hypothyroid.

On the other hand, a small study that accurately measured thyroid function in hypothyroid women revealed a successful outcome in nine of eleven pregnancies. The nine children revealed no physical or intellectual deficiencies.[2] All of the women in this study were able to become pregnant and maintain their pregnancies. Three of the women received no treatment during pregnancy, the others received thyroid hormone. One untreated patient had a stillborn infant with no abnormalities. This mother had preeclampsia, a complication usually of late pregnancy, which is characterized by high blood pressure (hypertension), protein in the urine (proteinuria), and swelling due to fluid retention (edema). This condition is risky to both the mother and the unborn child. Another mother gave birth to a child with Down Syndrome. Because the risk of bearing a child with Down Syndrome increases significantly in women who are 35 years or older when they give birth, her age of 41 years probably accounted for this genetic birth defect. Seven of the children were followed up to 2.7 years of age, and their thyroid function and

*above the 4% background risk

development continued to be normal. Longer follow-up studies are still needed before definitive conclusions about their intellectual function can be reached.

References:

[1]J. H. Mestman, Thyroid disease in pregnancy, *Clinics in Perinatology* 12 (1985): 651–67.
[2]M. Montoro, J. V. Collea, S. D. Frasier, and J. H. Mestman, Successful outcome of pregnancy in women with hypothyroidism, *Annals of Internal Medicine* 94 (1981): 31–34.

GENERIC NAME: **TIMOLOL**

Brand name: **(Blocadren)**

FDA Pregnancy Category: C

ESTIMATED RISK SUMMARY:
   Time of Exposure throughout pregnancy
   Risk Risk assessment is not possible
   Pregnancy Outcome uncertain
   Documentation unavailable

pre-conception	All or None		Organ Development – (in weeks)						Maturation – (in weeks)				
	1	2	3	4	5	6	7	8	9	10	12	20-36	38

conception   ←——Time of Greatest Risk——→   birth

Timolol belongs to a group of drugs that are classified as beta-adrenergic blocking agents (beta blockers). It is used to treat high blood pressure (hypertension). Currently there is no evaluation of the effects this drug might have on an unborn baby.

Some newborns exposed to beta-blocking agents near the time of delivery have evidence of a slower than normal heartbeat (bradycardia) and/or low blood pressure (hypotension) (see acebutolol, page 50, and atenolol, page 89). Although the effects of timolol are unknown, it is a beta blocker. For this reason, babies born to mothers using this drug should be observed for a couple of days for any evidence of these symptoms.

Long-term follow-up studies of children exposed before birth have not been located.

COMMON NAME: **TOXOPLASMOSIS**

Brand Name/Chemical Name: **not applicable**

FDA Pregnancy Category: not applicable

ESTIMATED RISK SUMMARY:

Time of Exposure throughout pregnancy, particularly 10 to 24 weeks

Risk Known risk,* when infection occurs for the first time during pregnancy

Pregnancy Outcome adverse

Documentation conclusive, based on current knowledge

← pre-conception ←	All or None		Organ Development – (in weeks)						Maturation – (in weeks)				
	1	2	3	4	5	6	7	8	9	10	12	20-36	38

conception   ←— Time of Greatest Risk —→   birth

Toxoplasmosis[1] is a very common infectious disease caused by a microscopic organism (toxoplasma gondii). It is transmitted to humans by the eating or handling of contaminated *raw* meat or by contact with the feces of an infected cat. Toxoplasmosis is usually symptomless, but when symptoms do occur they are often confused with other disease states such as a cold, the flu, or mononucleosis.

Infection confers immunity, so you need be concerned during pregnancy *only* if you've never had the infection before. Immunity also protects your developing baby from harm, even if you again come in contact with the infectious organism. Even though the infection is very common, an estimated 62 percent of women of childbearing age in the United States have not yet had toxoplasmosis. Approximately 3,300 newborns acquire toxoplasmosis from their mothers and are born with it each year in the United States.

Toxoplasmosis infection carries a risk for the developing baby throughout pregnancy, but the degree of risk is related to the time when infection occurs. In the last months of pregnancy the infection is most frequently transmitted to the fetus, but the newborn is usually symptomless. Earlier infection is less frequently transmitted to the fetus, but more often causes serious problems. Studies show that the highest risk period is from ten to twenty-four weeks of pregnancy.

*above the 4% background risk

The majority of infants born with toxoplasmosis infection have no symptoms; however, signs or symptoms of the disease can become apparent weeks or months later. Newborns who do show physical signs of the disease can have a variety of abnormalities including eye defects (chorioretinitis, blindness); enlarged head size related to accumulation of fluid within the baby's brain (hydrocephalus); convulsions, calcium deposits in the brain (cerebral calcifications); abnormally small head size (microcephaly); mental retardation; yellowing of the skin due to high levels of bilirubin in the blood (jaundice); and enlarged liver and spleen; as well as other complications, including deafness.

The disease could be virtually eliminated through prevention during pregnancy.

The most important information to remember about toxoplasmosis is (1) the birth defects it causes can be prevented by preventing infection during pregnancy, and (2) unnecessary worry can be prevented by determining whether or not you have already had the infection!

Prevention:

Wash hands with soap and water before eating.

Testing

- *Before* becoming pregnant, it is helpful to determine whether or not you've ever had toxoplasmosis. This can be accomplished by a test called a *titer*. A titer identifies antibodies, formed in response to a specific infection. If antibodies are present, you have had the infection and need not be concerned about being reinfected. The absence of these antibodies means that you are susceptible to infection.
- Once you become pregnant, titers are not always helpful. This is because it is not always possible to determine when the infection occurred and, most important, whether it occurred during your pregnancy. As some titers will detect an infection that occurred within three to four months, testing during early pregnancy could still provide helpful information. Because this issue can create a great deal of anxiety for you, discuss it with your health care provider, asking for a thorough explanation of your options.

Cats

The organism toxoplasma gondii can live in the intestines of cats and be passed in the cat's feces. Outdoor cats are more likely to be infected. Routine testing of cats for toxoplasmosis is not recommended. There is no reason to get rid of your household pet if you follow these preventive measures:

- *Completely avoid* contact with cat feces.
- Wash hands after contact with cats.
- Wear gloves when handling soil potentially contaminated by cat feces, as the organism toxoplasma gondii can live in such soil for over a year.
- If you have a cat, have someone else empty the litter box; if you must do this task, wear disposable gloves.

Food

Toxoplasmosis can also be acquired by eating uncooked meat, so:

- Wash hands with soap and water after handling raw meat.
- Avoid contact with mouth and eyes while handling raw meat.
- Cook meat thoroughly, until it changes color. Lamb is the meat to be most concerned about, although pork and beef can also be carriers of the organism.
- Avoid eating raw eggs.
- Wash fruit and vegetables before eating them.

Pregnant women are encouraged to discuss toxoplasmosis with their doctors. Recommendations and treatment considerations are the realm of the physician.

Reference:

[1] J. S. Remington and J. O. Klein (eds.), *Infectious Diseases of the Fetus and Newborn Infant* (2d ed). (Philadelphia: W. B. Saunders, 1983), pp. 144–263.

GENERIC NAME: **TRETINOIN**

Brand Name: **(Retin-A)**

FDA Pregnancy Category: B

ESTIMATED RISK SUMMARY:

Time of Exposure throughout pregnancy
Risk Risk assessment is not possible
Pregnancy Outcome uncertain
Documentation unavailable

← pre-conception	All or None		Organ Development – (in weeks)						Maturation – (in weeks)				
	1	2	3	4	5	6	7	8	9	10	12	20-36	38

conception   ← Time of Greatest Risk →   birth

Tretinoin is a vitamin A derivative used to control acne (see vitamin A, page 341). This product is for topical use only and is available in cream, gel, or liquid form.

Tretinoin is chemically related to two other vitamin A derivatives, etretinate and isotretinoin, both drugs are teratogenic in animals and in humans (see etretinate, page 157, and isotretinoin, page 206). Because etretinate and isotretinoin are taken orally, much greater doses are present in the mother's system and therefore more of the drug is available to her developing baby. It's important to keep in mind that, while related, tretinoin is used in a completely different manner than are etretinate and isotretinoin. Despite their chemical similarities, there are still very distinct differences among these three drugs.

It is reassuring to know that studies calculating the amount of tretinoin absorbed during its usual use estimate that prenatal vitamins provide about seven times the vitamin A activity than is provided by one topical application.[1]

Although controlled studies have not been conducted in pregnant women using tretinoin, I am not aware of any anecdotal evidence associating tretinoin with birth defects. Until information becomes available on the effect of this product on a developing baby, pregnant women should avoid using tretinoin.

Reference:

[1] G. Zbinden, Investigations on the toxicity of tretinoin administered systemically to animals, *Acta Dermatovener* (Stockhom) suppl.74 (1975): 36–39.

MEDICATION CLASSIFICATION: **TRICYCLIC ANTIDEPRESSANTS**

GENERIC NAMES: **AMITRIPTYLINE, AMOXAPINE, DE-SIPRAMINE, DOXEPIN, IMIPRAMINE, MAPROTY-LINE, NORTRIPTYLINE, TRIMIPRAMINE**

Brand Names: **(Adapin, Amitril, Asendin, Aventyl, Elavil, Emitrip, Endep, Janimine, Ludiomil, Norpramin, Pamelor, Pertofrane, Sinequan, SK-Pramine, Surmontil, Tipramine, Tofranil)**

FDA Pregnancy Category: matprotyline: B; all others: C

ESTIMATED RISK SUMMARY:

Time of Exposure throughout most of pregnancy
Risk No known risk*
Pregnancy Outcome appears favorable
Documentation inconclusive, based on minimal data

Time of Exposure near the time of delivery
Risk Suspected risk* for withdrawal symptoms
Pregnancy Outcome uncertain: favorable and adverse outcomes observed
Documentation inconclusive, based on minimal data

pre-conception	All or None		Organ Development – (in weeks)						Maturation – (in weeks)				
	1	2	3	4	5	6	7	8	9	10	12	20-36	38

conception   ← Time of Greatest Risk →   birth

Tricyclic antidepressants[1] are used to relieve symptoms of depression.

Isolated cases of defects, including limb abnormalities, in children prenatally exposed to tricyclic antidepressants (**amitriptyline, imipramine, nortriptyline**) have been reported. In contrast, several investigations, involving over half a million cases (161 of them first trimester exposures) have failed to show that these drugs are teratogenic. More specifically, they have not found them to be a major cause of congenital limb defects. Unfortunately, these results are not as helpful as they could be, because only 161 first trimester exposures were recorded, and this is the time when the arms and legs are developing. In other words, most of the collected information did not address the possible relationship between tricyclic antidepressants and limb abnormalities.

Some infants exposed before birth to tricyclic antidepressants (**desipramine,**

*above the 4% background risk

imipramine) have suffered withdrawal symptoms. These include breathlessness, rapid heart rate, muscle spasms, irritability, and feeding difficulties.

In one case, a newborn child's retention of urine was linked to the mother's taking **nortriptyline** while pregnant. Nortriptyline can also cause urinary retention in adults.

Long-term follow-up studies of children exposed before birth have not been located.

Reference:

[1]J. R. Calabrese and A. D. Gulledge, Psychotropics during pregnancy and lactation: A review, *Psychosomatics* 26 (1985): 413–26.

GENERIC NAMES: **TRIMETHADIONE (and PARAME-THADIONE)**

Brand names: **(Paradione, Tridione)**

FDA Pregnancy Category: D

ESTIMATED RISK SUMMARY:

Time of Exposure potentially throughout pregnancy

Risk Known risk*

Pregnancy Outcome adverse

Documentation conclusive, based on current knowledge

pre-conception	All or None		Organ Development – (in weeks)						Maturation – (in weeks)				
	1	2	3	4	5	6	7	8	9	10	12	20-36	38

conception　　　←—Time of Greatest Risk—→　　　birth

Trimethadione and *paramethadione*[1,2] are anticonvulsants—drugs that inhibit seizures or epilepsy.

Opinions differ about the specific risk of anticonvulsants. Many experts say there is two to three times the risk of major malformations in the children of epileptic women as in the general population. Some think the underlying disease is the cause. Others

*above the 4% background risk

believe this statistic reflects a population of women who are exposed more often to anticonvulsant drugs.

Trimethadione and paramethadione are both associated with a similar spectrum of defects, principally:

• *head and facial abnormalities*—short, upturned nose, low and broad nose bridge, a slightly flat midface area, prominent forehead with V-shaped eyebrows, low-set ears, and cleft lip and palate,
• *heart defects*
• *genital defects*—external sex organs not clearly male or female, enlarged clitoris, and hypospadias (abnormal placement of the urethral opening on the penis),
• *developmental delay,*
• *speech disorders,* and
• *prenatal onset growth deficiency.*
• The possibility of an increased frequency of miscarriages also exists.

Significant abnormalities are reported to occur in two out of every three children whose mothers take trimethadione and paramethadione during pregnancy.

Investigations have focused on women taking these drugs *throughout* pregnancy. As yet, no studies have been conducted on limited or first trimester exposures. This is important, because abnormalities can occur at various times within the embryonic and fetal periods. Trimethadione and paramethadione can harm organs that develop in the first trimester. They also affect growth early or late in pregnancy. And they can potentially damage the baby's brain anytime during pregnancy.

Theoretically, exposures limited to early pregnancy might affect only those organs that are already significantly developed. This would reduce the risk for growth retardation and mental deficiency.

Most women continue taking anticonvulsant medication during pregnancy, unless they have been seizure-free for many years. *Under no circumstances should you ever discontinue your anticonvulsant medication, unless under the direction and supervision of the prescribing physician.* Sudden withdrawal could cause a seizure. And while seizures are not known to cause malformations, they do present a possible risk to both you and your unborn baby.

Many women question how epilepsy or anticonvulsant medication in the father might affect their baby. Although not all scientists agree, most experts think this presents no increased risk. They believe that children fathered by men taking these drugs have the same chance of being normal and healthy as anyone else's, and well-conducted animal research confirms this belief.[3] (For more information on this, see Risks from Exposures in the Baby's Father, page 14.)

References:

[1]E. H. Zackai, W. J. Mellman, B. Neiderer, and J. W. Hanson, The fetal trimethadione syndrome, *Journal of Pediatrics* 87 (1975): 280–84.
[2]A. S. Goldman and S. J. Yaffe, Fetal trimethadione syndrome, *Teratology* (1978): 103–6.
[3]R. H. Finnell and J. F. Baer, Congenital defects among the offspring of epileptic fathers: Role of the genotype and phenytoin therapy in a mouse model, *Epilepsia* 25 (1986): 697–705.

GENERIC NAME: **TRIMETHOPRIM**

Brand Names: (◇ **Bactrim,** ◇ **Bethaprim SS,** ◇ **Cotrim, Proloprim,** ◇ **Septra,** ◇ **Sulfatrim, Trimpex)**

FDA Pregnancy Category: C

ESTIMATED RISK SUMMARY:

Time of Exposure throughout pregnancy

Risk No known risk,* although judicious use is still advised

Pregnancy Outcome appears favorable

Documentation inconclusive, based on minimal data

pre-conception	All or None		Organ Development – (in weeks)						Maturation – (in weeks)				
	1	2	3	4	5	6	7	8	9	10	12	20-36	38

conception ←— Time of Greatest Risk —→ birth

Trimethoprim, an anti-infective drug, may be used alone or in combination with a sulfonamide (sulfamethoxazole), another anti-infective. (see sulfonamides, page 305). Trimethoprim is used most commonly to treat urinary tract infections, but also for bacterial infections of the ear, lungs, and gastrointestinal tract.

Trimethoprim is classified as a folic acid antagonist. It works by blocking bacteria's use of folic acid. It does not have this effect on human cells. Although not specifically toxic to human cells, trimethoprim could cause folic acid deficiency. Folic acid, one of

◇ = contains sulfamethoxazole
*above the 4% background risk

the B vitamins, is required for fetal growth and development. For this reason, folic acid supplements are often recommended when trimethoprim is used in pregnancy.

While trimethoprim is teratogenic in rats, the human evidence from controlled studies and case reports shows no increased incidence of birth defects.[1,2,3]

Nevertheless, all folic acid antagonists remain suspect because one of the group, aminopterin, is a known human teratogen. (see chemotherapeutic drugs, page 103). *Unlike trimethoprim,* aminopterin can interfere with the growth of rapidly dividing human cells like cancer cells, fetal cells, and bone marrow. It is for these reasons that trimethoprim and other folic acid antagonists carry a warning about usage during pregnancy, particularly in the first trimester, when very rapid cell division takes place.

Long-term follow-up studies of children exposed before birth have not been located.

References:

[1]J. D. Williams, A. P. Condie, W. Brumfitt, and D. S. Reeves, The treatment of bacteriuria in pregnant women with sulfamethoxazole and trimethoprim, *Postgraduate Medical Journal* 45(suppl.) (1969): 71–76.

[2]W. Brumfitt and R. Pursell, Trimethoprim/sulfamethoxazole in the treatment of bacteriuria in women, *Journal of Infectious Diseases* 1(suppl.) (1973): S657–63.

[3]A. G. Ochoa, Trimethoprim and sulfamethoxazole in pregnancy, *Journal of the American Medical Association* 217 (1971): 1244.

MEDICATION CLASSIFICATION: **TUBERCULIN SKIN TEST**

Generic Name: **Purified Protein Derivative (PPD)**

Brand Names: **Aplitest, Sclavo Test-PPD, Tine Test PPD**

FDA Pregnancy Category: C

ESTIMATED RISK SUMMARY:
  Time of Exposure throughout pregnancy
  Risk No known risk*
  Pregnancy Outcome appears favorable
  Documentation inconclusive, based on minimal data

*above the 4% background risk

← pre-conception	All or None		Organ Development – (in weeks)						Maturation – (in weeks)				
	1	2	3	4	5	6	7	8	9	10	12	20-36	38

conception ←——— Time of Greatest Risk ———→ birth

This entry will not review the indications for tuberculosis screening during pregnancy, nor will it discuss the interpretations of the tests.

Tuberculin skin tests[1,2] are used to detect tuberculosis. Such tests performed during pregnancy are not known to cause birth defects. Tuberculosis screening often includes a chest X ray, but this information is no longer routinely required for prenatal screening. If, however, your skin test reaction is positive, a chest X ray might be needed. Happily, chest X rays deliver no measurable amount of radiation to your unborn baby (see X rays, page 347).

Long-term follow-up studies of children exposed before birth have not been located.

References:

[1] D. Snider, Pregnancy and tuberculosis, *Chest* 86 (1984): 10S–3S.
[2] J. J. Bush, Protocol for tuberculosis screening in pregnancy, *Journal of Obstetric, Gynecologic, and Neonatal Nursing* 15 (1986): 225–30.

COMMON NAME: **ULTRASOUND**

Brand Name/Chemical Name: **not applicable**

FDA Pregnancy Category: not applicable

ESTIMATED RISK SUMMARY:

Time of Exposure throughout pregnancy
Risk No measurable risk* for *diagnostic* ultrasound
Pregnancy Outcome favorable
Documentation conclusive, based on current knowledge

Time of Exposure throughout pregnancy
Risk Risk assessment is not possible for *therapeutic* ultrasound

*above the 4% background risk

Pregnancy Outcome uncertain
Documentation unavailable

← pre-conception	All or None	Organ Development – (in weeks)						Maturation – (in weeks)				
	1	2	3	4	5	6	7	8	9	10	12	20-36	38

conception   ← Time of Greatest Risk →   birth

Ultrasound[1] is the use of high-frequency sound waves to produce an image. Ultrasound does not produce ionizing radiation (X rays) (see X rays, page 347). Ultrasound is used during pregnancy to help a physician make a diagnosis and provide better care (see ultrasound, page 24). A "sound picture" of the baby is taken by a specialist called a sonographer and displayed on a TV-like monitor.

Diagnostic ultrasound has been used in obstetrics for more than twenty years. Studies to date have *not* implicated *diagnostic ultrasound* as being harmful to an unborn baby. Long-term follow-up studies, some of which are still in progress, have not revealed any adverse effects.[2] Rumors linking ultrasound to deafness or hearing loss remain unfounded, since no differences have been found in studies of exposed and unexposed children.

Despite its presumed safety, ultrasound should only be performed when there is some medical indication for the procedure and not to just view the unborn baby or to obtain a picture of it.

High energy or *therapeutic ultrasound,* which produces heat, is used in physical therapy to treat muscle soreness and back pain. The effect of ultrasonic heat treatments on a developing fetus has not been studied. It is reassuring to note that during the first trimester of pregnancy, the uterus is in the pelvis. Logic indicates that the fetus is seemingly well protected, as the maternal pubis and several centimeters of tissue will absorb much of the heat transmitted by the ultrasound. However, this has not been confirmed by studies in pregnant women. Because there is some concern about high temperatures during pregnancy, pregnant women are advised to avoid such exposures to *therapeutic* ultrasound, until it is actually investigated (see hyperthermia, page 197).

References:

[1]Public Health Service National Institutes of Health, Diagnostic ultrasound imaging in pregnancy, U.S.

department of Health and Human Services. February 6–8, 1984, Public Health Service National Institutes of Health (NIH Publication No. 84–667).

[2]C. R. Stark, M. Orleans, A. D. Havercamp, and J. Murphy, Short- and- long-term effects after exposure to diagnostic ultrasound in utero, *Obstetrics and Gynecology* 63 (1984): 194–200.

COMMON NAME: **URINARY TRACT INFECTION**

Brand Name/Chemical Name: **not applicable**

FDA Pregnancy Category: not applicable

ESTIMATED RISK SUMMARY:

>*Time of Exposure* throughout pregnancy
>*Risk* No known risk* when *treated*
>*Pregnancy Outcome* appears favorable
>*Documentation* inconclusive

>*Time of Exposure* throughout pregnancy
>*Risk* Known risk* when *untreated*
>*Pregnancy Outcome* adverse
>*Documentation* conclusive, based on current knowledge

pre-conception	All or None		Organ Development – (in weeks)						Maturation – (in weeks)				
	1	2	3	4	5	6	7	8	9	10	12	20-36	38

conception   ← Time of Greatest Risk →   birth

Urinary tract infections (UTI)[1] are the most common infectious complications of pregnancy. Somewhere between 2 percent to 7 percent of pregnant women have evidence of bacteria in their urinary tract but have no symptoms of infection. This condition is appropriately called asymptomatic bacteriuria (ASB). If left untreated, ASB will develop into a serious kidney infection (acute pylonephritis) about 20–40 percent of the time.

Kidney infections are likely to increase a pregnant woman's risk for premature labor and a low-birth-weight infant. The risk of infant death and illness shortly before and after birth is also increased with these infections. In addition, the high fever that so

*above the 4% background risk

often accompanies a kidney infection is an added concern, and perhaps even an added risk during pregnancy (see hyperthermia, page 197).

For these reasons, when women come in for their first prenatal care visit, health care providers, as a precaution, routinely screen the urine for any sign of bacteria. If necessary, antibiotic treatment is prescribed in order to prevent growth of the bacteria from posing a threat to the mother and her unborn baby. (For further information about antibiotics, read the entry about the medicine which has been prescribed for you.)

Receiving treatment for a urinary tract infection, including ASB, is therefore very important. But pregnant women are so often warned about the dangers of drug use that many are apprehensive about taking even prescribed antibiotics. This is often even more difficult for women with ASB, because they don't feel sick. Without the antibiotic, chances of illness, and perhaps serious illness, increase greatly. Under such circumstances, antibiotics would eventually be required anyway. It is also essential that you fully understand how important it is to take the entire prescription of medication; the reason is because some antibiotics are not immediately lethal to the bacteria and if the drug is withdrawn, the bacteria will usually resume growth.

Further reinforcing the need for treatment of urinary tract infections is an investigation that examined birth weight and infant weight and length at one, three, six, nine, and twelve months, and the development quotient at two years. No differences were found in children whose mothers were treated for bacteriuria compared with those whose mothers showed no evidence of bacteriuria.[2]

Last, if you are still unsure about the necessity of the treatment, seek another medical opinion.

References:

[1]G. D. V. Hankins and P. J. Whalley, Acute urinary tract infections in pregnancy, *Clincal Obstetrics and Gynecology* 28 (1985): 266–78.

[2]R. Gofin, H. Palti, and B. Adler. Bacteriuria in pregnancy and growth and development of the infants, *Early Human Development* 9 (1984): 341–46.

GENERIC NAME: **VALPROIC ACID**

Brand Names: **(Depakene, Depakote)**

FDA Pregnancy Category: D

ESTIMATED RISK SUMMARY:

Time of Exposure very early pregnancy (about 14 to 28 days postconception)

Risk Known risk* for spina bifida
Pregnancy Outcome adverse
Documentation conclusive, based on current knowledge

Time of Exposure difficult to be specific, possibly throughout most of pregnancy
Risk Suspected risk* for a variety of defects
Pregnancy Outcome uncertain: favorable and adverse outcomes observed
Documentation inconclusive, based on minimal data

← pre-conception ←	All or None		Organ Development – (in weeks)						Maturation – (in weeks)				
	1	2	3	4	5	6	7	8	9	10	12	20-36	38

conception   ←—Time of Greatest Risk—→   birth

Valproic acid is an anticonvulsant—a drug that inhibits recurrent seizures, or epilepsy.

Opinions differ about the specific risk of anticonvulsants. Many experts say there is two to three times the risk of major malformations in the children of epileptic women as in the general population. Some think the underlying disease is the cause. Others believe this statistic reflects a population of women who are exposed more often to anticonvulsant drugs.

The difference of opinion arises, in part, from the variation in types of defect, and in their incidence. The best explanation of this variation is the way the genetics of the mother and fetus influence drug reaction[1] (First Principle of Teratology page 33).

The various studies of anticonvulsants as teratogens are also hard to compare because they are designed so differently.

Malformations reported in infants born to mothers receiving valproic acid during pregnancy, include:[2,3,4,5,6]

• *Spina bifida*—a defect in the closure of the spinal cord,
• *peculiar facial appearance*—a small nose with a flat bridge and upturned nostrils, wide-spaced eyes, a relatively small mouth with downturned corners, and a long thin upper lip,
• *external ear abnormalities,*
• *skeleton defects,*

*above the 4% background risk

• *heart defects,* and
• *hypospadias*—abnormal placement of the urethral opening on the penis.

The facial alterations are the basis of the proposed "fetal valproate syndrome."[2] Some of these features resemble those observed with hydantoins, but differences do exist (see hydantoins, page 191).

Low birth weight and small head size have been reported in some children born to women taking valproic acid alone or with another anticonvulsant.[7,8] A small number of children so exposed before birth have also exhibited developmental delay.[7,9]

At the time of this writing, the only major malformation *known* to be *caused* by valproic acid is spina bifida. The risk for spina bifida is during the early first trimester, between the fourteen to the twenty-eight days (primarily 21–28 days) after conception, when the spinal cord is developing. Fortunately, prenatal diagnosis can usually detect its presence. Depending on certain circumstances, including the stage of your pregnancy and the severity of the spina bifida, diagnosis may require maternal alpha-fetoprotein test, amniocentesis or a Level II ultrasound (see Diagnosing and Treating Problem Pregnancies, page 21). The frequency of spina bifida in those exposed to valproic acid in the early first trimester is not known; however, after-the-fact studies indicate the incidence is between 1[10] and 1.5[11] percent.

The other abnormalities reported could occur at various times within the embryonic and fetal periods. Valproic acid might harm organs that develop in the first trimester. It might also affect growth early or late in pregnancy, and it may damage the brain, which is vulnerable throughout pregnancy. At the present, however, researchers are unsure about how many of these defects are actually caused by valproic acid, and if so, how often they occur.

In animals high concentrations of valproic acid increase the drug's teratogenic potential; this might also be true for humans. A small prospective study that included infants prenatally exposed to valproic acid *alone,* found that the number of minor malformations was related to the amount of valproic acid the mother received.[5] Fetal distress and low Apgar scores (a numeric expression of infant well-being at birth) were more common in those exposed only to valproic acid and most frequent in those exposed to the highest doses. In order to avoid dangerously high drug concentrations, the authors of this study recommend pregnant women have their blood levels of valproic acid monitored.

Most women continue taking anticonvulsant medication during pregnancy, unless they have been seizure-free for many years. *Under no circumstances should you ever discontinue your anticonvulsant medication, unless under the direction and supervision of the prescribing physician.* Sudden withdrawal could cause a seizure.

And while seizures are not known to be a direct cause of malformation, they do present a possible risk to both you and your unborn baby.

Many women question how epilepsy or anticonvulsant medication in the father might affect their baby. Although not all scientists agree, most experts think this presents no increased risk. They believe that children fathered by men taking these drugs have the same chance of being normal and healthy as anyone else's and well-conducted animal research confirms this belief.[12] (For more information on this see Risks From Exposures in the Baby's Father, page 14).

References:

[1]R. H. Finnell and G. F. Chernoff, Genetic background: The elusive component of the Fetal Hydantoin Syndrome, *American Journal of Medical Genetics* 19 (1984): 459–62.

[2]J. H. Di Liberti, P. A. Farndon, N. R. Dennis, C. J. R. Curry, The fetal valproate syndrome, *American Journal of Medical Genetics* 19 (1984): 473–81.

[3]P. M. Jeavons, Non-dose related side effects of valproate, *Epilepsia* 25(suppl.) (1984): 50S–55S.

[4]A. S. Garden, R. J. Benzie, E. M. Hutton, and D. J. Gare, Valproic acid therapy and neural tube defects, *Canadian Medical Association Journal* 132 (1985): 933–36.

[5]E. Jäger-Roman, A. Deichl, S. Jakob, A. M. Hartman, S. Koch, D. Rating, R. Steldinger, H. Nau, and H. Helge, Fetal growth, major malformations, and minor anomalies in infants born to women receiving valproic acid, *Journal of Pediatrics* 108 (1986): 997–1004.

[6]E. J. Lammer, L. E. Sever, and G. P. Oakley, Jr., Teratogenic Update: Valproic Acid, *Teratology* 35 (1987): 465–73.

[7]H. Nau, D. Rating, S. Koch, I. Häuser, and H. Helge, Valproic acid and its metabolities: Placental pharmacokinetics, transfer via mother's milk and clinical status in neonates of epileptic mothers, *Journal of Pharmacology and Experimental Therapeutics* 219 (1981): 768–77.

[8]I. Tein and D. L. MacGregor, Possible valproate teratogenicity, *Archives of Neurology* 42 (1985): 291–93.

[9]S. A. Clay, R. McVie, H. Chen, Possible teratogenic effect of valproic acid, *Journal of Pediatrics* 99 (1981): 828.

[10]D. Lindhout and D. Schmidt, In-utero exposure to valproate and neural tube defects, *Lancet* 1 (1986): 1392–93.

[11]T. Bjerkedal, A. Czeizel, J. Goujard, B. Kallen, P. Mastroiacova, N. Nevin, G. Oakley, and E. Robert, Valproic acid and spina bifida, *Lancet* 2 (1982): 1096.

[12]R. H. Finnell and J. F. Baer, Congenital defects among the offspring of epileptic fathers: Role of the genotype and phenytoin therapy in a mouse model, *Epilepsia* 25 (1986): 697–705.

GENERIC NAME: **VANCOMYCIN**

Brand Name: **(Vancocin)**

FDA Pregnancy Category:—

ESTIMATED RISK SUMMARY:

Time of Exposure throughout pregnancy

Risk Risk assessment is not possible

Pregnancy Outcome uncertain

Documentation insufficient

← pre- conception →	All or None		Organ Development – (in weeks)						Maturation – (in weeks)				
	1	2	3	4	5	6	7	8	9	10	12	20-36	38

conception   ←—— Time of Greatest Risk ——→   birth

Vancomycin is an antibiotic usually reserved to treat very serious infections. To date there is only one report on the effects of this drug when used during pregnancy. A woman who received an intravenous dose of vancomycin one hour before delivery experienced a drop in blood pressure.[1] The fetus exhibited an abnormally slow heartbeat (bradycardia), which persisted for only a matter of minutes. No further adverse effects were observed in this newborn.

Reference:

[1] L. M. Hill, Fetal distress secondary to vancomycin-induced maternal hypotention, *American Journal of Obstetrics and Gynecology* 153 (1985): 74–75.

COMMON NAME: **VARICELLA (CHICKEN POX)**

Brand Name/Chemical name: **not applicable**

FDA Pregnancy Category: not applicable

ESTIMATED RISK SUMMARY:

    Time of Exposure primarily during the first 20 weeks of gestation,** and within four days or less of delivery.

    Risk Known risk*

    Pregnancy Outcome adverse

    Documentation conclusive, based on current knowledge

    **The term *gestation* is often used to describe the time from the first day of the last menstrual period to birth, rather than the period from conception to birth.

    *above the 4% background risk

		All or None	Organ Development – (in weeks)						Maturation – (in weeks)				
← pre- conception ←		1	2	3	4	5	6	7	8	9	10	12	20-36	38

conception　　　　←—Time of Greatest Risk—→　　　　birth

Varicella (chicken pox)[1,2] is a common infectious disease of childhood, affecting more than 80 percent of children under 10 years of age. Varicella and the related infection herpes zoster ("shingles") are both caused by the varicella-zoster virus (see herpes zoster, page 190). Women who have never had varicella before can get the infection from contact with an individual who has either one of these infections.

Varicella infection is very rare during pregnancy, but when contracted it can pose a risk to both the mother and her unborn baby. Maternal complications associated with this infection include pneumonia and premature labor, and although it is infrequent, death can also occur.[3] Infection, primarily during the first twenty weeks of gestation, can cause a recognizable pattern of defects in the baby termed the "varicella syndrome." As many as thirty infants with the so-called varicella syndrome have been reported in the medical literature.[4] Most of these cases were the result of maternal infection during the first eight to nineteen weeks of gestation.[5] Affected infants may have severe skin scarring, limb defects, eye abnormalities, mental deficiency, and retarded growth (particularly low birth weight). How often these problems occur in the infants of infected mothers can only be approximated. Data collected from three prospective evaluations indicate that the incidence of observable problems in an infant from a first trimester varicella infection is low (4.9%, three of sixty-one babies).[3]

Birth defects associated with varicella infection in the latter part of pregnancy are extremely rare. Infections occurring primarily after twenty-one weeks of gestation are more often linked to the development of herpes zoster in early or late infancy.[4] It is reassuring to note that zoster tends to be mild in these infants.

The highest risk from varicella during pregnancy is for those infants *born* during the four-day period after their mothers developed the infection. Since these newborns apparently don't have the chance to receive protective antibodies from their mothers, they are at a high risk of developing a severe life-threatening varicella infection.

There is some evidence that the risk to the fetus and newborn might be reduced by administering certain concentrated solutions of antibodies (pooled immune serum globulin [SG] or zoster immune globulin [ZIG] to the pregnant mother.[1,5] Unfortunately there are no adequate studies of ISG or ZIG for the treatment of varicella during pregnancy or in treatment or prevention of varicella in the newborn baby. Your physician can give you more specific information about the benefits and limitations of these products.

References:

J. S. Remington and J. O. Klein, (eds.), *Infectious Diseases of the Fetus and Newborn Infant*, 2d ed. (Philadelphia, W. B. Saunders, 1983), pp. 376–402.

[2]W. S. Chosos, Varicella and pregnancy: Report of a case and review of the literature, *Journal of the American Osteopathic Association* 81 (1982): 644–46.

[3]S. G. Paryani, and A. M. Arvin, Intrauterine infection with varicella-zoster virus after maternal varicella, *New England Journal of Medicine* 314 (1986): 1542–46.

[4]K. Higa, K. Dan, and H. Manabe, Varicella-zoster virus infections during pregnancy: Hypothesis concerning the mechanisms of congenital malformations, *Obstetrics and Gynecology* 69 (1987): 214–22.

[5]G. Enders, Varicella-zoster virus infection in pregnancy, *Progress in Medical Virology* 29 (1984): 166–96.

COMMON NAME: **VARICELLA VACCINE**

Brand Name/Chemical name: **not applicable**

FDA Pregnancy Category: not applicable

ESTIMATED RISK SUMMARY:

Time of Exposure throughout pregnancy

Risk Risk assessment is not possible

Pregnancy Outcome uncertain

Documentation insufficient; no information is available

← pre-conception	All or None		Organ Development – (in weeks)						Maturation – (in weeks)				
	1	2	3	4	5	6	7	8	9	10	12	20-36	38

conception   ←——Time of Greatest Risk——→   birth

At the time of this writing the *varicella vaccine* has not been licensed for use in the United States. It is hoped that it will one day be possible to vaccinate susceptible women before they are pregnant, thereby eliminating the risks varicella infection (chicken pox) presents during pregnancy (see varicella, page, 336).

GENERIC NAME: **VERAPAMIL**

Brand Names: **(Calan, Isoptin)**

FDA Pregnancy Category:—

ESTIMATED RISK SUMMARY:

Time of Exposure throughout pregnancy
Risk Risk assessment is not possible
Pregnancy Outcome uncertain
Documentation insufficient

← pre-conception ←	All or None		Organ Development – (in weeks)						Maturation – (in weeks)				
	1	2	3	4	5	6	7	8	9	10	12	20-36	38

conception   ←—Time of Greatest Risk—→   birth

Verapamil is used in the treatment of abnormal heartbeat rhythms (arrhythmias). Experience with the use of verapamil in pregnant women is very limited, and while teratogenic effects have not been located, further study is required before its safety in pregnancy can be established.

Verapamil crosses the placenta into the unborn child's bloodstream. It has recently been administered to a pregnant woman to return her unborn baby's rapid heartbeat (tachycardia) to normal.[1]

Low blood pressure has been observed in some patients who receive verapamil intravenously. This raises the *theoretical* concern that blood flow between the uterus and the placenta could be reduced, thereby interfering with the amount of oxygen the unborn child receives. Confirmation is required before this concern can be interpreted as an actual risk.

Long-term follow-up studies of children exposed before birth have not been located.

Reference:

[1] F. Wolf, K. H. Breuker, K. H. Schlensker, and A. Bolte, Prenatal diagnosis and therapy of fetal heart rate anomalies: With a contribution on the placental transfer of verapamil, *Journal of Perinatal Medicine* 8 (1980): 203–8.

COMMON NAME: **VIDEO DISPLAY TERMINALS (VDT, CRT)**

Brand name/Chemical name: **not applicable**

FDA Pregnancy Category: not applicable

ESTIMATED RISK SUMMARY:
  Time of Exposure throughout pregnancy
  Risk No known risk*
  Pregnancy Outcome appears favorable
  Documentation inconclusive

← pre-conception ←	All or None		Organ Development – (in weeks)						Maturation – (in weeks)				
	1	2	3	4	5	6	7	8	9	10	12	20-36	38

conception   ←—— Time of Greatest Risk ——→   birth

The computer age is here! By the end of this century, an estimated 40 million people will be using *video display terminals (VDTs)*[1] in their occupations.

The mechanism of a VDT is exactly the same as that of your color television set. Prior to 1970 some television sets emitted X rays in excess of the established safety limits. All sets manufactured after this time are in compliance with current safety standards.

The cathode ray tube (CRT) component of the VDT emits X rays. But the screen of the VDT completely absorbs this radiation! In fact, no X rays have been detected in investigations conducted by safety agencies in several countries. VDTs also emit non-ionizing radiation, such as microwaves and radio waves, but they are not known to be harmful to life either.

The first investigation into the effects of VDTs on pregnancy was launched in 1980, after four women working at a Toronto newspaper gave birth to children with birth defects. It is important to remember the 4 percent incidence of birth defects in our population and that some birth defects do occur by chance; nevertheless, this cluster of defects warranted investigation. The Ontario ministry of Labor checked the terminals for emission of any ionizing radiation (X rays) and detected none. The investigation

*above the 4% background risk

also revealed that each affected child had a completely different birth defect. One was born with a club foot; one had an underdeveloped eye; another had a cleft palate; and one child was born with a heart defect. Reviewing the principles of teratology, we find that individuals affected by the same teratogen usually share a similar pattern of abnormality (see Fourth Principle of Teratology, page 39). Therefore, the diversity of the defects makes any link between the VDTs and the reported abnormalities very unlikely.

Other clusters of birth defects and miscarriages among VDT operators have also been reported. However, in no instance were the defects uniform. Some of the problems labeled as malformations were later correctly identified as premature births, respiratory illness, and bronchitis. Unfortunately, much of the publicity on the issue of VDT-related birth defects does not make clear the many scientific inconsistencies of each incident. Currently the number of abnormal births reported by VDT operators are well within the expected 4 percent general population incidence of birth defects, and are attributed to chance.

Long-term follow-up studies of children exposed before birth have not been located.

Finally, psychological stress, neck and back pain, eyestrain, and other discomforts are not uncommon among VDT workers. I wrote this book using a computer, so I'm sympathetic to how annoying these problems can be. I find it helpful to take frequent breaks, move around a bit (stretching or taking a short walk—even if it's just down the hall) to get that circulation going! This is particularly important for pregnant women, who tend to feel uncomfortable after sitting for long periods of time. When I don't actually get up, I roll my head around in place and move my shoulders in circular shrugging motions. Twisting gently from side to side is beneficial, as is sticking the legs straight out in front of you and tensing, then relaxing them. Four or five deep breaths can work wonders too. Sometimes I just close my eyes for a minute or two—it helps a lot.

Reference:

[1]Reproductive Toxicology, a medical letter on Environmental Hazards to Reproduction, Video display terminals and human reproduction, Reproductive Toxicology Center, Washington, D. C., 3(1)(1984): 1–3.

GENERIC NAME: **VITAMIN A**

Brand names: **(various)**

FDA Pregnancy Category: —

ESTIAMTED RISK SUMMARY:

Time of Exposure throughout pregnancy

Risk No measurable risk* in doses within the RDA

Pregnancy Outcome favorable

Documenttion conclusive, based on current knowledge

Time of Exposure at least during the first trimester. (Evidence from animal studies suggests potential sensitivity throughout pregnancy.)

Risk Suspected risk* in doses significantly higher than the RDA

Pregnancy Outcome uncertain: favorable and adverse outcomes observed

Documentation inconclusive, based on minimal data

pre-conception		All or None		Organ Development – (in weeks)						Maturation – (in weeks)				
		1	2	3	4	5	6	7	8	9	10	12	20-36	38

conception   ⟵ Time of Greatest Risk ⟶   birth

Vitamin A[1] or *retinol* is a fat-soluble vitamin. This means that unused amounts are not readily excreted from your system; instead, they are stored in your body fat. Because high levels of fat-soluble vitamins can build up in the body, excessive doses can be toxic (poisonous). For this reason it is a good idea to stay within the Recommended Dietary Allowances (RDA) for these substances. The National Research Council's Committee on Dietary Allowances suggests the daily RDA for vitamin A during pregnancy is 1,000 retinol equivalents (RE). This is the same as 3,300 International Units (IU) of vitamin A obtained from a supplement as retinol, or 5,000 IU of vitamin A obtained from the typical American diet. The U.S. Food and Drug Administration's RDA for vitamin A during pregnancy is 8,000 IU. (Toxic effects from vitamin A probably occur at 20–30 times the RDA.)

Food sources of vitamin A include liver, eggs, kidney, milk, cream, ice cream, butter, margarine, orange and dark green vegetables, fish and liver oils.

Animal studies have linked vitamin A deficiency to birth defects; it was the first nutritional substance so associated. Excessive amounts of vitamin A are also known to cause birth defects in laboratory animals. Drugs similar in chemical structure to vitamin A (excluding tretinoin, page 322), have been proven to cause abnormalities in both animals and in humans. (see etretinate, page 157 and isotretinoin, page 206) All of these observations have led to much speculation on the potential teratogenicity of

*above the 4% background risk

vitamin A in humans. Unfortunately, very little information is available on what risks, if any, are associated with too much or too little of this vitamin during pregnancy.

Only three isolated cases of birth defects—all some type of eye problem or eye abnormality—associated with **severe vitamin A deficiency** have been located. This is very interesting, since Vitamin A is necessary for normal vision.

By December of 1986, the U.S. Food and Drug Administration was aware of 22 cases of birth defects which coincided with **excessive or "mega" doses of vitamin A** taken during pregnancy. The abnormalities observed in these children include defects of the skeleton, heart, urinary tract, central nervous system, and of the head and face (abnormally small head, small eyes, small chin, cleft lip, cleft palate, and various ear abnormalities). These babies were prenatally exposed to doses equal to or greater than 25,000 IU of vitamin A per day; only one mother took less (18,000 IU daily). Some of these babies were also exposed to high doses of other vitamins (vitamins D and E). In all but one case, the mothers continued taking high doses of vitamin A for quite some time beyond conception, usually throughout pregnancy. The only exception was a woman who accidentally swallowed a poisonous amount of oily vitamin A solution (10 ml) during the first month of her pregnancy.[2] In this instance, the woman gave birth to a child with Goldenhar syndrome (characterized by malformations of the face and neck).

These cases are few in number, but they do underscore the potential adverse effects of high doses of vitamin A during pregnancy. Pregnant women are therefore advised to restrict their intake of vitamin A to within the Recommended Dietary Allowances. If you routinely take mega doses of this vitamin, immediately inform your health care provider.

Long-term follow-up studies of children exposed before birth have not been located.

References:

[1] F. W. Rosa, A. L. Wilk, and F. O. Kelsey, Teratogen update: Vitamin A congeners, *Teratology* 33 (1986): 355–64.

[2] R. L. Mounoud, D. Klein, and F. Weber, A propos d'un cas de syndrome de goldenhar: Intoxication aiguë à la vitamine A chez la mère pendant la grossesse, *Journal de Génétique Humaine* 33 (1975): 135–54.

MEDICATION CLASSIFICATION: **VITAMINS**

GENERIC NAMES: **VITAMIN A, B-COMPLEX, C, D, E, K**

Brand Name/Chemical Name: **various**

FDA Pregnancy Category:—

ESTIMATED RISK SUMMARY:

Time of Exposure throughout pregnancy

Risk No measurable risk* when doses are within the RDA

Pregnancy Outcome favorable

Documentation conclusive, based on current knowledge

← pre-conception	All or None		Organ Development – (in weeks)						Maturation – (in weeks)				
	1	2	3	4	5	6	7	8	9	10	12	20-36	38

conception   ←——Time of Greatest Risk——→   birth

Vitamins are nutrients that are necessary, in small amounts, for the proper functioning of the body. The recommended dietary allowances (RDA) of vitamins, determined by the National Research Council, are not known to cause birth defects. However, deficiencies and excessive doses of some vitamins have been linked to problems during pregnancy. For this reason, women are advised to stay within the RDA for vitamin intake during pregnancy. This can be accomplished by taking prenatal vitamin supplements. Most doctors recommend these for their pregnant patients anyway, because vitamins and minerals promote good health in both the mother and her developing baby.

Vitamin A is discussed separately (see page 341). The other vitamins are grouped here.

There are two classes of vitamins: fat soluble and water soluble. The fat-soluble vitamins—A, D, E, and K—will be stored in the body fat of people who take amounts above those needed. Water-soluble vitamins—the B complex and vitamin C—are not stored. The body uses what it needs from the amount taken in every day, and excretes the rest. Even so, very large or "mega" doses of water-soluble vitamins can have toxic effects, can interact with other vitamins or with drugs, and may even lead to dependency. Beause they are not stored in the body, water-soluble vitamins cross the placental barrier to the developing child more easily than fat-soluble vitamins do.

B Vitamins

Thiamine (vitamin B₁). In pregnancy, the RDA is 1.4 mg. per day for women over the age of 23, and 1.5 mg. for those 22 and younger. Thiamine is found

---

*above the 4% background risk

in red meat, liver, grains, peas, and beans. It is important for turning the calories you eat into energy.

Riboflavin. In pregnancy, the RDA is 1.5 mg. per day for women 23 and over, and 1.6 mg. for those 22 and younger. Good sources of riboflavin are liver, milk, and grains. It assists in energy metabolism and in your body's use of protein.

Niacin. In pregnancy, the RDA is 16 mg. per day for women 23 and over, and 16 milligrams for those 22 and younger. Fish, meat, legumes, and grains are good sources of niacin. Your body uses it to trigger energy and protein metabolism.

Pyridoxine (B$_6$). In pregnancy, the RDA is 2.6 mg. per day for women 15 and older, and 17 mg. for those 14 and younger. Good sources of vitamin B$_6$ are grains and meat. Necessary for protein metabolism, vitamin B$_6$ also is important for the growth of the unborn child.

Vitamin B$_6$ has been used frequently to treat nausea and vomiting associated with early pregnancy. It was also a component in the drug Bendectin, which was specifically used for this purpose (see doxylamine, page 148). An increased risk for birth defects has been linked to the mother's use of this vitamin alone or as a component in Benedectin.

Overuse of vitamin B$_6$ can lead to dependency, and withdrawal problems when it is discontinued. Case reports have been cited of babies with seizures born to women who took high doses of the vitamin while pregnant. Abnormal vitamin B$_6$ metabolism has been the suggested cause of these problems.

Folic acid or folacin. In pregnancy, the RDA is 800 micrograms per day. Folic acid is found in raw leafy vegetables and in liver. It is for the production of hemoglobin, the principal component of red blood cells.

Larger than normal amounts of folic acid are not known to harm unborn babies. However, some studies have found that deficiencies are related to miscarriage and to neural tube defects (spina bifida and anencphaly). Such observations have led to research on the role of vitamin supplementation in the prevention of birth defects. Many investigations have found no relationship between children born with abnormalities and folic acid deficiency or low levels of any other vitamin in their mothers. Definitive conclusions about this matter have not yet been reached. Some anticonvulsants and anticancer drugs are known to reduce the unborn child's levels of folic acid. Severe folic acid deficiency can lead to anemia and low blood platelet count, both of which can cause problems in pregnancy and in the child shortly before and after birth.

Cobalamin (B$_{12}$). In pregnancy, the RDA is 4 micrograms per day. Dairy products, eggs, meat, and liver are all good sources of vitamin B$_{12}$.

Severe vitamin B_{12} deficiency can lead to megaloblastic anemia, a condition associated with infertility. Fortunately, this condition responds well to vitamin B_{12} therapy. Normal pregnancies have been recorded after treatment.

There is no evidence of harmful effects to the unborn child from large doses of vitamin B_{12}.

Vitamin C

In pregnancy, the RDA for vitamin C is 80 mg. daily for women 15 and over, and 70 mg for those 14 and younger. It is found in citrus and other fruits, leafy vegetables, broccoli, and tomatoes. It is necessary for maintaining the structure of various body tissues, and it makes the body absorb iron more efficiently.

People who discontinue taking large amounts of vitamin C sometimes develop the deficiency disease scurvy, called "rebound scurvy," in these circumstances. There have been reports of scurvy among children whose mothers took megadoses of vitamin C while pregnant. However, most experts believe that lower than normal, normal, and high doses of vitamin C are not harmful to the unborn child.

Vitamin D

The RDA for vitamin D in pregnancy is 10 micrograms (400 IU) daily for women 23 and older, 12.5 micrograms (500 IU) for those between 19 and 22, and 15 micrograms (600 IU) for those 18 and younger. This vitamin is found principally in fish and fortified milk. It is vital for the body's making the most efficient use of its calcium supply.

Large amounts of vitamin D have been suspected to contribute to the infantile Hypercalcemic* syndrome, which is characterized by structural defects of the skull and face, mental retardation, growth retardation, defective tooth enamel, and narrowing of the major arteries of the heart and lungs (supravalvular aortic and pulmonary stenosis). But there is no actual proof of this. Vitamin D deficiency has been linked to slowed growth of the unborn child, and hypocalcemia, rickets, and poor tooth structure in the newborn child.

Vitamin E

The RDA for vitamin E during pregnancy is 10 mg. Good sources of this vitamin are leafy vegetables, cereals, eggs, dairy products, and meat.

No harm to the unborn child has been associated with vitamin E, in either normal, high, or low doses.

Hypercalcemia means excessive amounts of calcium.

COMMON NAME: **X rays**

Brand name/Chemical name: **not applicable**

FDA Pregnancy Category: not applicable

ESTIMATED RISK SUMMARY:

Time of Exposure throughout pregnancy

Risk no measurable risk* for birth defects when the dose received to the uterus is below 5 to 10 Rads

Pregnancy Outcome favorable

Documentation conclusive, based on current knowledge

Time of Exposure throughout pregnancy

Risk Known risk* for birth defects when dose received by the uterus exceeds 10 Rads

Pregnancy Outcome adverse

Documentation conclusive, based on current knowledge

← pre-conception	All or None		Organ Development – (in weeks)						Maturation – (in weeks)				
	1	2	3	4	5	6	7	8	9	10	12	20-36	38

conception   ←— Time of Greatest Risk —→   birth

Universally misunderstood by both health professionals and lay individuals, the concern for *X-ray*-related[1,2] birth defects has caused more unnecessary panic and unwarranted anxiety than any single issue in teratology. The X ray is one of the earliest identified teratogens, and information on the harmful affects of X rays during pregnancy has been widely distributed in an effort to minimize exposures during pregnancy and thus avoid damage to the unborn baby.

Unfortunately, the education campaign omitted informing people that the adverse effects of radiation are dose related (see the Third Principle of Teratology, page 39). In the past, high levels of radiation were used for cancer treatment during pregnancy. This practice resulted in an increase in abnormalities in the exposed infants. Today the questions about X rays most often relate to diagnostic procedures rather than therapeutic treatment. Happily, most diagnostic procedures deliver little, if any,

*above the 4% background risk

scattered radiation to the uterus. In fact, with rare exceptions, diagnostic X rays during pregnancy *do not* increase the risk of birth defects.

It is helpful to understand that the concern for X rays is related to the amount of radiation that reaches the uterus (fetus). The farther away the procedure is from the uterus, the less likely the fetus is to be exposed. Studies conducted in laboratory animals and information gathered from procedures performed on pregnant women suggest that exposures exceeding 10 rads (a rad is a measure of radiation) are risky. That is, doses over 10 rads to a pregnant woman's uterus may increase the risk of embryonic death and birth defects, specifically: an abnormally small head size, (microencephaly), mental retardation, and eye malformations. X rays delivering over 5 rads to the unborn baby may raise some concern. The most serious effects of radiation during pregnancy have occurred at levels of 50 to 100 rads and greater.

(For information on the estimated radiation doses delivered to the uterus from various diagnostic procedures, see Table 5–4 on page 350).

Suspicions about the unborn's susceptibility to radiation-induced cancer were first raised by a study examining the prebirth X-ray history of children dying of cancer. Healthy children were not evaluated in this investigation, which biased the results by finding only sick children born to women who were X-rayed during pregnancy. Another problem with this and other studies investigating this issue is that mothers were X-rayed only when there was a medical need for the examination.

The rate of leukemia in children whose mothers received about 2 rads to the uterus, increased to 1 in 2,000 from the expected incidence of 1 in 3,000 in unexposed children. Both of these rates are significantly less than the incidence of leukemia in brothers and sisters of children with this cancer (1 in 720 per ten years). Interestingly, *unexposed* brothers and sisters of the leukemic children in this study had a greater incidence of both leukemia and other cancers than did the brothers and sisters in the unexposed control group.[3] This observation seems to indicate that some other environmental or genetic factor might have been more related to the production of cancer in these children than were the X rays they received before birth. A number of subsequent investigations have failed to link X rays during pregnancy with childhood cancers, casting further doubt on the plausibility of a cause-and-effect.[4] Currently the possible risk for radiation-induced cancer from X rays before birth is low enough to justify reassurance.

I want to end this entry emphasizing the importance of avoiding unnecessary X-ray exposures whether you are pregnant or not. When you must receive an X ray, be certain to inquire about being protected by a lead shield during the process. The lack of demonstrated ill effects from small radiation doses during pregnancy is not to be taken as license for unnecessary exposures!

Carol Ann's Story:

At two and one-half months, my pregnancy was going along normally. In fact, I felt great! Unlike during my previous pregnancies I didn't even have morning sickness. Then one day during lunch an incredible pain occurred in my tooth while having some hot soup. It happened again that evening while drinking some hot herbal tea. My tooth throbbed throughout the night, and the next day I saw my dentist. She informed me that my symptoms revealed a dying nerve in my tooth and that I needed a root canal. My tooth hurt so badly, I knew I couldn't wait another six and one-half months before receiving treatment.

I was scared to death. It wasn't the procedure I was afraid of—friends who had had root canal therapy reassured me it wouldn't hurt. What I feared were the X rays that had to be taken, I was afraid the X rays would hurt my developing baby.

Before having the procedure I asked my obstetrician and the root canal specialist a lot of questions. I knew it would be best to ask such questions now rather than worry about it later! They both reassured me that today's X-ray machines focus the X rays on the structure that's being filmed, and that no detectable amount of radiation would reach my baby from dental X rays. They also explained that, in general, dental X rays put out very little radiation. For extra protection, a lead shield would be placed over me. This would prevent any possible scattered radiation from getting through. They did remind me that only certain doses of radiation have been associated with harmful effects, but regardless of whether you're pregnant, it's a good idea not to subject yourself to unnecessary radiation. For this reason, using lead shields are the standard of care.

I was surprised to hear all of this—I always thought that any amount of radiation during pregnancy could cause a birth defect. In fact a friend of mine who had a chest X ray not knowing she was pregnant, contemplated an abortion for fear of what the X ray had done. Happily, she continued the pregnancy. At birth her baby was just fine and now her child acts like any 2-year-old—tearing up the house.

References:

[1] R. L. Brent, The effects of embryonic and fetal exposure to X-Ray, microwaves and ultrasound. *Clinical Obstetrics and Gynecology* 26 (1983): 484–510.

[2] H. M. Swartz and B. A. Reichling, Hazards of radiation exposure for pregnant women, *Journal of the American Medical Association* 239 (1978): 1907–8.

[3] A. Stewart and G. W. Kneale, Radiation dose effects in relation to obstetric X-rays and childhood cancers, *Lancet* 1 (1970): 1185–88.

[4] B. E. Oppenheim, M. L. Griem, and P. Meier, The effects of diagnostic X-Ray exposure on the human fetus: An examination of the evidence, *Radiology* 114 (1975): 529–34.

Table 5–4
Estimated Radiation to the Uterus from Diagnostic Procedures:[1]

Procedure	Dose (rads)
Dental	unmeasurable
Chest	unmeasurable
Skull	unmeasurable
Cervical Spine	unmeasurable
Full Spine (chiropractic)*	0.40
Upper Gastrointestinal (GI) tract	0.15
Intravenous Pylogram (IVP)*	0.60
Abdomen*	0.50
Pelvis*	0.25
Lower GI tract* (with barium enema and 5 min. fluoroscopy)	1.60

*The dose received may vary for these procedures. Therefore it is imperative that your doctor or a radiology department be consulted to calculate the exact amount of scattered radiation your uterus received.

Reference

[1]Public Health Service Food and Drug Administration, handbook of doses for Projections Common in Diagnostic Radiology, U.S. Department of Health, Education, and Welfare (adapted from HEW Publication [FDA] 76–8030, *Organ Doses in Diagnostic Radiology,* May 1976, Rockville, Md.).

GENERIC NAME: **YELLOW FEVER VACCINE**

Brand name: **(YF-VAX)**

FDA pregnancy Category: C

ESTIMATED RISK SUMMARY:

Time of Exposure throughout pregnancy

Risk Risk assessment is not possible

Pregnancy Outcome uncertain

Documentation unavailable

← pre-conception ←	All or None		Organ Development – (in weeks)						Maturation – (in weeks)				
	1	2	3	4	5	6	7	8	9	10	12	20-36	38

conception   ←—Time of Greatest Risk—→   birth

Yellow fever vaccine[1] contains the live virus, which has been made noninfectious—what is called a live attenuated vaccine. Because yellow fever, a very serious and deadly disease, occurs primarily in Africa and South America, there is no indication for the use of yellow fever vaccine in the United States.

No information is available on any effects of yellow fever vaccine on the unborn child. Pregnant women are advised to postpone travel to areas where yellow fever is present. If travel cannot be avoided, being vaccinated poses fewer theoretical risks than does contracting the yellow fever infection itself.

Some foreign countries require yellow fever vaccination before entry, and not because of the risk of infection. In this case, you should obtain a waiver letter from your physician, in order to enter without the vaccination.

Reference:

[1]Centers for Disease Control, Yellow fever vaccine, *Morbidity and Mortality Weekly Report* 32 (1984): 679–88.

* SIX *

Helpful Sources of Information

Many of you may have specific or individual questions that are beyond the power of this book to answer. Fortunately, some states have services for the specific purpose of answering your questions, if you are a resident or, in some cases, live in the region. These information centers are listed here. Unless noted, they serve only the regions shown with the phone numbers.

There is also such a service in Canada.

If your region does not have a teratogen information center, the information may still be available. Call the department of genetics at your nearest medical center. The people there may be able to answer your question, or refer you to someone who can. Or people at a neighboring teratogen center may be able to refer you to a source of information, even if they cannot provide it themselves. Your local March of Dimes chapter is another excellent referral source.

UNITED STATES

ARIZONA
Arizona Teratogen Information Program
Arizona Health Sciences Center, Tucson
1-800/362-0101 (Arizona only)
602/626-6016 (local)

CALIFORNIA
California Teratogen Registry
University of California, San Diego
1-800/532-3749 (California only)

619/294-6084 (local)
No out-of-state calls accepted.

COLORADO

Genetics Unit/Teratology Service
University of Colorado Health Sciences Center, Denver, CO
303/394-8742 (Colorado)

CONNECTICUT

Connecticut Pregnancy Exposure Information Service
University of Connecticut Health Center, Farmington, CT
1-800/325-5391 (Connecticut only)
203/679-2676 (local)

FLORIDA

Genetics Division/The Teratology Service
University of Miami School of Medicine, Miami, FL
305/547-6006 (Florida)
Does answer questions from public and professionals over the phone,
but is primarily a clinical service.

MASSACHUSETTS

Pregnancy/Environmental Hotline
National Birth Defects Center
Kennedy Memorial Hospital, Brighton, MA
1-800/322-5014 (Massachusetts only)
617/787-4957 (local)

NEW JERSEY

Teratology Information Network
University of Medicine and Dentistry of New Jersey
School of Osteopathic Medicine, Camden, NJ
609/757-7869 (New Jersey)

NEW YORK

Luther K. Robinson, M.D.
Chief Clinical Genetics

Children's Hospital of Buffalo
716/878-7530

Dr. Robinson is in the process of developing a teratogen service that will primarily serve the Western New York area.

PENNSYLVANIA
Pregnancy Healthline
Pennsylvania Hospital, Philadelphia, PA
215/829-KIDS
Serves Pennsylvania, primarily Philadelphia, and New Jersey.

Department of Reproductive Genetics
Magee-Women's Hospital, Pittsburgh, PA
412/647-4168
Provides information in Pennsylvania, West Virginia, and eastern Ohio

Pregnancy Safety Hotline
Western Pennsylvania Hospital, Pittsburgh, PA
412/687-SAFE
Serves Pennsylvania, and parts of West Virginia and Ohio.

TEXAS
Genetic Screening and Counseling Service
Texas State Department of Mental Health and Mental Retardation
Denton, TX
817/383-3561
Primarily counsels Texas residents and those of communities in bordering states using its services.

UTAH
Pregnancy Risk Line
University of Utah Medical Center, Salt Lake City, UT
1-800/822-BABY (Utah only)
801/583-2229
Utah and Montana

VERMONT

Vermont Teratogen Information Network
University of Vermont, Burlington, VT
1-800/531-9800 (Vermont only)
802/658-4310 (local)

WASHINGTON

Washington State Poison Control Network
1-800/732-6985 (Washington state only)
206/526-2121 (also accepts calls from Alaska)
with Central Laboratory for Human Embryology
206/543-3373

WISCONSIN

Wisconsin Teratogen Project
University of Wisconsin, Madison, WI
1-800/362-3020 (Wisconsin only)
608/262-4719

Focus is clinical and callers are often asked to come to the clinic for evaluation. Primarily a service for Wisconsin, though also sees patients from northern Illinois and Michigan's upper peninsula.

Teratogen Hotline
Birth Defects Center, Children's Hospital of Milwaukee
Milwaukee, WI
414/931-4172 (local)

CANADA

TORONTO

Motherisk
Division of Pharmacology, Hospital for Sick Children
Toronto, Ontario
416/598-5781

Glossary

Amebiasis—the state of being infected with amebae (one-celled organisms).

Amniotic fluid—the fluid within the uterus in which the developing child lives before birth.

Amoebic dysentery—an infectious intestinal disease, caused by amoebae, resulting in loose, bloody bowel movements and loss of body fluids. It occurs much more frequently in the tropics than in temperate climates.

Anencephaly—a malformation of the developing brain resulting in the absence of the top of the head and a portion of the brain. Anencephaly is a neural tube defect.

Angina—a heart condition that causes pain and a feeling of suffocation.

Anomaly—deviation from normal, a malformation.

Antagonist—a substance that counteracts another substance.

Antiemetic—a substance that counteracts nausea.

Apgar scores—a numeric expression of infant well-being at birth.

Arrythmia—abnormal heartbeat rhythm.

Auditory nerve (eighth nerve)—responsible for hearing and balance.

Bilirubin—a pigment from red blood cells, too much of which can lead to *jaundice.*

Bradycardia—a slower than normal heartbeat.

Carcinogenic—cancer-causing.

Cardiac—referring to the heart.

Cardiac arrythmia—abnormal heartbeat rhythm.

Central nervous sytem—the part of the nervous system that contains the brain and spinal cord

Chromosome—rodlike bodies within every cell that contain the DNA (genetic material) inherited from the person's parents.

Chronic or long-term hypertension—the presence of persistent hypertension in the mother from any cause occurring before the twentieth week of gestation or persisting after the forty-second day after birth. This condition can be risky to both the mother and the unborn or newborn child.

Cleft lip—an opening in the lip resulting from a failure of the lip to fuse during the embryo's development. Also called "harelip." This malformation occurs with or without cleft palate in about 1 per 1,000 births.

Cleft palate—an opening in the palate (roof of the mouth) resulting from a failure of the palate to fuse during the embryo's development. This malformation occurs alone in about 1 per 2,500 births.

Cochleovestibular—meaning part of the ear.

Congenital—a condition present at birth and usually during prenatal development.

Eclampsia—the occurrence of seizure activity or coma in a patient with *preeclampsia*. This condition can be risky to both the mother and the unborn or newborn child.

Edema—the presence of abnormal amounts of fluid in body tissues.

Electrocardiogram (ECG)—a graphic record of heart muscle action.

Folic acid, or folate—a water-soluble B-complex vitamin. The need for folate increases greatly during pregnancy, as this vitamin is required for fetal growth and development.

Genitalia—the reproductive organs.

Gestation—the time of the baby's development, beginning with conception and ending with birth. However, some use this term to encompass the time beginning with the first day of a woman's last menstrual period and ending with birth.

Gestational hypertension—pregnancy-induced *hypertension* without *edema* or *proteinuria* that usually develops in the mother after twenty weeks of gestation or in the first ten days after birth. This condition can be risky to both the mother and the unborn or newborn child.

Goiter, congenital—enlargement of the thyroid gland that is present at birth.

Hemolytic anemia—anemia (low blood cell count) due to shortened survival of red blood cells and the inability of bone marrow to compensate for this reduced survival.

Hydrocephalus—enlargement of the cerebral ventricles related to the accumulation of fluid within the baby's brain.

Hyperglycemia—abnormally high blood sugar.

Hyperreflexia—abnormal muscle movements.

Hypertension—high blood pressure.

Hyperthermia—an abnormally high body temperature.

Hypertonicity—increased muscle tone.

Hypoglycemia—low blood sugar.

Hypokalemia—a decrease in potassium level in the body.

Hyponatremia—too low a level of salt in the body.

Hypoplasia—incomplete or underdevelopment of a body part.

Hypoprothrombinemia—deficiency of a coagulation factor in the blood.

Hypospadias—malplacement of the urethral opening on the male penis.

Hypothermia—an abnormally low body temperature.

Infertility—inability to reproduce.

IUGR = intrauterine growth retardation—growth retardation occurring in the uterus.

Jaundice—yellowing of the eye whites or skin, caused by liver damage or by too much *bilirubin* in the blood.

Kernicterus—a severe neurological disorder occurring when there are high levels of *bilirubin* in the blood.

Labia—skin folds located on either side of the vaginal opening.

Microcephaly—abnormally small head size.

Mutagenic—able to alter genetic material.

Neonatal—the first four weeks after birth.

Neural tube defects—birth defects arising from an error in the prenatal development of the brain and spinal cord. Neural tube defects occur in our population in about 1 of 1,000 live births. *Spina bifida* and *anencephaly* each account for about 50 percent of these defects.

Optic nerve hypoplasia—incomplete development of the nerve of sight.

Oral clefts—include cleft lip with or without cleft palate or cleft palate alone.

Patent ductus arteriosis—a common heart defect resulting from failure of a passageway in the fetal heart to close soon after birth.

Perinatal—the period shortly before *and* after birth (includes both the unborn child and the infant).

Perinatal loss—death of a child shortly before or after birth.

Postpartum—the time for the mother after childbirth.

Preeclampsia—pregnancy-induced *hypertension* in the mother with *proteinuria* and/or *edema* that usually develops after twenty weeks of gestation. This condition can be risky to both the mother and the unborn or newborn child.

Prenatal—the period before birth.

Prophylaxis—preventative.

Prospective studies—studies conducted before the birth outcome is known.

Proteinuria—the presence of excess proteins in the urine.

Pyloric stenosis—a severe narrowing (stenosis) of the pyloric canal, which is in the stomach. This defect occurs in 1 of 150 males and 1 of 750 females.

Retina—a part of the eyeball.

Retrospective studies—studies conducted after the pregnancy outcome is known.

Spina bifida—a defect in the closure of the developing spinal cord that may be open or closed. Spina bifida is a neural tube defect.

Spontaneous abortion—loss of an unborn child during the first twenty weeks of gestation.

Stillbirth—loss of an unborn child during the last twenty weeks of gestation.

Tachycardia—a rapid heart rate.

Teratogen—any drug, chemical, pollutant, infection, physical agent or material physical state (like diabetes) that can interfere with the normal development of an unborn baby.

Thrombocytopenia—a decrease in blood platelets; platelets are essential for blood coagulation.

Toxemia—a term including the conditions of *preeclampsia* and *eclampsia*.

Toxic—another term for poison.

Tracheoesophageal fistula—an abnormal link between the trachea and the esophagus.

Trichomonas vaginalis—a parasitic protozoa found in the vagina, which can cause infection that produces an unusual discharge.

Trichomoniasis—an infection with *Trichomonas.*

Trimester—a period of three months.

Tumorogenic—something that gives rise to tumors in the body.

Index